PSYCHOLOGICAL TREATMENT OF BIPOLAR DISORDER

Psychological Treatment of Bipolar Disorder

Edited by

SHERI L. JOHNSON
ROBERT L. LEAHY

THE GUILFORD PRESS
New York   London

© 2004 The Guilford Press
A Division of Guilford Publications, Inc.
72 Spring Street, New York, NY 10012
www.guilford.com

Printed in the United States of America

This book is printed on acid-free paper.

Last digit is print number: 9 8 7 6 5 4 3 2

Library of Congress Cataloging-in-Publication Data

Psychological treatment of bipolar disorder / edited by Sheri L.
Johnson, Robert L. Leahy.
    p. cm.
Includes bibliographical references and index.
  ISBN 1-57230-924-5 (alk. paper)
  1. Manic–depressive illness—Treatment. I. Johnson, Sheri L. II.
Leahy, Robert L.
  RC516.P795 2004
  616.89′506—dc22
                                            2003015343

*To the many people with bipolar disorder
who have shared their experiences with us.*

ABOUT THE EDITORS

Sheri L. Johnson, PhD, is Associate Professor of Psychology and Psychiatry at the University of Miami. Over the past decade, she has conducted research on psychosocial facets of bipolar disorder. Her work has been funded by the National Alliance for Research on Schizophrenia and Depression and by the National Institute of Mental Health, and her findings have been published in a number of journals, including the *Journal of Abnormal Psychology* and the *American Journal of Psychiatry*. More information about her work is available at *http://www.psy.miami.edu/faculty/sjohnson/*.

Robert L. Leahy, PhD, is President of the International Association for Cognitive Psychotherapy, Founder and Director of the American Institute for Cognitive Therapy in New York City (*www. CognitiveTherapyNYC.com*), Professor of Psychology in Psychiatry at Weill–Cornell University Medical School, and former Editor of the *Journal of Cognitive Psychotherapy*. Dr. Leahy's recent books include *Cognitive Therapy: Basic Principles and Applications, Practicing Cognitive Therapy, Treatment Plans and Interventions for Depression and Anxiety Disorders* (with Stephen J. Holland), *Overcoming Resistance in Cognitive Therapy, Bipolar Disorder: A Cognitive Therapy Approach* (with Cory F. Newman, Aaron T. Beck, Noreen A. Reilly-Harrington, and Laslo Gyulai), *Clinical Applications of Cognitive Psychotherapy* (edited with E. Thomas Dowd), *Psychology and the Economic Mind, Cognitive Therapy Techniques: A Practitioner's Guide,* and *Roadblocks in Cognitive-Behavioral Therapy: Transforming Challenges into Opportunities for Change.*

CONTRIBUTORS

Edward Altman, PsyD, Department of Psychiatry, University of Illinois at Chicago, Chicago, Illinois

Monica Ramirez Basco, PhD, Division of Psychology, Department of Psychiatry, University of Texas Southwestern Medical Center at Dallas, Dallas, Texas

Mark S. Bauer, MD, Department of Psychiatry and Human Behavior, Brown University Medical School, Providence, Rhode Island

Amy N. Cohen, PhD, Department of Veterans Affairs Desert Pacific Mental Illness Research, Education, and Clinical Center (MIRECC), West Los Angeles Veterans Healthcare Center, Los Angeles, California

Norah Feeny, PhD, Department of Psychiatry, Case Western Reserve University, Cleveland, Ohio

Robert L. Findling, MD, Division of Child and Adolescent Psychiatry, Case Western Reserve University, Cleveland, Ohio

Ellen Frank, PhD, Western Psychiatric Institute and Clinic, University of Pittsburgh Medical Center, Pittsburgh, Pennsylvania

Joseph F. Goldberg, MD, Department of Psychiatry, Zucker Hillside Hospital, North Shore–Long Island Jewish Health System, Glen Oaks, New York

Constance Hammen, PhD, Department of Psychology, University of California at Los Angeles, Los Angeles, California

Sheri L. Johnson, PhD, Department of Psychology, University of Miami, Coral Gables, Florida

Robert L. Leahy, PhD, American Institute for Cognitive Therapy and Department of Psychiatry, Weill–Cornell University Medical School, New York, New York

Harriet P. Lefley, PhD, Department of Psychiatry and Behavioral Sciences, University of Miami School of Medicine, Miami, Florida

Noelle McDonald, BS, Division of Psychology, Department of Psychiatry, University of Texas Southwestern Medical Center at Dallas, Dallas, Texas

Megan Merlock, BA, Division of Psychology, Department of Psychiatry, University of Texas Southwestern Medical Center at Dallas, Dallas, Texas

Björn Meyer, PhD, School of Psychology and Therapeutic Studies, University of Surrey Roehampton, London, United Kingdom

David J. Miklowitz, PhD, Department of Psychology, University of Colorado at Boulder, Boulder, Colorado

Cory F. Newman, PhD, Center for Cognitive Therapy, University of Pennsylvania School of Medicine, Philadelphia, Pennsylvania

Jan Scott, MD, Division of Psychological Medicine, Institute of Psychiatry, London, United Kingdom

Holly A. Swartz, MD, Western Psychiatric Institute and Clinic, University of Pittsburgh Medical Center, Pittsburgh, Pennsylvania

Suzanne Vogel-Scibilia, MD, Western Psychiatric Institute and Clinic, Beaver, Pennsylvania

Eric A. Youngstrom, PhD, Department of Psychology, Case Western Reserve University, Cleveland, Ohio

PREFACE

While there are several excellent treatment manuals and edited volumes on bipolar disorder, we recognized that practicing clinicians did not have a single updated resource that would provide them with an understanding of the diagnostic, social, and clinical issues involved in providing therapy for bipolar disorder. More than for any other psychiatric disorder, there is a significant need for a comprehensive—as well as integrative—treatment approach for bipolar disorder. Although many practitioners may still be limited by their view that medication is the only method of treatment, the contributors to this volume make clear that a multifaceted approach is now available.

The book begins with a discussion of diagnostic issues. Even experienced clinicians can easily miss the nuanced issues in differential diagnosis or the early signs of bipolar disorder unfolding during adolescence. Unfortunately, many patients will finally receive an accurate diagnosis only after they have suffered years of unnecessary depressions and manias. Because few people complain about hypomanic symptoms, such as "feeling especially good," inappropriate monodrug treatments can exacerbate symptoms.

Beyond diagnosis, this volume covers psychosocial approaches to supplement medication management. Many of the chapters share commonalities in the targets of treatment. For example, psychoeducation and strategies to improve medication adherence are a major part of all of these treatments. However, there are important differences in emphasis and strategies. The great advantage that practicing clinicians have is the freedom to integrate these approaches with one another to provide comprehensive treatment.

Bipolar disorder does not occur in a vacuum. There is considerable evidence that psychosocial variables, including impaired occupational functioning, social conflicts, and life stressors, can be unfortunate consequences of this disorder and in fact catalyze future episodes. Fortunately, these variables can be modified, and this volume provides an array of insights into how to do so.

Although medication approaches dramatically reduce the symptoms of bipolar disorder, relapse remains the normative experience for patients with bipolar disorder, even when they are taking medications. Most of us treasure our emotional reactions as a reflection of our core values. Bipolar disorder forces people to question their emotional reactions and exacts a powerful toll on their self-confidence. Moreover, the unpredictable timing of relapse forces people to consider how to live a full life during periods of wellness, even though episodes could return. These issues help place the suicidality associated with bipolar disorder in context. On the other hand, the hopelessness that contributes to suicidality can be challenged by noting the empirical evidence—reported herein—that psychosocial treatments, when offered along with medication, improve the course of this illness.

In assembling the chapters for this book, our aim was to provide chapters that covered the basic problems associated with bipolar disorder, drawing on the empirical literature as a foundation. We are encouraged that so many researchers are working on solutions to these problems. We are cautiously optimistic that clinical science and practice are moving toward important new treatments that can offer greater hope and empowerment to individuals with bipolar disorder and their families.

CONTENTS

I. Overview of Bipolar Disorder

II. Therapy and Treatment Issues

III. Special Issues in Treatment

Appendices

PART I

OVERVIEW OF BIPOLAR DISORDER

CHAPTER ONE

DEFINING BIPOLAR DISORDER

SHERI L. JOHNSON

Bipolar disorder, formerly known as manic–depressive disorder, has intrigued scholars dating back to ancient Greece, yet it remains enigmatic in many ways. Hypomania, with its euphoria, energy, and productivity, has been described as a powerful elixir, and there is no other psychiatric condition in which people report craving the return of symptoms. Literature, arts, and history have been shaped by the remarkable creativity of individuals with bipolar disorder, including Vincent van Gogh, Martin Luther, Robert Schumann, Pytor Illyich Tchaikovsky, and the Pulitzer Prize winners John Berryman, Amy Lowell, and Anne Sexton (Goodwin & Jamison, 1990; Jamison, 1996). In popular imagery, mania remains an alluring, powerful, and mysterious condition. Indeed, mania has been chosen as the name for a perfume. It is unlikely that any other psychiatric condition will ever be used in that way. Despite mesmerizing stereotypes, however, bipolar disorder is one of the most severe of psychiatric disorders.

In this chapter, I begin by defining bipolar disorder, then briefly review its diagnostic criteria, epidemiology, course, and biological foundations. Next I examine the rationale for the use of psychosocial treatments for this disorder. Finally, I briefly highlight the major topics that are covered in the remaining chapters of this volume.

DEFINITIONS OF BIPOLAR DISORDER

Kraepelin (1921) described the course of this illness systematically more than 80 years ago. He noted the heterogeneity in the types of symptoms, the pattern of episodes, and the level of functioning. His descriptions of symptoms are strikingly concordant with the terms used to describe bipolar

3

disorder in DSM-IV-TR, and many of his diagnostic distinctions remain well supported today. Similarly, issues he raised regarding the heterogeneity of this diagnosis remain prominent.

Diagnostic Criteria

Diagnostic errors are common with this disorder. One survey suggested that, on average, bipolar disorder was not diagnosed for 8 years after onset (Lish, Dime-Meenan, Whybrow, Price, & Hirschfeld, 1994). The most common misdiagnosis is unipolar depression: Approximately 40% of persons with bipolar disorder are misdiagnosed with unipolar disorder (Ghaemi, Boiman, & Goodwin, 2000; Ghaemi, Sachs, Chiou, Pandurangi, & Goodwin, 1999). Even though approximately 10% of people with major depression have a history of mania, three-quarters of practitioners fail to screen for mania routinely among individuals reporting depression (Brickman, LoPiccolo, & Johnson, 2002). When treated with antidepressants without mood-stabilizing medication, as many as one-fourth of individuals with bipolar disorder experience iatrogenic manic symptoms (Ghaemi, Lenox, & Baldessarini, 2001). In one managed care organization, failure to consistently note a history of mania was associated with a doubled risk of hospitalization (Johnson, Eisdorfer, LoPiccolo, & Brickman, 2003). Hence, differential diagnosis of bipolar disorder remains an important challenge in health care systems today.

Although researchers have proposed myriad subtypes of depression (i.e., bipolar III, bipolar II½), there are two major subtypes of disorder in DSM-IV-TR: bipolar I and bipolar II. Bipolar I disorder is diagnosed on the basis of a single lifetime manic or mixed episode. Despite the name "bipolar disorder," depression is not a diagnostic criterion. The symptoms of mania can vary a great deal from person to person.

Even though the lay public tends to think of mania as involving euphoria, it is important to note that the cardinal mood symptoms can include either euphoria and expansiveness or anger and irritability. In addition to a distinct change in mood, the diagnostic criteria for mania include at least three of seven symptoms (four, if irritability is the major mood state). The symptoms of mania include inflated self-esteem, decreased need for sleep, pressured speech, flight of ideas or racing thoughts, distractibility, increased goal-directed activity, and increased involvement in pleasurable activities with a high potential for negative consequences (American Psychiatric Association, 2000). Symptoms must be present for 1 week or require hospitalization. In addition to symptoms, marked functional impairment must be present. A mixed episode includes symptoms of depression and mania. That is, symptoms meet severity criteria for a manic episode and a depressed episode for at least 1 week, and marked functional impairment is present. Although diagnostic criteria provide an objective definition, clinicians looking for subjective descriptions of mania and depression often find autobiographies by Kay Jamison on bipolar disorder or Robert Lowell on depression helpful (see Appendix 4 for recommended autobiographies).

Bipolar II disorder is diagnosed on the basis of a single lifetime episode of hypomania (in the absence of mania) and at least one lifetime episode of major depression. Hypomanic episodes require the presence of at least three of the symptoms of mania described above (again, four if irritability is the major mood state). Unlike the definition of mania, hypomanic episodes do not include severe impairment and only need to be present for 4 days. Notably, lifetime episodes of hypomania in the absence of depressive episodes do not meet criteria for any diagnosis. Few individuals are expected to seek treatment for brief periods of increased mood, activity, energy, and confidence that fail to cause severe impairment and are not associated with depression. Some people believe that periods of hypomania may underlie the increased productivity and artistic endeavors seen within bipolar disorder (see Weisberg, 1994, for a discussion).

DSM-IV-TR also includes a range of bipolar spectrum conditions, including cyclothymia (milder but frequent symptoms of hypomania and depression) and substance-induced mood disorders (e.g., manic episodes triggered by antidepressants or other substances). In addition, DSM-IV-TR includes a diagnosis of bipolar disorder not otherwise specified. This diagnostic category may be useful for individuals who report atypical manic symptoms, manic symptoms lasting less than 4 days, or hypomanic symptoms in the absence of depressive episodes. For more detail on differential diagnosis of bipolar spectrum conditions, see Altman (Chapter 3, this volume).

Psychotic symptoms can co-occur with either manic or depressive episodes. In studies of relatively severe samples, psychotic symptoms have been reported by approximately one-third to one-half of those with bipolar I disorder (Judd et al., 2002; Lenzi, Rinaldi, Bianco, Balestri, & Marazziti, 1996). However, these symptoms tend to be brief—they tend to present for only one or two weeks per year (Judd et al., 2002)—and they are much more likely to accompany mania than depression (Black & Nasrallah, 1989). Psychotic symptoms that occur for 2 weeks or more outside the context of a mood episode are an indicator of schizoaffective disorder. Because schizoaffective disorder may represent the expression of underlying genetic vulnerabilities for both psychosis and mood disorders (Cardno, Rijsdijk, Sham, Murray, & McGuffin, 2002), more intensive and specialized treatment is likely to be required in these cases.

Epidemiology

Lifetime prevalence rates for bipolar disorder are approximately 0.8% (Kessler, 1994; Weissman et al., 1996), and the prevalence rate appears comparable crossculturally (cf. Faravelli, Degl'Innocenti, Aiazzi, & Incerpi, 1990). Bipolar spectrum disorders (cyclothymia and bipolar II) are more common. Although the median age of onset of bipolar I disorder was estimated to occur in the early 20s (Loranger & Levine, 1978; Kessler, Rubinow, Holmes, Abelson, & Zhao, 1997), recent research has documented a much higher rate of bipolar disorder among adolescents than was previously believed (Geller & Luby, 1997). In one epidemiological survey, a rate of 1% was documented during adolescence (Lewinsohn, Klein, & Seeley, 1995). Community studies of this issue are difficult to conduct, however, as standard epidemiological surveys may fail to reliably diagnose as many as 50% of cases (Kessler et al., 1997). Youngstrom and his colleagues (Chapter 4, this volume) provide extensive discussion of the expression and recognition of bipolar disorder in children and adolescents.

Course of Disorder

There is tremendous heterogeneity in the course of bipolar symptoms over time. Some individuals experience a single episode during their lifetime, and others can go for years or even decades free of symptoms. However, most people with the disorder experience frequent and severe episodes, despite the powerful reduction in symptoms from the use of lithium and other mood-stabilizing medications. Results from one major study suggested that most persons taking recommended doses of lithium alone relapsed within 5 years (Keller et al., 1992). In a naturalistic study of individuals treated at a tertiary care center, those with bipolar disorder reported symptoms during at least 50% of the weeks. In one naturalistic study of lithium monotherapy that included persons who were not medication adherent, less than 10% remained symptom free for a full year (Sachs, Lafer, Truman, Noeth, & Thibault, 1994). Hence, relapse is normative, even among people who are taking mood-stabilizing medications.

Many of the relapses experienced by persons with bipolar disorder result in hospitalization. In one study of 20,350 patients with mood disorders, hospitalization rates were found to become more frequent over the life course (Kessing, Andersen, Mortenson, & Bolwig, 1998). Bipolar disorder accounts for a major portion of inpatient care costs (Kent, Fogartee, & Yellowless, 1995). In one study of a major mental health managed care organization, bipolar disorder accounted for 45% of the inpatient care costs, even though only 8% of the treated population met criteria for bipolar disorder (Johnson et al., 2003). In 1991, the annual direct and indirect costs associated with bipolar disorder in the United States were estimated at $45.2 billion (Wyatt & Henter, 1995), due in part to the disproportionately high treatment costs (Sajatovic, Popli, & Semple, 1996; Simon & Unuetzer, 1999).

As noted earlier, depression is not a diagnostic criterion for bipolar disorder. Indeed, in community samples, as many as 20–33% of people with bipolar disorder report no lifetime episodes of major depression (Depue & Monroe, 1978; Karkowski & Kendler, 1997; Kessler et al., 1997; see Johnson & Kizer, 2002, for discussion). Because people are more likely to seek treatment for depression than mania, however, the vast majority of patients in treatment will report depression as well as mania. Indeed, in one follow-up survey of tertiary care patients, depressive symptoms were more than three times as frequent as manic symptoms (Judd et al., 2002). Hence, the base rates of depression among persons with bipolar disorder can be expected to vary, depending on the setting.

Beyond major episodes, it is important to attend to the course of subsyndromal and prodromal symptoms. Prodromal symptoms of depression and mania may unfold in a matter of days to weeks (Smith & Tarrier, 1992). Given this possible speed of symptom onset, strong psychoeducational programs for identifying prodromal symptoms are important when treating persons with this disorder (Lam, Wong, & Sham, 2001).

Many people will experience symptoms that do not conform to the classic pattern of clear episodes of mania and depression separated by full recovery. Indeed, some authors have begun to challenge the stereotype of clear-cut episodes within this disorder. Individuals in one National Institute of Mental Health (NIMH) study of bipolar disorder had a median of six changes in symptom levels per year (Judd et al., 2002), and subsyndromal symptoms were three times as common (29.9 weeks of the year) as full-blown episodes (11.2 weeks of the year).

Comorbidity

The presence of comorbid conditions appear to be the rule rather than the exception in people with bipolar disorder (Kessler et al., 1997). Lifetime estimates of (1) comorbid alcohol or substance abuse are as high as 50% (Brown, Suppes, Adinoff, & Thomas, 2001; Chengappa, Levine, Gershon, & Kupfer, 2000; Zarate & Tohen, 2001), (2) anxiety disorders as high as 60% (Goodwin & Hoven, 2002; Tamam & Ozpoyraz, 2002), and (3) personality disorders ranging from 33–50% (Uecok, Karaveli, Kundakci, & Yazici, 1998). Although studies are not entirely consistent, obsessive–compulsive disorder, simple phobia, social phobia, and panic disorder appear to be the most common anxiety conditions associated with bipolar disorder (Kessler, Stang, Wittchen, Stein, & Walters, 1999; Tamam & Ozpoyraz, 2002). The most common personality disorders include those from Cluster B (antisocial, borderline, histrionic, and narcisstic personality disorders) and Cluster C (avoidant, dependent, and obsessive–compulsive personality disorders) (Brieger, Ehrt, & Maneros, 2003). Each of these comorbid conditions has been found to be associated with a poorer course over time, including longer time to recovery, faster time to relapse, poor medication adherence, and suicidality (Dunayevich et al., 2000; Frangou, 2002; Uecok et al., 1998; Vieta et al., 2001). An important intake goal is to capture the presence of comorbid conditions.

Biological Basis of the Disorder

It is well established that bipolar disorder is a genetically influenced condition—heritability has been estimated to be as high as 80% (Veh-manen, Kaprio, & Loennqvist, 1995). Indeed, the only psychiatric disorders with comparable heritability estimates appear to be autism and attention-deficit/hyperactivity disorder (Hinshaw, 2002). Mania is unusual among individuals without a family history of mood disorder; both mania and unipolar depression are overrepresented in the pedigrees of individuals with bipolar disorder (Plomin, DeFries, McClearn, & Rutter, 1997; Winokur & Tsuang, 1996). First-degree relatives of individuals with bipolar disorder have a risk of approximately 10% of developing bipolar disorder and a comparable risk for unipolar depression (Plomin et al., 1997). Despite the compelling evidence for a genetic etiology, discovering the genes responsible for the disorder is a complex task. Unlike disorders such as Huntington's chorea, which is inherited in a one-gene Mendelian fashion, bipolar disorder is likely to be a polygenic disorder, involving a combination of several genes.

This genetic vulnerability likely involves dysregulation of neurotransmitters. During periods of depression and mania, persons with bipolar disorder display functional changes in the activity of several amines, including dopamine, serotonin, and, to some extent, norepinephrine. Many of these neurotransmitter correlates appear to normalize between episodes, but current models emphasize difficulties in maintaining homeostasis within these systems. Hence, systems that modulate neurotransmitter levels at the cellular level, such as g-proteins, as well as neurotransmitters that seem to modulate the catecholamine functioning, such as gamma-aminobutyric acid (GABA), have received increasing research attention. One exciting line of research has focused on how symptoms unfold in the face of neurobiological challenges, such as sleep deprivation (Barbini et al., 1998). Congruent with a model of biological dysregulation, persons with bipolar disorder are much more vulnerable to developing manic symptoms after sleep deprivation.

Bipolar disorder is not associated consistently with substantial changes in the number or density of neurons in any particular brain region, although lower density of glial cells has been found in some postmortem studies (Vawter, Freed, & Kleinman, 2000). Compared to research on structural abnormalities, more focus is being placed on understanding the level of activity in different brain regions, particularly during episodes. Mania appears to be tied to increases in activity throughout the frontal cortex (George, Ketter, Kimbrell, & Post, 1998). People with bipolar depression, like those with unipolar depression, show changes in the activation levels of the amygdala, prefrontal cortex, and anterior cingulate during tasks involving emotionally relevant stimuli (Drevets, 2001). To date, no biological assay has proven helpful in diagnosing bipolar disorder.

Pharmacological Approaches

Given the genetic vulnerability to this disorder and the neurotransmitter correlates of its expression, it is not surprising that medications form the bedrock of its treatment (see Goldberg, Chapter 6, this volume). Lithium remains the treatment with the strongest research support, and the APA Practice Guidelines (Hirschfeld et al., 2002; see *http://www.psych.org/ clin_res/bipolar_revisebook_index.cfm*) recommend lithium as the first-choice treatment. Beyond evidence from double-blind randomized trials of reductions in symptoms and episodes (Prien et al., 1984), lithium is the only treatment shown to reduce suicidality (cf. Bocchetta et al., 1998; Jamison, 1999), and lithium discontinuation is a major predictor of rehospitalization (Johnson & McFarland, 1996). However, approximately three-quarters of people report side effects from lithium, which most commonly include excessive thirst, frequent urination, memory problems, tremor, weight gain, drowsiness, and diarrhea (Goodwin & Jamison, 1990). Antiseizure medications, such as Depakote, have fewer side effects and have been shown to reduce symptoms. Mood-stabilizing medications (i.e., lithium and antiseizure medications) have been found to be less effective in reducing depressive symptoms compared to manic symptoms (Hlastala et al., 1997). Psychotherapy may be particularly important in helping to alleviate residual depressive symptoms. It is common for patients to be prescribed antidepressants and antipsychotic medications along with mood-stabilizing medications. Other novel medication treatments are receiving increasing attention (Rivas-Vazquez, Johnson, Rey, & Blais, 2002). However, *psychotherapy should always be an adjunct to medication approaches.*

RATIONALE FOR ADJUNCTIVE PSYCHOSOCIAL TREATMENTS

Beyond symptom reduction and basic psychoeducation for bipolar and comorbid conditions, psychosocial interventions can target several other goals, including improving adherence, addressing secondary consequences of the disorder, and reducing the impact of psychosocial variables related to relapse. I briefly review the literature on the relevance of these issues.

Nonadherence

In one community survey, only 20% of people with bipolar disorder reported receiving outpatient treatment in the past year (Kessler et al., 1997). Even among those receiving outpatient treatment, as many as 75% have been found to experience disruptions in consistent medication maintenance within a 1-year period (Unuetzer, Simon, Pabiniak, Bond, & Katon, 2000). Because high rates of nonadherence are common to many medical treatments, some issues in nonadherence are likely to be general across disorders. Other issues may be specific to bipolar disorder; for example, accepting the bipolar diagnosis is likely to be a difficult process for many individuals (see Basco, Merlock, & McDonald, Chapter 12, this volume). These issues are particularly important to address, because poor medication adherence is one of the most robust predictors of hospitalization as well as suicide (Baldessarini, Tondo, & Hennen, 1999; Coppen & Farmer, 1998). Indeed, Nilsson (1999) found that suicide mortality was 77% higher among patients who were not receiving ongoing lithium treatment compared to those who were receiving it.

Psychosocial Consequences of the Disorder

One of the most striking features of this disorder is the dramatic variability in functioning, both across time and across individuals. Whereas the enormous creative output of some persons with this disorder is noteworthy, the normative profile appears to include substantial difficulty with work and relationships (see Hammen & Cohen, Chapter 2, this volume). One-third of individuals remain unemployed a full year after hospitalization for mania (Harrow, Goldberg, Grossman, & Meltzer, 1990). Bipolar disorder is projected to become the sixth leading medical cause of disability-adjusted life years worldwide by the year 2020 (Murray & Lopez, 1996). Because functioning is impaired even during asymptomatic periods, strategies to improve functioning are of vital importance (see Bauer, Chapter 10, this volume).

Some of the difficulty in maintaining strong social relationships and occupational stability may relate to the stigma still surrounding the disorder. Although awareness of mental health issues has increased dramatically over the past several decades, a recent survey suggests that most mental health consumers report stigma from family members, employers, and even within their religious organizations (Wahl, 1999). Hence, isolation and self-esteem consequences of this disorder are very important (see Hinshaw, 2002, for a biographical account that covers these issues well). As an antidote to the negative attitudes toward persons with mental illness, consumer support groups may provide an important context for normalization and acceptance (see Lefley & Vogel-Scibilia, Chapter 14, this volume).

Given the high rates of subsyndromal symptoms, relapse, and the difficulties in maintaining employment and social relationships, it is not surprising that hopelessness and demoralization are common in this population. Rates of completed suicides are approximately 12–15 times those of the general population (Angst, Stassen, Clayton, & Angst, 2002; Harris & Barraclough, 1997). Indeed, after cardiovascular events, suicide is the most likely cause of death for individuals with bipolar disorder (Angst et al., 2002). Suicide attempts are reported by approximately one-third to one-half of individuals with bipolar disorder (Chen & Dilsaver, 1996; Goodwin & Jamison, 1990). In response to these alarming statistics, this volume includes one chapter dedicated specifically to this topic (see Newman, Chapter 13).

Psychosocial Predictors of Course

Although biological models remain the central focus of research and treatment in bipolar disorder, and genes are the central determinant of onset, few biological variables have been identified that predict the course of the disorder (Prien & Potter, 1990). In contrast, there is substantial evidence that psychosocial variables predict the course of the disorder (see Johnson & Meyer, Chapter 5, this volume). Drawing on these psychosocial predictors, there is a strong rationale for reducing family conflict, life stress, and social isolation as a way to protect against symptoms (see Frank & Swartz, Chapter 8, and Miklowitz, Chapter 9, this volume).

In addition to high rates of environmental stressors, bipolar disorder may be related to a propensity to think about the self and the world more negatively, particularly during depression (Johnson & Kizer, 2002). In contrast, overly optimistic cognitions may be correlates of mania. Treatments specifically focused on addressing these maladaptive cognitions are an important part of the toolkit for any clinician working in this area (see Leahy, Chapter 7, this volume).

SUMMARY

Psychosocial approaches as adjuncts to pharmacological treatment of bipolar disorder are important for several reasons; they (1) provide psychoeducation regarding symptoms, (2) promote adherence with medication regimens, (3) address comorbid conditions, (4) ameliorate the stigma and self-esteem consequences of the diagnosis, (5) promote greater social and occupational adjustment, (6) help reduce the risk of suicide, and (7) identify and reduce psychosocial triggers that may intensify the risk for relapse, including family conflict and life stressors. Perhaps the most important reason to consider adjunctive psychotherapy, however, is that recent outcome trials provide evidence that these treatments alleviate and prevent symptoms (see Scott, Chapter 11, this volume).

Fortunately, the last decade has seen the publication of a series of treatment manuals designed to address these issues in bipolar disorder.

More broadly, biological and psychosocial research on the topic has expanded rapidly. Indeed, the explosion in knowledge is remarkable, given the underrepresentation of bipolar disorder in the NIMH portfolio (Hyman, 2000). Overall, these are exciting times in the effort to understand and treat bipolar disorder.

In the context of the rapidly expanding knowledge base concerning treatment and basic science, it is impossible to cover all of the advances within one book. There are several recent treatments that provide focused analyses of specific topics, including specific interventions to improve adherence (Davidoff, Forester, Ghaemi, & Bodkin, 1998), address comorbid substance abuse (Weiss, Najavits, & Greenfield, 1999), and help regulate sleep cycles (Wehr et al., 1998; Wirz-Justice, Quinto, Cajochen, Werth, & Hock, 1999). Similarly, novel approaches to setting standards for care at a community level are being developed (Kashner, Rush, & Altshuler, 1999; Suppes et al., 2000). Throughout the volume, as well as in the Appendices, we have tried to provide direction for those seeking more detailed information. Persons who seek more in-depth coverage of the basic research literature may find Goodwin and Jamison's (1990) encyclopedic volume, *Manic–Depressive Illness*, to be helpful. Similarly, many treatment manuals are now available, which provide more detailed insights than can be found within a single treatment chapter. Increasingly sophisticated web resources are becoming available as well.

This book provides on overview of resources for providing psychosocial assessment and treatment. Part I covers basic findings on the psychosocial predictors and outcomes associated with bipolar disorder, as well as chapters reviewing assessment strategies. Part II covers treatment approaches that have empirical support. Part III is devoted to chapters on specific treatment issues, such as suicide and adherence. We hope that this volume provides a starting point for understanding the important problems faced by individuals with bipolar disorder and the array of treatment approaches that may help solve these problems.

ACKNOWLEDGMENTS

Special thanks to Amy Kizer, Camilo Ruggero, and Charles Carver for their helpful comments regarding this chapter.

REFERENCES

American Psychiatric Association. (2000). *Desk reference to the diagnostic criteria from DSM-IV-TR*. Washington, DC: Author.

Angst, F., Stausen, H. H., Clayton, P. J., & Angst, J. (2002). Mortality of patients with mood disorders: Follow-up over 34 to 38 years. *Journal of Affective Disorders, 68,* 167–181.

Baldessarini, R. J., Tondo, L., & Hennen, J. (1999). Effects of lithium treatment and its discontinuation on suicidal behavior in bipolar manic–depressive disorders. *Journal of Clinical Psychiatry, 60*(Suppl. 2), 77–84.

Barbini, B., Colombo, C., Benedetti, F., Campori, E., Bellodi, L., & Smeraldi, E. (1998). The unipolar–bipolar dichotomy and the response to sleep deprivation. *Psychiatry Research, 79,* 43–50.

Black, D. W., & Nasrallah, A. (1989). Hallucinations and delusions in 1,715 patients with unipolar and bipolar affective disorders. *Psychopathology, 22,* 28–34.

Bocchetta, A., Ardau, R., Burrai, C., Chillotti, C., Quesada, G., & Del Zompo, M. (1998). Suicidal behavior on and off lithium prophylaxis in a group of patients with prior suicide attempts. *Journal of Clinical Psychopharmacology, 18,* 384–389.

Brickman, A., LoPiccolo, C., & Johnson, S. L. (2002). Screening for bipolar disorder by community providers [Letter to the editor]. *Psychiatric Services, 53,* 349.

Brieger, P., Ehrt, E., & Maneros, A. (2003). Frequency of comorbid personality disorders in bipolar and unipolar affective disorders. *Comprehensive Psychiatry, 44,* 28–34.

Brown, E. S., Suppes, T., Adinoff, B., & Thomas, N. R. (2001). Drug abuse and bipolar disorder: Comorbidity or misdiagnosis? *Journal of Affective Disorders, 65,* 105–115.

Cardno, A. G., Rijsdijk, F. V., Sham, P. C., Murray, R. M., & McGuffin, P. (2002). A twin study of genetic relationships between psychotic symptoms. *American Journal of Psychiatry, 159,* 539–545.

Chen, Y. W., & Dilsaver, S. C. (1996). Lifetime rates of suicide attempts among subjects with bipolar and unipolar disorders relative to subjects with other Axis I disorders. *Biological Psychiatry, 39,* 896–899.

Chengappa, K. N. R., Levine, J., Gershon, S., & Kupfer, D. J. (2000). Lifetime prevalence of substance or alcohol abuse and dependence among subjects with bipolar I and II disorders in a voluntary registry. *Bipolar Disorders, 2,* 191–195.

Coppen, A., & Farmer, R. (1998). Suicide mortality in patients on lithium maintenance therapy. *Journal of Affective Disorders, 50,* 261–267.

Davidoff, S. A., Forester, B. P., Ghaemi, S. N., & Bodkin, J. A. (1998). Effect of video self-observation on development of insight on psychotic disorders. *Journal of Nervous and Mental Diseases, 186,* 697–700.

Depue, R. A., & Monroe, S. M. (1978). The unipolar–bipolar distinction in the depressive disorders. *Psychological Bulletin, 85,* 1001–1029.

Drevets, W. C. (2001). Integration of structural and functional imaging: Examples in depression research. In D. D. Dougherty & S. L. Rauch (Eds.), *Psychiatric neuroimaging research: Contemporary strategies* (pp. 249–290). Washington, DC: American Psychiatric Association Press.

Dunayevich, E., Sax, K. W., Keck, P. E., Jr., McElroy, S. L., Sorter, M. T., McConville, B. J., & Strakowski, S. M. (2000). Twelve-month outcome in bipolar patients with and without personality disorders. *Journal of Clinical Psychiatry, 61,* 134–139.

Faravelli, C., Degl'Innocenti, B. G., Aiazzi, L., & Incerpi, G. (1990). Epidemiology of mood disorders: A community survey in Florence. *Journal of Affective Disorders, 20,* 135–141.

Frangou, S. (2002). Predictors of outcome in a representative population of bipolar disorder. *Bipolar Disorders, 4*(Suppl. 1), 41–42.

Geller, B., & Luby, J. (1997). Child and adolescent bipolar disorder: A review of the past 10 years. *Journal of the American Academy of Child and Adolescent Psychiatry, 36,* 1168–1176.

George, M. S., Ketter, T. A., Kimbrell, T. A., & Post, R. M. (1998). Brain imaging. In P. J. Goodnick (Ed.), *Mania: Clinical and research perspectives* (pp. 191–238). Washington, DC: American Psychiatric Association.

Ghaemi, S. N., Boiman, E. E., & Goodwin, F. K. (2000). Diagnosing bipolar disorder and the effect of antidepressants: A naturalistic study. *Journal of Clinical Psychiatry, 61,* 804–808.

Ghaemi, S. N., Lenox, M. S., & Baldessarini, R. J. (2001). Effectiveness and safety of long-term antidepressant treatment in bipolar disorder. *Journal of Clinical Psychiatry, 62*, 565–569.

Ghaemi, S. N., Sachs, G. S., Chiou, A. M., Pandurangi, A. K., & Goodwin, F. K. (1999). Is bipolar disorder still underdiagnosed? Are antidepressants overutilized? *Journal of Affective Disorders, 52*, 135–144.

Goodwin, F. K., & Jamison, K. R. (1990). *Manic–depressive illness*. Oxford, UK: Oxford University Press.

Goodwin, R. D., & Hoven, C. W. (2002). Bipolar–panic comorbidity in the general population: Prevalence and associated morbidity. *Journal of Affective Disorders, 70*, 27–33.

Harris, E. C., & Barraclough, B. (1997). Suicide as an outcome for mental disorders: A meta-analysis. *British Journal of Psychiatry, 170*, 205–228.

Harrow, M., Goldberg, J. F., Grossman, L. S., & Meltzer, H. Y. (1990). Outcome in manic disorders: A naturalistic follow-up study. *Archives of General Psychiatry, 47*, 665–671.

Hinshaw, S. P. (2002). *The years of silence are past: My father's life with bipolar disorder*. New York: Cambridge University Press.

Hirschfeld, R. M. A., Bowden, C. L., Gitlin, M. J., Keck, P. E., Suppes, T., Thase, M. E., & Perlis, R. H. (2002). TI: Practice guidelines for the treatment of patients with bipolar disorder (2nd ed.). In American Psychiatric Association, *American Psychiatric Association practice guidelines for the treatment of psychiatric disorders: Compendium 2002* (pp. 547–634). Washington, DC: American Psychiatric Association.

Hlastala, S. A., Frank, E., Mallinger, A. G., Thase, M. E., Ritenour, A. M., & Kupfer, D. J. (1997). Bipolar depression: An underestimated treatment challenge. *Depression and Anxiety, 5*, 73–83.

Hyman, S. E. (2000). Goals for research on bipolar disorder: The view from NIMH. *Biological Psychiatry, 48*, 436–441.

Jamison, K. R. (1996). *Touched with fire: Manic–depressive illness and the artistic temperament*. New York: Free Press.

Jamison, K. R. (1999). *Night falls fast: Understanding suicide*. New York: Knopf.

Johnson, R. E., & McFarland, B. H. (1996). Lithium use and discontinuation in a health maintenance organization. *American Journal of Psychiatry, 153*, 993–1000.

Johnson, S. L., Eisdorfer, C., LoPiccolo, C., & Brickman, A. (2003). *Disregarding a prior diagnosis of mania predicts hospitalization in a managed care setting*. Manuscript submitted for publication.

Johnson, S. L., & Kizer, A. (2002). Bipolar and unipolar depression: A comparison of clinical phenomenology and psychosocial predictors. In I. H. Gotlib & C. L. Hammen (Eds.), *Handbook of depression* (pp. 141–165). New York: Guilford Press.

Judd, L. L., Akiskal, H. S., Schettler, P. J., Endicott, J., Maser, J., Solomon, D. A., Leon, A. C., Rice, J. A., & Keller, M. B. (2002). The long-term natural history of the weekly symptomatic status of bipolar I disorder. *Archives of General Psychiatry, 59*, 530–538.

Karkowski, L. M., & Kendler, K. S. (1997). An examination of the genetic relationship between bipolar and unipolar illness in an epidemiological sample. *Psychiatric Genetics, 7*, 159–163.

Kashner, T. M., Rush, A. J., & Altshuler, K. Z. (1999). Measuring costs of guideline-driven mental health care: The Texas medication algorithm project. *Journal of Mental Health Policy and Economics, 2*, 111–121.

Keller, M. B, Lavori, P. W., Kane, J. M, Gelenberg, A. J., Rosenbaum, J. F., Walzer, E. A., & Baker, L. A. (1992). Subsyndromal symptoms in bipolar disorder: A comparison of standard and low serum levels of lithium. *Archives of General Psychiatry, 49*, 371–376.

Kent, S., Fogarty, M., & Yellowlees, P. (1995). A review of studies of heavy users of psychiatric services. *Psychiatric Services, 46,* 1247–1253.

Kessing, L. V., Andersen, P. K, Mortensen, P. B., & Bolwig, T. G. (1998). Recurrence in affective disorder: I. Case register study. *British Journal of Psychiatry, 172,* 23–28.

Kessler, R. C. (1994). The National Comorbidity Survey of the United States. *International Review of Psychiatry, 6,* 8–19.

Kessler, R. C., Rubinow, D. R., Holmes, C., Abelson, J. M., & Zhao, S. (1997). The epidemiology of DSM-III-R bipolar I disorder in a general population survey. *Psychological Medicine, 27,* 1079–1089.

Kessler, R. C., Stang, P., Wittchen, H. U., Stein, M., & Walters, E. E. (1999). Lifetime comorbidities between social phobia and mood disorders in the U.S. National Comorbidity Survey. *Psychological Medicine, 29,* 555–567.

Kraepelin E. (1921). *Manic–depressive insanity and paranoia.* Edinburgh, Scotland: Livingstone.

Lam, D., Wong, G., & Sham, P. (2001). Prodromes, coping strategies and course of illness in bipolar affective disorder: A naturalistic study. *Psychological Medicine, 31,* 1397–1402.

Lenzi, A., Rinaldi, A., Bianco, I., Balestri, C., & Marazziti, D. (1996). Psychotic symptoms in mood disorders: Evaluation of 159 inpatients. *European Psychiatry, 11,* 396–399.

Lewinsohn, P. M., Klein, D. N., & Seeley, J. R (1995). Bipolar disorders in a community sample of older adolescents: Prevalence, phenomenology, comorbidity, and course. *Journal of the American Academy of Child and Adolescent Psychiatry, 34,* 454–463.

Lish, J. D., Dime-Meenan, S., Whybrow, P. C., Price, R. A., & Hirschfeld, R. M. (1994). The National Depressive and Manic–Depressive Association (DMDA) survey of bipolar members. *Journal of Affective Disorders, 31,* 281–294.

Loranger, A. W., & Levine, P. M. (1978). Age at onset of bipolar affective illness. *Archives of General Psychiatry, 35,* 1345–1348.

Murray, J. L., & Lopez, A. D. (1996). *The global burden of disease: A comprehensive assessment of mortality and disability from diseases, injuries, and risk factors in 1990 and projected to 2020.* Boston: Harvard University Press.

Nilsson A. (1999). Lithium therapy and suicide risk. *Journal of Clinical Psychiatry, 60* (Suppl. 2), 85–88.

Plomin, R., DeFries, J. C., McClearn G. E., & Rutter, M. (1997). *Behavioral genetics* (3rd ed.). New York: Freeman.

Prien, R. F., Kupfer, D. J., Mansky, P. A., Small, J. G., Tuason, V. B., Voss, C. B., & Johnson, W. B. (1984). Drug therapy in the prevention of recurrences in unipolar and bipolar affective disorders: Report of the NIMH Collaborative Study Group comparing lithium carbonate, imipramine, and a lithium carbonate–imipramine combination. *Archives of General Psychiatry, 41,* 1096–1104.

Prien, R. F., & Potter, W. Z. (1990). NIMH workshop report on treatment of bipolar disorder. *Psychopharmacology Bulletin, 26*(4), 409–427.

Rivas-Vazquez, R., Johnson, S. L., Rey, G. J., & Blais, M. A. (2002). Current treatments for bipolar disorder: A review and update for psychologists. *Professional Psychology: Research and Practice, 33,* 212–223.

Sachs, G. S., Lafer, B., Truman, C. J., Noeth, M., & Thibault, A. B. (1994). Lithium monotherapy: Miracle, myth and misunderstanding. *Psychiatric Annals, 24,* 299–306.

Sajatovic, M., Popli, A., & Semple, W. (1996). Ten-year use of hospital-based services by geriatric veterans with schizophrenia and bipolar disorder. *Psychiatric Services, 47,* 961–965.

Simon, G. E., & Unuetzer, J. (1999). Health care utilization and costs among patients treated for bipolar disorder in an insured population. *Psychiatric Services, 50,* 1303–1308.

Smith, J. A., & Tarrier, N. (1992). Prodromal symptoms in manic–depressive psychosis. *Social Psychiatry and Psychiatric Epidemiology, 27*, 245–248.

Suppes, T., Dennehy, E. B., Swann, A. C., Bowden, C. L., Calabrese, J. R., Hirschfeld, R. M. A., Keck, P. E., JR., Sachs, G. A., Crismon, M. L., Toprac, M. G., & Shon, S. P. (2002). Report of the Texas consensus conference panel on medication treatment of bipolar disorder 2000. *Journal of Clinical Psychiatry, 63*, 288–299.

Tamam, L., & Ozpoyraz, N. (2002). Comorbidity of anxiety disorder among patients with Bipolar I Disorder in remission. *Psychopathology, 35*, 203–209.

Uecok, A., Karaveli, D., Kundakci, T., & Yazici, O. (1998). Comorbidity of personality disorders with bipolar mood disorders. *Comprehensive Psychiatry, 39*, 72–74.

Unuetzer, J., Simon, G., Pabiniak, C., Bond, K., & Katon, W. (2000). The use of administrative data to assess quality of care for bipolar disorder in a large staff model HMO. *General Hospital Psychiatry, 22*, 1–10.

Vawter, M. P., Freed, W. J., & Kleinman, J. E. (2000). Neuropathology of bipolar disorder. *Biological Psychiatry, 48*, 486–504.

Vehmanen, L., Kaprio, J., & Loennqvist, J. (1995). Twin studies of bipolar disorder. *Psychiatria Fennica, 26*, 107–116.

Vieta, E., Colom, F., Corbella, B., Martinez, A. A., Reinares, M., Benabarre, A., & Gasto, C. (2001). Clinical correlates of psychiatric comorbidity in bipolar I patients. *Bipolar Disorders, 3*, 253–258.

Wahl, O. F. (1999). Mental health consumers' experience of stigma. *Schizophrenia Bulletin, 25*, 467–478.

Wehr, T. A., Turner, E. H., Shimada, J. M., Lowe, C. H., Barker, C., & Leibenluft, E. (1998). Treatment of a rapidly cycling bipolar patient by using extended bed rest and darkness to stabilize the timing and duration of sleep. *Biological Psychiatry, 43*, 822–828.

Weisberg, R. W. (1994). Genius and madness?: A quasi-experimental test of the hypothesis that manic–depression increases creativity. *Psychological Science, 5*, 361–367.

Weiss, R. D., Najavits L. M., & Greenfield, S. F. (1999). A relapse prevention group for patients with bipolar and substance use disorders. *Journal of Substance Abuse Treatment, 16*, 47–54.

Weissman, M. M., Bland, R. C., Canino, G. J., Faravelli, C., Greenwald, S., Hwu, H. G., Joyce, P. R., Karam, E. G., Lee, C. K., Lellouch, J., Lepine, J. P., Newman, S. C., Rubio-Stipec, M., Wells, J. E., Wickramaratne, P. J., Wittchen, H., & Yeh, E. K. (1996). Cross-national epidemiology of major depression and bipolar disorder. *Journal of the American Medical Association, 276*, 293–299.

Winokur, G., & Tsuang, M. T. (1996). *The natural history of mania, depression, and schizophrenia*. Washington, DC: American Psychiatric Press.

Wirz-Justice, A., Quinto, C., Cajochen, C., Werth, E., & Hock C. (1999). A rapid-cycling bipolar patient treated with long nights, bedrest, and light. *Biological Psychiatry, 45*, 1075–1077.

Wyatt, R. J., & Henter, I. (1995). An economic evaluation of manic–depressive illness— 1991. *Social Psychiatry and Psychiatric Epidemiology, 30*, 213–219.

Zarate, C. A., Jr., & Tohen, M. F. (2001). Bipolar disorder and comorbid substance use disorders. In J. R. Hubbard & P. R. Martin (Eds.), *Substance abuse in the mentally and physically disabled* (pp. 59–75). New York: Dekker.

CHAPTER TWO

PSYCHOSOCIAL FUNCTIONING

CONSTANCE HAMMEN
AMY N. COHEN

Although most studies of patients with bipolar disorder focus mainly on clinical course, including episodes and symptoms, there has been a growing interest in assessment and characterization of psychosocial role functioning. Such focus is an important development, deserving emphasis across several forms of major mental illness (e.g., Hirschfeld et al., 2000; Weissman, 1997). It is critical to acknowledge that disorders occur in the context of human lives, and that context and illness mutually affect one another.

Quality of life for those with bipolar disorder is undeniably affected by their ability to perform the roles of parent or relative, marital partner, friend, and coworker. Unfortunately, it is becoming increasingly evident from research that level of functioning in these roles is often compromised, even in the absence of currently diagnosable episodes. Moreover, impairments in role performance may negatively affect many other people in addition to the person diagnosed with bipolar disorder; a "ripple effect" extends to marital partners and intimates, children, family members, friends and associates, and to the wider community. Ultimately, social and occupational dysfunction contribute to a stressful personal environment, a context that itself may be conducive to clinical exacerbation and relapse. This chapter is the first of two focusing on psychosocial aspects of bipolar disorder; we discuss functioning and its predictors, whereas Chapter 5 discusses psychosocial predictors of clinical course.

First we provide a brief overview of bipolar symptomatology and its capacity to disrupt psychosocial role performance, noting empirical evidence of the sizable proportion of patients with bipolar disorder who function poorly, relatively independent of treatment efforts and clinical status.

Subsequently, we review studies investigating several role areas: work, marital, parental, and social support. We attempt to identify clinical, demographic, and psychosocial predictors of functioning, although admittedly the data are relatively sparse in most of these topics. We conclude with implications for treatment and recommendations for further research.

OVERVIEW OF FUNCTIONAL IMPAIRMENT

The symptoms of mania, such as grandiosity often to the point of psychosis, excessive activity, distractibility, impulsiveness, and poor judgment, obviously interfere with role performance. Even hypomanic symptoms of excessive extroversion, high energy, impatience, and irritability can be impairing to the person and bothersome to others (e.g., Depue et al., 1981). Similarly, major depressive episodes, with their low energy, cognitive dysfunction, dispirited mood, low motivation, and hopelessness, are well known to disrupt interpersonal (e.g., review in Joiner, 2002) and work functioning (Mintz, Mintz, Arruda, & Hwang, 1992); even milder depressive states are associated with impairment (e.g., Judd et al., 2000; Wells et al., 1989).

In addition to the obvious impact of symptoms on role functioning, however, are two additional issues: (1) Individuals with bipolar disorder are at risk for significant impairment *independent of episodes*, and (2) there is enormous variation among patients in their levels of psychosocial functioning, with insufficient understanding of the causes of the variability.

Recent naturalistic follow-up studies of patients with bipolar disorder have shown that, as a group, these individuals display functional impairment across multiple domains (e.g., Coryell et al., 1993; Dion, Tohen, Anthony, & Waternaux, 1988; Gitlin, Swendsen, Heller, & Hammen, 1995; Goldberg, Harrow, & Grossman, 1995; Solomon et al., 1996; Strakowski et al., 1998; Tohen, Waternaux, & Tsuang, 1990). Moreover, although perhaps one-third of patients with bipolar disorder appear to have a relatively good level of adjustment, a substantial number (ranging from perhaps 15–40%, depending on sample and outcome variables) has significant if not profound impairment across different roles, despite clinical improvement (Goldberg & Harrow, 1999). Even during stable, euthymic periods, impairment may be pronounced. Cooke, Robb, Young, and Joffe (1996) identified a sample of patients with bipolar disorder who were euthymic—free of recent substance abuse, personality disorder, or medical illness. They found that the patients with bipolar disorder scored lower than the medically ill patients on social functioning, broadly defined, on the self-report scales of the Medical Outcomes Study. Similarly, Bauwens, Tracy, Pardoen, Vander Elst, and Mandlewicz (1991) found worse overall functional outcomes in patients with bipolar disorder compared to controls during remission.

It might be noted that indicators of functional impairment (e.g., work, marital/family adjustment) are generally related to each other; that is, individuals who are impaired in one area tend to be impaired in others. However, research is sketchy on whether such patterns reflect measurement issues (e.g., similar scales), clinical factors (i.e., illness parameters impact all areas of functioning), or whether the role areas are themselves functionally related. For instance, Hammen, Gitlin, and Altshuler (2000) found that good quality of close relationships was a predictor of good work adjustment over time, controlling for clinical factors. Further studies are needed to explore the nature of relationships among functional outcomes. In the following sections we examine in greater detail the functioning of individuals with bipolar disorder in specific adult roles.

OCCUPATIONAL IMPAIRMENT

The work lives of people with bipolar disorder are as varied as their clinical histories, ranging from excellent functioning in high-level professions to those who have never worked due to marked disability—or who do work but at levels significantly below their training and qualifications. In the following sections we describe the relatively sparse data on occupational functioning in people with bipolar disorders, both cross-sectionally and over time, and discuss research on predictors of work adjustment.

Occupational Functioning

Cross-sectional studies paint a relatively pessimistic picture of work adjustment. It appears that the majority of adults with bipolar disorder has difficulty sustaining employment positions. The large-scale Stanley Foundation Bipolar Treatment Outcome Network compiled data on outpatients with bipolar I ($n = 211$) or bipolar II ($n = 42$) disorder and reported on their current employment status (Suppes et al., 2001). Only 33% worked full-time outside the home, and 9% worked part-time; 21% reported that they were unable to work, but this figure is probably actually higher, given the large percentage (36%) of additional patients who reported that they did volunteer work, were unemployed, or worked in sheltered or rehabilitation settings. Suppes et al. (2001) also found that nearly one-fourth of those working full-time indicated working at a level below their qualifications. The UCLA Bipolar I study (methods reported in Cohen, Hammen, Henry, & Daley, 2003) of 64 outpatients assessed during remission similarly found that only 31% worked full-time, and 17% worked part-time; 34% were unemployed (a figure that may include volunteer work). Several other studies similarly reported that only a minority of patients with bipolar disorder was working, even including the number working only part-time or employed at levels below his or her training (Dion et al., 1988; Kusznir, Cooke, & Young, 2000).

Apart from rates of employment, several studies have evaluated current occupational functioning in various ways, similarly presenting a picture of considerable impairment. Hammen et al. (2000) interviewed 52 patients with bipolar I disorder at 3-month intervals and rated level of job functioning on a 5-point scale. Averaged over two years, 44% scored fair or poor job functioning, and only 15% scored in the excellent range (others scored midway, indicating average and good functioning). Solomon et al. (1996) reported a lower rate of fair–poor baseline work functioning (22%), but their sample was recruited for a medication treatment study and excluded those who had rapid cycling or recent drug/alcohol use—conditions that typically reduce occupational functioning.

Overall, the studies of work functioning indicate relatively high rates of occupational maladjustment. A further fact of occupational activity is clarified by longitudinal studies: Occupational success appears to decline over time for many patients with bipolar disorder, and dysfunction is relatively independent of remission. Coryell et al. (1993) reported on a 5-year followup of patients with bipolar disorder in the Collaborative Study of the Psychobiology of Depression ($n = 148$). Fifty-five percent showed decreased occupational status from their lifetime best, and about one-third showed decreased income over time. The changes were significantly worse than those of a comparison group, despite the fact that the groups did not differ on initial levels of occupational status. Dion et al. (1988) found that 6 months after hospitalization, only 43% of patients with bipolar disorder were working despite the fact that the majority were symptom free or only mildly symptomatic. Dion et al. (1988) also observed an apparent downward trend in employment in those with first admissions compared to patients with multiple admissions. In a 2-year follow-up Hammen et al. (2000) found that work functioning status was independent of whether the individual had experienced an episode during the follow-up period. The researchers (Hammen, Cohen, & Henry, 2000) observed similar results in a separate sample of patients (the UCLA Bipolar I study) over a 1-year follow-up.

Overall, results of a handful of studies suggest a puzzling picture: Work status and impairment are quite variable within samples (although indicating, overall, that the majority fail to function well), but even in cases of clinical remission, many adults with bipolar disorder may not be working at levels consistent with their education and qualifications. What clues do we have about the predictors of work functioning?

Predictors of Work Adjustment

A few studies have examined clinical, demographic, or psychosocial predictors of occupational functioning. It would seem obvious that clinical features of the bipolar course likely would impede work capability, but the data are somewhat ambiguous. Dion et al. (1988) found that greater number of previous hospital admissions correlated with poorer work functioning, and Tohen et al. (1990), who studied mostly the same sample reported by Dion and colleagues, found that those with one or more admissions had worse work outcomes at 4 years compared to first admissions. However, Hammen et al. (2000) and Kusznir et al. (2000) did not find significant predictive associations with number of episodes or hospitalizations. On the other hand, several studies consistently found that subsyndromal symptoms, especially depressive symptoms—even in the absence of episode recurrence—were significantly associated with worse job functioning (Bauer, Kirk, Gavin, & Williford, 2001; Dion et al., 1988; Gitlin et al., 1995). Other clinical features that appeared to predict worse job functioning included (1) history of alcohol abuse (Kusznir et al., 2000; Tohen et al., 1990), (2) high levels of anxiety (Kusznir et al., 2000), and (3) psychotic features (Tohen et al., 1990).

Relatively few studies have examined possible demographic characteristics predictive of worse job adjustment. Hammen et al. (2000) found that younger patients with bipolar disorder demonstrated worse job adjustment, but Dion et al. (1988) and Kusznir et al. (2000) found no association with age. Tohen et al. (1990) reported that males displayed worse functioning than females, but Kusznir et al. (2000) found no gender differences, whereas Bauer et al. (2001) studied only male veterans. Socioeconomic status (SES; including education) would seem to be a potentially important predictor, but generally this variable has not been examined. Exceptions include Dion et al. (1988), who found no correlation with job functioning, and Strakowski et al. (1998), who found that higher SES was related to superior functional recovery among those hospitalized with a first episode. Conversely, lower SES was predictive of slower recovery or nonrecovery during the 12-month follow-up.

Finally, the relatively inconsistent or low–moderate associations of clinical and demographic factors with work adjustment seem to suggest the importance of personal, psychosocial variables. However, only Hammen et al. (2000) have explored the contribution of psychosocial variables to work functioning. These researchers found that two personality features were significantly correlated with work adjustment: Greater neuroticism and interpersonal dependency were associated with worse job functioning. Also, the latter traits were highly correlated with self-reported personality disorder symptoms on the Personality Disorder Questionnaire (PDQ; Hyler et al., 1988). When the PDQ was entered in a regression equation, along with clinical variables to predict work functioning, it emerged as a significant predictor—along with a measure of quality of functioning in close relationships. When the psychosocial variables were added to the equation, clinical factors, including recent symptomatology, hospitalizations, and relapse, were nonsignificant predictors of occupational functioning during the follow-up period. Thus, personality and interpersonal characteristics, rather than clinical history features, were predictive of work adjustment.

MARITAL FUNCTIONING

Studies have clearly linked depression with marital distress, both as a cause and consequence of depression (e.g., reviewed in Whisman, 2001). Indeed, Zlotnick, Kohn, Keitner, and Della Grotta (2000) analyzed data from the National Comorbidity Survey and found that marital problems were strongly and specifically linked to current depressive disorders. Moreover, the relative negativity was especially pronounced in depressed individuals' attitudes toward their romantic relationships but not in their attitudes toward their friendships. Although numerous studies have been conducted on the associations between marital functioning and depression, relatively less information is available on these variables in relation to persons with bipolar disorder. In the following sections we summarize the small amount of information that is available.

Marital Functioning

Marital status rates appear to indicate high risk of failure to sustain intimate relationships among people with bipolar disorder. In their 5-year follow-up, Coryell and colleagues (1993) studied 148 patients with bipolar I disorder and found that they were only one-half as likely to be married by the end of the follow-up period as matched non-ill controls (45% divorced compared to 18% among controls; 32% never married, compared to 15% of the controls). Similarly, the Stanley Foundation Bipolar Treatment Outcome Network reported rates of divorce/separation or single status among those with bipolar disorder that were higher than among U.S. national norms (Suppes et al., 2001). It should be noted, however, that there is no evidence that divorce rates are higher among those with bipolar disorder than those with unipolar depression.

Additionally, research overall suggests that the *quality* of marital relationships may be impaired. In a study of children of mothers with mood disorders, Radke-Yarrow (1998) interviewed the mothers and found that those with bipolar disorder (a mix of bipolar I and II) reported higher rates of marital discord at all follow-up assessments (62–76%) compared to non-ill mothers (7–13%) or mothers with unipolar depression (53–59%). In another study Bauwens et al. (1991) collected Social Adjustment Scale information on 27 remitted patients with bipolar disorder, 24 patients with remitted unipolar depression, and 25 control individuals. They found that those with bipolar disorder scored midway between the unipolar (worst) and control (best) subjects in overall marital adjustment.

A small body of research has examined the nonbipolar spouses' attitudes toward the marriage. Levkovitz, Fennig, Horesh, Barak, and Treves (2000) collected reports from 34 spouses of patients with bipolar or unipolar disorder during remission, compared to 34 non-ill control spouses of non-ill wives. Unfortunately, results were not reported separately for the two diagnoses, but, overall, indicated that patients' spouses reported significantly more negative characteristics of their marriages, lower marital satisfaction, more negative partner traits, and fewer positive traits compared to the control spouse reports.

A somewhat related topic concerns caregiver burden—the experience of significant others, often spouses, in dealing with the problems posed by life with an individual who has bipolar disorder. A classic study by Targum, Dibble, Davenport, and Gershon (1981), based on a small sample ($n = 19$ patients with bipolar disorder and their spouses), asked whether the nonbipolar spouses would have married their spouses with bipolar disorder if they had known more about manic–depressive illness. Whereas 5% of the patients said they would not have married, 53% of their spouses said they would not have married the person had they understood bipolar illness. Both the patients and their spouses reported that violence was the most worrisome part of mania, although spouses also expressed concerns about impulsive spending, overtalkativeness, and decreased need for sleep. Spouses reported that suicidality during depression was the major worry, and they were also bothered by the depressive social withdrawal.

The most recent study of caregiver burden among spouses of patients with bipolar disorder ($n = 41$) was conducted by Dore and Romans (2001) in New Zealand. The caregivers were partners or parents, for the most part, and virtually all reported that the person with bipolar disorder was difficult and irritable or hard to be close to during an episode, and that this behavior caused them considerable distress. Nearly half reported experience with or concern about violence when the patient was in an episode. Marital difficulties were common and sometimes persistent. Sixty-two percent of the partners said they would probably not have entered the relationship if they had had more knowledge and understanding of the illness beforehand. Nevertheless, most caregivers felt that the relationship was good when the person was in remission.

Predictors of Marital Adjustment

There is very little information about the predictors of marital/intimate functioning in subjects with bipolar disorder. It would certainly be logical to hypothesize that substantial impediments to marital stability and satisfaction in both the patient and spouse are the severity and frequency, and perhaps predictability, of mood episodes—as well as interepisode symptomatology and role functioning. However, there is little direct empirical evidence. Bauwens et al. (1991) reported that frequency of hospitalizations per year tended to be correlated with poorer marital adjustment. However, there was no indication of which specific features of the course of illness might be more associated with marital difficulties. Similarly, Levkovitz et al. (2000) found that more negative views of non-ill spouses toward the partner were associated with partners' unemployment status or prior history of suicide attempts, but generally there were no associations with clinical features of the disorder. The Lish, Dime-Meenan, Whybrow, Price, and Hirschfeld (1994) survey of National Manic Depressive Association (NMDA) members found that marital difficulties and divorce were associated with both early onset (childhood or adolescence) as well as more frequent recurrences.

Assortative mating (i.e., marrying others with similar conditions/disorders/attributes) is an intriguing aspect of the marriages of those with bipolar disorder. Merikangas and Spiker (1982) found a higher degree of assortative mating among patients with bipolar than unipolar disorder in a sample of 56 married inpatients with primary mood disorders. They noted high concordance between patients and spouses for both affective disorders and alcoholism. The effects could not be attributed to spouses' symptomatic reactions to marriage to a partner with bipolar disorder, because the nonbipolar spouses appeared to have a predisposition to disorders based on elevated rates of psychiatric and mood disorders in their own relatives. Colombo, Cox, and Dunner (1990) studied assortative mating in a large sample of over 1,000 patients with mood or anxiety disorders. They observed that although patients with bipolar illness were less likely to marry, overall, than those with unipolar disorder, there was a specific assortative mating pattern such that men with bipolar disorder were more likely to marry women with mood disorders than were the controls.

A recent meta-analysis by Mathews and Reus (2001), based on the six best-designed studies, confirmed the commonly reported finding of assortative mating for individuals with bipolar disorder, with higher rates than for those with unipolar depression. Specific analyses based on husbands and wives were inconclusive (due to limited data) but suggested that there are much more robust data supporting marriage of men with bipolar disorder to women with mood disorders than of women with bipolar disorder married to men with mood disorders.

The implications of assortative mating are enormous, certainly including genetic risk to offspring. Such dual-disorder pairings are likely to lead to increased marital discord and instability due to the concomitant increases in stress in the home environments and the potentially problematic styles of dealing with interpersonal disputes.

An important predictor of marital functioning among individuals with bipolar disorder might be spouses' attitudes about the ill mate's degree of control over symptoms. Research by Hooley, Richters, Weintraub, and Neale (1987) included ratings of marital satisfaction by spouses of patients with schizophrenia, depression, and bipolar disorder. Marital adjustment was significantly better in cases where spouses had florid "positive" symptoms, including psychotic symptoms, grandiosity, and thought disorder, than when ill spouses were primarily characterized by "negative" or deficit symptoms, including depression, withdrawal, inactivity, and flat emotion. The authors speculated that non-ill spouses may view the severe, florid symptoms to be the product of an illness process beyond the affected person's control but erroneously believe that deficit symptoms are willful or controllable. Such attributions to personality and volition may lead to greater anger and resentment and, hence, marital dissatisfaction. Spouse interpretations of the relatively milder symptoms of hypomania and most symptoms of depression, in particular, may be frequently viewed as within the patient's realm of control, leading to negative attitudes toward the person with the disorder.

PARENTAL FUNCTIONING

Research on parental role functioning by those with bipolar disorder is even more sparse than studies of marital adjustment. Interest in the development of the children of parents with mood disorders has focused largely on those with unipolar depression, yielding a wealth of information on the parental dysfunctions of those who have depressive disorders or symptoms (e.g., reviewed in Goodman & Gotlib, 1999). However, studies of high-risk offspring of bipolar parents, especially those providing information on parental functioning, have been relatively few, although there is recent evidence of increased interest in children at risk for bipolar disorders, so more information may become available in the near future.

It is safe to say that depression is associated with significant impairments in parental functioning, whether the parent has relatively mild but enduring episodes or diagnosable and recurrent episodes (e.g., Beardslee, Versage, & Gladstone, 1998; Downey & Coyne, 1990; Gelfand & Teti, 1990). It is evident that depressive symptoms may impair a parent's ability to sustain calm, patient, and positive engagement with a child. However, it is not so clear whether the enduring parental disabilities are primarily caused by (1) the depressive symptoms themselves (e.g., irritability, low motivation, reduced ability to experience pleasure, withdrawal), (2) the stressful conditions in which depressive experiences are often embedded, or (3) preexisting interpersonal deficiencies that serve as vulnerabilities to experience depressive reactions (e.g., Hammen & Brennan, 2002; Hammen, Shih, & Brennan, 2003).

In recent years several studies have reported on offspring outcomes of parents with bipolar disorder. Overall, a review of these high-risk studies (Lapalme, Hodgins, & LaRoche, 1997) indicates that approximately 52%

of the offspring of parents with bipolar disorder met criteria for a diagnosis of some disorder, compared to 29% of children of parents with no disorders. Overall, 26.5% of the offspring had an affective disorder (i.e., major, minor, or intermittent depression or dysthymia; mania, hypomania, cyclothymia, or hyperthymia states) compared to 8.3% of children of non-ill parents. Bipolar disorder occurred in 5.4% of the offspring, whereas none of the children of non-ill parents was bipolar.

Regarding parenting quality, studies are rare. Only three studies have examined the quality of parenting in mothers with bipolar disorder. Radke-Yarrow (1998) and her colleagues reported on several observations of women with bipolar disorder, interacting with their young children over a 10-year period. The researcher noted that women in both the bipolar and comparison unipolar groups were often irritable and angry with their youngsters (42%), and some of the women with bipolar disorder displayed an overall uninvolved or unavailable style (19%). Women with bipolar disorder also were seen as displaying boundary issues, "unstable enthusiasms," and impulsive behavior in their interactions (61–69%). Overall, dysfunctional maternal styles were predictive of maladaptive outcomes in the children; 58% of the children had received diagnoses by adolescence (chiefly, depression and anxiety disorders, but also disruptive behavior disorders). It should be noted that since most of the women suffered from bipolar II disorder, their symptoms were mainly depressive, and the specific role of mania was not examined.

Hipwell and Kumar (1996) examined mother–infant interactions when the mothers were hospitalized for bipolar disorder, unipolar depression, or schizophrenia. Initially, all the women showed erratic or dysfunctional interactions, but with clinical improvement the majority of women with bipolar disorder or depression displayed normal interactions, compared with a much lower percent of women with schizophrenia.

Gordon et al. (1989), in the UCLA High Risk study, observed mother–child interactions of women with bipolar disorder, unipolar disorder, or medical illness, as well as non-ill controls during discussions of typical family disagreements with school-age children, conducted while the women were in remission. These investigators found that the women with bipolar disorder mostly resembled the normal comparison women in their interaction styles, whereas the women with unipolar depression were significantly more negative, critical, and withdrawn from the discussion task with their children. Overall, depression was a strong predictor of maternal behavior (Hammen, 1991). Regardless of diagnosis, women with more severe depressive symptoms had more disturbances in their interactions with their children, and their children were less well adjusted in various roles. Women with bipolar disorder had significantly fewer depressive episodes over the course of the study (3 years) than did the women with unipolar depression, and thus the phenomenology of the family experiences was quite different for the two groups with mood disorders.

It might be speculated that children's and other family members' reactions to depression and mania would be quite different. A manic episode may be seen as more clearly beyond the individual's control and perhaps more likely to elicit alternative caretaking for children. In contrast, as noted earlier, chronic or recurrent depression is often erroneously attributed to personality deficiencies and seen as within the individual's control. Moreover, children might believe that they are the cause the distress. Obviously the parent's state between episodes is likely to be a strong predictor of the child's adjustment, so that stable and euthymic periods may help to repair disruptions created by periods of symptomatology. Thus, the specific effects of depression and mania as well as the level of chronicity or recovery *between* major episodes may be of considerable predictive significance in understanding overall parenting behavior.

SOCIAL FUNCTIONING

Early reports of the social functioning of individuals with bipolar disorder were almost exclusively limited to descriptive data included as part of a study sample's demographic data. Recently, information on social functioning has been collected systematically, using interviews and questionnaires. Typically, information on social functioning is reported as a global measure of functioning that combines marital, parental, and work functioning, relationships with extended family, friendships, and participation in leisure activities. On a rare occasion, quantity and quality of friendships have been reported separately. The limited information on social functioning among those with bipolar disorder and predictors of social functioning are discussed below.

Research Descriptions of Social Functioning

Reports on the social functioning of individuals with bipolar disorder consistently indicate a limited number of established friendships and social contacts. Kennedy, Thompson, Stancer, Roy, and Persad (1983) elicited patient self-report and found that significantly fewer people with bipolar I disorder had confiding relationships compared to controls with medical illness just prior to a hospital admission. It also has been reported that even during remission, outpatients with bipolar disorder reported fewer social contacts with friends (Bauwens et al., 1991). Gitlin et al. (1995) followed outpatients over 2 years and found that the majority (61%) showed only fair to poor social functioning, indicating limited and impaired contacts with friends. Consistent with that finding, the UCLA Bipolar I study of 64 outpatients found that the majority (58%) reported only occasional social activities, and 16% reported being very isolated.

Despite better developed interpersonal skills compared to patients with schizophrenia, those with bipolar disorder were indistinguishable from stable outpatients with schizophrenia in terms of the number of social activities attended and frequency of social contacts (Dickerson, Sommerville, Origoni, Ringel, & Parente, 2001). According to data collected across several diagnostic groups, the typical number of social outings per month for outpatients with bipolar disorder, unipolar depression, schizoaffective disorder, or schizophrenia were all limited, ranging from one to three occasions a month (Grossman, Harrow, Goldberg, & Fichtner, 1991).

The quality of the friendships and social contacts made by individuals with bipolar disorder has been found, almost exclusively, to be more impaired than normal control comparison groups. Outpatients reported significantly less available support and less adequate support from both close and acquaintance relationships when compared to a random community sample. Only 55% of the outpatients with bipolar disorder described their closest friendship as adequate, whereas 84% of the normal controls described an adequate relationship with their best friend (Romans & McPherson, 1992). In the UCLA Bipolar I study the typical finding was that outpatients had a close friend and reported being satisfied in that relationship, but interviewers' ratings of those relationships indicated that many (30%) had significant problems (e.g., patients with bipolar disorder displayed nonconfiding, unstable, or contentious, behavior and poor conflict-resolution skills). In the Collaborative Study of the Psychobiology of Depression, patients with either bipolar or unipolar disorder reported an equal degree of impairment in their relationships with friends, which was significantly worse than the functioning of the comparison group (Coryell et al., 1993). Johnson, Winett, Meyer, Greenhouse, and Miller (1999) also found that outpatients' perceived social support from friends was substantially lower than that of a normative sample.

In contrast, one study found no difference between outpatients with bipolar disorder and controls on the quality of their friendships (Staner et al., 1997). This discrepant finding may be due to the small sample size of each diagnostic group (*n* = 16 with bipolar I disorder), which required data to be pooled for patients with bipolar I and bipolar II disorder. Clinically, it seems possible that individuals with bipolar II disorder may exhibit better social functioning than individuals with bipolar I disorder, raising the social functioning of the combined group with bipolar disorder to a level similar to the functioning of the control group.

Although limited in number, the consensus of the studies on social functioning by those with bipolar disorder indicates considerable impairment. It is possible that this impairment is almost exclusively related to the affective episode, resolving quickly after remission, or alternatively, that the impairment is present irrespective of mood symptomatology. Although only longitudinal studies can establish the course of the social impairment in bipolar disorder, many cross-sectional studies provide information by interviewing participants when they are euthymic. Almost all of the researchers presented in this section interviewed their sample of people with bipolar disorder when the patient's mood was euthymic or limited to a very few symptoms. Therefore, the collection of studies reviewed lends support to the conclusion that social impairment in bipolar disorder is not directly related to mood symptomatology; rather it persists despite a resolution of symptoms. The Chicago Longitudinal Follow-Up Study is the only one that has reported both global and social functioning of outpatients at two time points. Findings indicated that although global functioning improved over a 3-year-period from index hospitalization, social impairments worsened over the same period (Goldberg et al., 1995; Grossman et al., 1991).

Predictors of Social Functioning

Clinically it seems reasonable to hypothesize that poor social functioning could be a consequence, at least in part, of the nature of bipolar disorder. The disorder typically has an onset around 20 years old, a time of establishing adult friendships and practicing social skills. Additionally, the disorder has a chronic, episodic course that is likely to alienate friends over time.

The data from the few available studies are ambiguous as to the relationship between illness parameters and social functioning. Two studies have reported that illness parameters, including age of onset, illness severity, number of previous episodes, and number of hospital admissions, are unrelated to amount of social contact and level of perceived support (Bauwens et al., 1991; Johnson et al., 1999). Yet, in two other studies, illness parameters have been related to social functioning, although the correlations have been low. Those with bipolar disorder who had been ill longer reported fewer available supports (Romans & McPherson, 1992) but reported better functioning in their existing relationships (UCLA Bipolar I study).

Despite finding that the *number* of previous episodes is unrelated to social functioning, the *type* of previous episodes does seem to be related. Precisely which type of affective episode causes more distress or impairment in social relationships has only been examined in two studies, and the results are contradictory. The results from the Romans and McPherson (1992) study suggested a statistical trend that patients with bipolar disorder, whose course had been dominated by manic episodes, had less adequate and less available support compared to those whose course had been dominated by depressive episodes. Although only a statistical trend, it contradicts later findings by Gitlin et al. (1995) who found that depressive episodes had a more impairing effect on social relationships compared to manic episodes. Due to these mixed findings, it remains unclear which type of affective episode is more damaging to supportive relationships. Future studies may benefit from examining the causal attributions of patients' behaviors made by friends. These attributions, in turn, may be a more reliable and consistent determinant of the symptoms that most impact friendships, as has been found in marital satisfaction and adjustment studies (see Hooley et al., 1987).

In terms of demographic predictors of social functioning, the UCLA Bipolar I study found that age did not predict social functioning, whereas Romans and McPherson (1992) found a low correlation between age and social functioning, such that older patients with bipolar disorder reported fewer available and less adequate close supports.

The almost exclusive research focus on symptomatic course and outcome among those with bipolar I disorder has restricted both the collection and report of data on psychosocial functioning in this population. Furthermore, when investigating types of psychosocial functioning, marital and parental functioning has often taken precedence over the examination of friendships. However, the importance of friendships and social network integration is self-evident, and as Chapter 5 indicates, social support may be an important predictor of symptomatic outcome.

CONCLUSIONS: IMPLICATIONS AND DIRECTIONS FOR FUTURE RESEARCH

Bipolar disorder is associated with work and interpersonal difficulties that are somewhat puzzling in several ways. First, the difficulties in occupational stability, marital status and quality, parental functioning, and social integration are enormously varied from one person to another. With a range encompassing homelessness, on the one hand, to outstanding personal accomplishments despite lifelong bipolar I disorder, on the other, the seemingly same disorder is remarkably different in its social manifestations. We need to understand more about the predictors of diverse levels of functioning.

Second, the dysfunctions in typical roles are not readily explained simply by clinical features of the disorder. This conclusion is admittedly based, in part, on the limitations in the amount and quality of available research. There is considerable need for research that clearly explores the role of various clinical parameters, including experiences of both mania and depression, age of onset, extent of developmental disruption of skills for social adjustment, as well as changes over time as a function of intervening clinical states. In addition, too little is known about clinical features such as psychosis and comorbid substance abuse. Moreover, most research has paid scant attention to the quality of the individual's personal attributes, as resources for coping with bipolar disorder—not to mention the overlooked arena of extent of exposure to parental mental health or illness. Thus, more research on traits, values, coping behaviors, family history, personality pathology, and even neuropsychological functioning is needed to shed light on further aspects of performance in social roles.

Finally, a critical issue is the extent to which functional impairment becomes part of the illness process itself. As Chapter 5 suggests, social impairment likely contributes to the recurrence of episodes and symptomatology. The mechanisms of such processes, probably involving stress and the ability to cope with adversity, require further study. A related question is the extent to which stressful lives and circumstances, along with the bipolar episodes, contribute to a potentially progressive neurobiological process in which poor adjustment and further symptomatology become even more pronounced—in a manner similar to the hypotheses of Post (1992).

Issues concerning psychosocial impairment clearly have considerable implications for treatment of bipolar disorder. Just as the treatment of schizophrenia has increasingly emphasized psychosocial rehabilitation, there is growing acceptance of the need for psychological interventions to supplement those of psychopharmacology in treatment of bipolar disorder (e.g., Goodwin & Ghaemi, 1999). More and more, investigators are studying the impact of treatments aimed at improving family understanding of and communication with the person with bipolar disorder (e.g., Miklowitz & Goldstein, 1997). Interpersonal and cognitive-behavioral interventions may be critical tools with which to address the marital, social, occupational, and parental difficulties encountered by those with bipolar disorder (see Chapter 10, this volume). It is to be hoped that such treatments will improve the lives of people with bipolar disorder and their families, and also improve the course of their disorder.

REFERENCES

Bauer, M. S., Kirk, G. F., Gavin, C., & Williford, W. O. (2001). Determinants of functional outcome and healthcare costs in bipolar disorder: A high-intensity follow-up study. *Journal of Affective Disorders, 65*, 231–241.

Bauwens, F., Tracy, A., Pardoen, D., Vander Elst, M., & Mandlewicz, J. (1991). Social adjustment of remitted bipolar and unipolar out-patients. *British Journal of Psychiatry, 159*, 239–244.

Beardslee, W. R., Versage, E. M., & Gladstone, T. R. (1998). Children of affectively ill parents: A review of the past 10 years. *Journal of the American Academy of Child and Adolescent Psychiatry, 37*, 1134–1141.

Cohen, A., Hammen, C., Henry, R., & Daley, S. (2003). *Effects of stress and social support on recurrence in bipolar disorder.* Manuscript submitted for publication.

Colombo, M., Cox, G., & Dunner, D. L. (1990). Assortative mating in affective and anxiety disorders: Preliminary findings. *Psychiatric Genetics, 1*, 35–44.

Cooke, R. G., Robb, J. C., Young, L. T., & Joffe, R. T. (1996). Well-being and functioning in patients with bipolar disorder assessed using the MOS 20–ITEM short form (SF-20). *Journal of Affective Disorders, 39*, 93–97.

Coryell, W., Scheftner, W., Keller, M., Endicott, J., Maser, J., & Klerman, G. L. (1993). The enduring psychological consequences of mania and depression. *American Journal of Psychiatry, 150,* 720–727.

Depue, R. A., Slater, J. F., Wolfstetter-Kausch, H., Klein, D., Goplerud, E., & Farr, D. (1981). A behavioral paradigm for identifying persons at risk for bipolar depressive disorder: A conceptual framework and five validation studies. *Journal of Abnormal Psychology, 90,* 381–439.

Dickerson, F. B., Sommerville, J., Origoni, A. E., Ringel, N.B., & Parente, F. (2001). Outpatients with schizophrenia and bipolar I disorder: Do they differ in their cognitive and social functioning? *Psychiatry Research, 102,* 21–27.

Dion, G. L., Tohen, M., Anthony, W. A., & Waternaux, C. S. (1988). Symptoms and functioning of patients with bipolar disorder six months after hospitalization. *Hospital and Community Psychiatry, 39,* 652–657.

Dore, G., & Romans, S. E. (2001). Impact of bipolar affective disorder on family and partners. *Journal of Affective Disorders, 67,* 147–158.

Downey, G., & Coyne, J. C. (1990). Children of depressed parents: An integrative review. *Psychological Bulletin, 108,* 50–76.

Gelfand, D. M., & Teti, D. M. (1990). The effects of maternal depression on children. *Clinical Psychology Review, 10,* 329–353.

Gitlin, M., Swendsen, J., Heller, T., & Hammen, C. (1995). Relapse and impairment in bipolar disorder. *American Journal of Psychiatry, 152,* 1635–1640.

Goldberg, J. F., & Harrow, M. (Eds.). (1999). *Bipolar disorders: Clinical course and outcome.* Washington, DC: American Psychiatric Press.

Goldberg, J. F., Harrow, M., & Grossman, L. S. (1995). Course and outcome in bipolar affective disorder: A longitudinal follow-up study. *American Journal of Psychiatry, 152,* 379–384.

Goodman, S., & Gotlib, I. (1999). Risk for psychopathology in the children of depressed mothers: A developmental model for understanding mechanisms of transmission. *Psychological Review, 106,* 458–490.

Goodwin, F., & Ghaemi, N. (1999). Bipolar disorder: State of the art. *Dialogues in Clinical Neuroscience, 1,* 41–51.

Gordon, D., Burge, D., Hammen, C., Adrian, C., Jaenicke, C., & Hiroto, D. (1989). Observations of interactions of depressed women with their children. *American Journal of Psychiatry, 146,* 50–55.

Grossman, L. S., Harrow, M., Goldberg, J. F., & Fichtner, C. G. (1991). Outcome of schizoaffective disorder at two long-term follow-ups: Comparisons with outcome of schizophrenia and affective disorders. *American Journal of Psychiatry, 148,* 1359–1365.

Hammen, C. L. (1991). *Depression runs in families: The social context of risk and resilience in children of depressed mothers.* New York: Springer-Verlag.

Hammen, C., & Brennan, C. (2002). Interpersonal dysfunction in depressed women: Impairments independent of depressive symptoms. *Journal of Affective Disorders, 72,* 145–156.

Hammen, C., Cohen, A., & Henry, R. (2000). *Predictors of work and social functioning in bipolar I disorder.* Presented at the annual meeting of the Society for Research in Psychopathology, Boulder, CO.

Hammen, C., Gitlin, M., & Altshuler, L. (2000). Predictors of work adjustment in Bipolar I patients: A naturalistic longitudinal follow-up. *Journal of Consulting and Clinical Psychology, 68,* 220–225.

Hammen, C., Shih, J., & Brennan, P. (2003). *Intergenerational transmission of depression: Tests of an interpersonal stress model in a community sample.* Manuscript submitted for publication.

Hipwell, A. E., & Kumar, R. (1996). Maternal psychopathology and prediction of outcome based on mother–infant interaction ratings (BMIS). *British Journal of Psychiatry, 169,* 655–661.

Hirschfeld, R. M. A., Montgomery, S. A., Keller, M. B., Kasper, S., Schatzberg, A. F., Moller, H.-J., Healy, D., Baldwin, D., Humble, M., Versiani, M., Montenegro, R., & Bourgeois, M. (2000). Social functioning in depression: A review. *Journal of Clinical Psychiatry, 61*, 268–275.

Hooley, J. M., Richters, J. E., Weintraub, S., & Neale, J. M. (1987). Psychopathology and marital distress: The positive side of positive symptoms. *Journal of Abnormal Psychology, 96*, 27–33.

Hyler, S., Rieder, R., Williams, J., Spitzer, R., Hendler, J., & Lyons, M. (1988). The Personality Diagnostic Questionnaire: Development and preliminary results. *Journal of Personality Disorders, 2*, 229–237.

Johnson, S. L., Winett, C. A., Meyer, B., Greenhouse, W. J., & Miller, I. (1999). Social support and the course of bipolar disorder. *Journal of Abnormal Psychology, 108*(4), 558–566.

Joiner, T. E., Jr. (2002). Depression in its interpersonal context. In C. L. Hammen & I. H. Gotlib (Eds.), *Handbook of depression* (pp. 295–313). New York: Guilford Press.

Judd, L. L., Akiskal, H. S., Zeller, P. J., Paulus, M., Leon, A. C., Maser, J. D., Endicott, J., Coryell, W., Kunovac, J. L., Mueller, T. I., Rice, J. P., & Keller, M. B. (2000). Psychosocial disability during the long-term course of unipolar major depressive disorder. *Archives of General Psychiatry, 57*, 375–380.

Kennedy, S., Thompson, R., Stancer, H. C., Roy, A., & Persad, E. (1983). Life events precipitating mania. *British Journal of Psychiatry, 142*, 398–403.

Kusznir, A., Cooke, R. G., & Young, L. T. (2000). The correlates of community functioning in patients with bipolar disorder. *Journal of Affective Disorders, 61*, 81–85.

Lapalme, M., Hodgins, S., & LaRoche, C. (1997). Children of parents with bipolar disorder: A meta-analysis of risk for mental disorders. *Canadian Journal of Psychiatry, 42*, 623–631.

Levkovitz, V., Fennig, S., Horesh, N., Barak, V., & Treves, I. (2000). Perception of ill spouse and dyadic relationship in couples with affective disorder and without. *Journal of Affective Disorders, 58*, 237–240.

Lish, J. D., Dime-Meenan, S., Whybrow, P. C., Price, R. A., & Hirschfeld, R. M. A. (1994). The National Depressive and Manic–Depressive Association (DMDA) survey of bipolar members. *Journal of Affective Disorders, 31*, 281–294.

Mathews, C. A., & Reus, V. I. (2001). Assortative mating in the affective disorders: A systematic review and meta-analysis. *Comprehensive Psychiatry, 42*, 257–262.

Merikangas, K. R., & Spiker, D. G. (1982). Assortative mating among in-patients with primary affective disorder. *Psychological Medicine, 12*, 753–764.

Miklowitz, D. J., & Goldstein, M. J. (1997). *Bipolar disorder: A family-focused treatment approach.* New York: Guilford Press.

Mintz, J., Mintz, L., Arruda, M., & Hwang, S. (1992). Treatments of depression and the functional capacity to work. *Archives of General Psychiatry, 49*, 761–768.

Post, R. M. (1992). Transduction of psychosocial stress into the neurobiology of recurrent affective disorder. *American Journal of Psychiatry, 149*, 999–1010.

Radke-Yarrow, M. (1998). *Children of depressed mothers: From early childhood to maturity.* Cambridge, UK: Cambridge University Press.

Romans, S. E., & McPherson, H. M. (1992). The social networks of bipolar affective disorder patients. *Journal of Affective Disorders, 25*, 221–228.

Solomon, D. A., Ristow, W. R., Keller, M. B., Kane, J. M., Gelenberg, A. J., Rosenbaum, J. F., & Warshaw, M. G. (1996). Serum lithium levels and psychosocial function in patients with Bipolar I disorder. *American Journal of Psychiatry, 153*, 1301–1307.

Staner, L., Tracy, A., Dramaix, M., Genevrois, C., Vander Elst, M., Vilane, A., Bauwens, F., Pardoen, D., & Mendlewicz, J. (1997). Clinical and psychosocial predictors of recurrence in recovered bipolar and unipolar depressives: A one-year controlled prospective study. *Psychiatry Research, 69*, 39–51.

Strakowski, S. M., Keck, P. E., McElroy, S. L., West, S. A., Sax, K. W., Hawkins, J. M.,

Kmetz, G. F., Upadhyaya, V. H., Tugrul, K. C., & Bourne, M. L. (1998). Twelve-month outcome after a first hospitalization for affective psychosis. *Archives of General Psychiatry, 55*, 49–55.

Suppes, T., Leverich, G. S., Keck, P. E., Nolen, W. A., Denicoff, K. D., Altshuler, L. L., McElroy, S. L., Rush, A. J., Kupka, R., Frye, M. A., Bickel, M., & Post, R. M. (2001). The Stanley Foundation Bipolar Treatment Outcome Network II. Demographics and illness characteristics of the first 261 patients. *Journal of Affective Disorders, 67*, 45–59.

Targum, S. D., Dibble, E., Davenport, Y. B., & Gershon, E. S. (1981). The Family Attitudes Questionnaire: Patients' and spouses' views of bipolar illness. *Archives of General Psychiatry, 38*, 562–568.

Tohen, M., Waternaux, C. M., & Tsuang, M. T. (1990). Outcome in mania: A 4–year prospective follow-up of 75 patients utilizing survival analysis. *Archives of General Psychiatry, 47*, 1106–1111.

Weissman, M. M. (1997). Beyond symptoms: Social functioning and the new antidepressants. *Journal of Psychopharmacology, 11*, S5–S8.

Wells, K. B., Stewart, A., Hays, R. D., Burnam, A., Rogers, W., Daniels, M., Berry, S., Greenfield, S., & Ware, J. (1989). The functioning and well-being of depressed patients. *Journal of the American Medical Association, 262*, 914–919.

Whisman, M. A. (2001). The association between depression and marital dissatisfaction. In S. R. H. Beach (Ed.), *Marital and family processes in depression: A scientific foundation for clinical practice* (pp. 3–24). Washington, DC: American Psychological Association.

Zlotnick, C., Kohn, R., Keitner, G., & Della Grotta, S. A. D. (2000). The relationship between quality of interpersonal relationships and major depressive disorder: Findings from the National Comorbidity Survey. *Journal of Affective Disorders, 59*, 205–215.

CHAPTER THREE

DIFFERENTIAL DIAGNOSIS AND ASSESSMENT OF ADULT BIPOLAR DISORDER

EDWARD ALTMAN

Bipolar disorder, characterized by mania (bipolar I) or hypomania (bipolar II), alternating or intermingling with episodes of depression, presents one of the most dramatic presentations among the major psychiatric disorders. Because this disorder frequently involves episodes of both mania and depression, an understanding of the interplay between these affective states is important for diagnosis and treatment. Thus, for example, depression may *precede* an episode of mania or hypomania, *intermingle* with manic symptoms during an episode, *follow* a manic or hypomanic phase, or occur as a distinct episode within the pattern of manic or hypomanic episodes.

ASSOCIATED FEATURES AND COMORBIDITY

Approximately one-third of individuals with bipolar disorder have a comorbid substance abuse disorder, and the rates of concomitant alcohol and drug abuse may exceed 50% in younger men. In addition to complicating the natural history of bipolar disorder and undermining treatment response, substance abuse may increase the risk of suicide and lead to medical and neurological complications.

In a longitudinal epidemiological study, Angst (1998) demonstrated that comorbidity of brief hypomania (a proposed variant of bipolar II disorder) was found primarily with panic disorder, social phobia, substance abuse/dependence, somatization disorder, personality disorders, suicidality, and delinquency. Other associations have included generalized anxiety disorder, obsessive–compulsive disorder, Tourette syndrome, and eating disorders.

Psychotic symptoms may develop in some individuals and usually recur in subsequent manic episodes. Rosen, Rosenthal, Dunner, and Fieve (1983) compared psychotic and nonpsychotic manic patients on a number of clinical outcome and demographic variables and found that the psychotic group had a significantly poorer outcome in terms of social functioning. The presence of psychosis is also associated with poorer interepisode recovery.

During a manic episode, mood may shift quickly to anger or depression, which may last hours or even days. Not uncommonly, depressive and manic symptoms may occur simultaneously. In cases where the DSM-IV (American Psychiatric Association, 1994) criteria are met for both a manic *and* a major depressive episode every day for at least one week, the episode is then classified as *mixed*.

DIFFERENTIAL DIAGNOSIS

Bipolar disorder can be divided into *primary* and *secondary* types. *Secondary* types are those that develop as a consequence of various medical conditions or substances that may alter brain structure or function. These may include stroke, neoplasms, epilepsy, infections (e.g., HIV), and metabolic or endocrine disturbances. In these cases, the proper DSM-IV diagnosis would be *mood disorder due to a general medical condition*. This determination should be based on a comprehensive history, physical examination, and/or laboratory findings. A late onset of a first manic episode (e.g., after age 55) may suggest the possibility of an etiological general medical condition or substance.

Manic-like disturbances also may be induced by medications (e.g., stimulants, steroids, antidepressants), drugs of abuse (e.g., alcohol, cocaine, heroin, PCP), and somatic treatments for depression (e.g., light therapy, ECT), in which case the correct DSM-IV diagnosis is *substance-induced mood disorder*. A substance-induced mood disorder may be distinguished from a *primary* mood disorder by considering the onset, course, and other factors. For drugs of abuse, there should be evidence from the history, physical examination, or laboratory findings of intoxication or withdrawal. The temporal relationship between the use of a substance and the development of mood symptoms is critical. Substance-induced mood disorders arise only in association with intoxication or withdrawal states, whereas *primary* mood disorders may precede the onset of substance use or may occur during times of sustained abstinence. Other diagnostic considerations for a primary mood disorder include whether or not symptoms persist well after cessation of the substance, and whether the symptoms are substantially in excess of what would be expected given the type, amount, or duration of the substance used.

It is also important to note that comorbid occurrence of substance and alcohol abuse disorders is significantly higher in patients with bipolar disorder than in the general population, and increases the risk of suicide in these individuals (Regier et al., 1990). As Janicak, Davis, Preskorn, and Ayd (2001) point out, it is important to ascertain whether an episode of bipolar disorder is (1) drug- or alcohol-induced, (2) an attempt by the patient to self-medicate, or (3) unrelated to the current exacerbation. Concurrent substance abuse may complicate diagnosis, undermine the potential benefits of treatment, and adversely affect the course of the illness.

Manic episodes (bipolar I disorder) can be distinguished from *hypomanic* episodes (bipolar II disorders) by severity. Although both disorders can display similar symptoms, hypomanic episodes are not severe enough to cause marked impairment in social or occupational functioning, or to require hospitalization. Furthermore, delusions and hallucinations are not present in hypomania.

Psychotic disorders (e.g., schizophrenia, schizoaffective disorder, and delusional disorders) may be difficult to distinguish from bipolar I disorder, primarily because both disorders share a number of clinical symptoms (e.g., irritability, agitation, grandiose and/or persecutory delusions). It may not be possible to make a definitive diagnosis until the course of the illness is followed over a period of time. Review of personal and family history may provide information to help differentiate between these disorders. In general, psychotic disorders are characterized by the presence of psychotic symptoms that occur in the absence of prominent mood symptoms for at least 2 weeks. When mood symptoms are present in schizophrenia or schizoaffective disorder, they rarely occur with sufficient intensity, number, or duration to meet criteria for a manic episode or a major depressive episode. However, for DSM-IV *schizoaffective disorder*, there must be a mood episode concurrent with the active symptoms of schizophrenia, and such symptoms must be present for a significant portion of the total duration of the disturbance. In addition, psychotic symptoms must be present for at least 2 weeks in the absence of prominent mood symptoms. Schizoaffective disorder can be further subtyped as either bipolar (if the disturbance includes a manic or mixed episode) or depressed (if the disturbance includes a major depressive episode). Mood symptoms in *schizophrenia* typically are brief, relative to the total duration of the disturbance, or occur only during the prodromal or residual phases and are not sufficient to meet the full criteria for an episode. Other considerations include the proclivity of bipolar patients to demonstrate pressured speech, flight of ideas, and grandiosity.

Delusions are more common than hallucinations in both mania and depression, and they tend to have more religious and grandiose schemes.

The DSM-IV distinguishes between psychotic features that are either mood-congruent or mood-incongruent. However, the clinical and diagnostic usefulness of this distinction remains unproven. For example, Pope and Lipinski (1978) reported that psychotic symptoms were evident in 20–50% of manic patients and that many of the delusions were mood-incongruent (i.e., delusions of persecution, catatonic symptoms, formal thought disorder, and auditory hallucinations not consistent with mood state). In addition, Schneiderian first-rank symptoms, once regarded as pathonomonic of schizophrenia, have been reported in a significant proportion of manic patients (Carpenter, Strauss, & Muleh, 1973; Taylor & Abrams, 1973).

In *cyclothymic disorder*, a chronic condition of at least 2 years duration, the hypomanic and depressive symptoms are not sufficient in severity, number, or pervasiveness to meet the full criteria for a manic episode. The course is typically marked by fluctuating mood disturbances involving numerous periods of hypomanic symptoms and numerous periods of depressive symptoms. This DSM-IV designation is made only if the initial 2-year episode is free of major depressive, manic, or mixed episodes. Furthermore, this diagnosis can only be given if there are no more than 2 months of symptom-free intervals during the 2-year period. Following the initial episode, manic, mixed, or major depressive episodes may be superimposed on the ongoing symptoms of cyclothymic disorder.

Bipolar I disorder also may resemble *attention-deficit/hyperactivity disorder*. Both disorders may involve excessive activity, impulsive behavior, poor judgment, and lack of insight. However, attention-deficit/hyperactivity disorder differs from bipolar I disorder by its early onset (i.e., before age 7 years), chronic as opposed to episodic course, absence of relatively clear onsets and offsets, and the absence of overly expansive or elevated mood or psychotic features.

Janowsky, El-Yousef, and Davis (1974) have shown that patients with mania display interpersonal styles suggestive of borderline or antisocial personality disorders; these styles fluctuate with the course of their illness. These patients may elicit anger from others, project responsibility onto others, test limits, and exploit or attack others' weaknesses. The authors further noted that these behaviors occurred primarily when patients were in a manic phase and often improved with lithium therapy.

As Janicak et al. (2001) note, characterological traits or disorders should be considered in the differential diagnosis. For example, some criteria for DSM-IV *borderline personality disorder* overlap with symptoms of mania or hypomania, such as impulsivity, affective instability, irritability or inappropriate anger, and unstable interpersonal relationships. When these individuals are followed longitudinally, some eventually may be reclassified as having a bipolar disorder, a subsyndromal variant, or an atypical presentation. Dunayevich et al. (2000) have shown that the co-occurrence of personality disorders and bipolar disorders is associated with poorer outcome after discharge from the hospital for an acute manic episode.

Finally, Akiskal (1987) discussed *subsyndromal* or *subclinical mood* disorders, which are characterized by milder bipolar symptoms, abrupt biphasic shifts, and troubled interpersonal relationships. Individuals with these features may be misdiagnosed as having personality disorders and referred for long-term therapy, which typically is ineffective. Akiskal noted that if these individuals are properly diagnosed and treated with mood stabilizers, their overall functioning often improves.

DIAGNOSIS AND ASSESSMENT OF BIPOLAR DISORDERS

Diagnostic Instruments

Schedule for Affective Disorders and Schizophrenia

Prior to the advent of DSM-III in 1980, the Research Diagnostic Criteria (RDC; Spitzer, Endicott, & Robins, 1979) was the primary instrument for diagnosing major psychiatric disorders in the United States. The RDC provides clear inclusion and exclusion criteria for a current episode. Information required for making an RDC diagnosis is gathered through a clinical interview using the Schedule for Affective Disorders and Schizophrenia (SADS; Endicott & Spitzer, 1978). The SADS contains structured interview questions and guidelines that allow clinicians to obtain clinical information in a standardized manner. It can be used to assess both the presence and severity of each symptom. Several versions of the SADS were developed for specific uses. For example, a change version (SADS-C; Spitzer & Endicott, 1978) is available for assessing outcome in treatment studies, and a lifetime version (SADS-L; Spitzer & Endicott, 1977) is available for diagnosing past episodes.

Structured Clinical Interview for DSM

The RDC was last revised in 1989 and subsequently replaced with the Structured Clinical Interview for DSM (SCID; Spitzer, Williams, Gibbon, & First, 1992). The SCID follows the structured format of the SADS but is intended for diagnosis only; it does not assess severity. It was designed to provide clinicians with a standard diagnostic instrument for deriving DSM-III diagnoses. It has been modified to incorporate changes in subsequent revisions of the DSM. Both the SADS and the SCID require some degree of clinical training and practice to ensure reliable administration. The SCID is available in different formats—for example, a clinician version for Axis I disorders (SCID-I), personality disorders (SCID-PD), and for family members or nonpatients (SCID-NP).

Diagnostic Interview Schedule

An alternative diagnostic instrument, developed primarily for use in epidemiological studies, is the Diagnostic Interview Schedule (DIS; Robins, Helzer, Croughan, & Radcliff, 1981). The DIS was designed to be administered by lay interviewers after 1 week of intensive training. Although other investigators have used the DIS for nonepidemiological studies, the SCID is still the preferred diagnostic instrument for clinical research.

Instruments to Assess the Course of Illness

With respect to assessing the course of bipolar disorder, there are few standardized methods for doing so. Past research has involved retrospective studies, prospective follow-up studies, and naturalistic studies. Post, Roy-Bryne, and Uhde (1988) encouraged the use of retrospective and prospective historical graphing as a method for tracking the disorder's progression and response to therapy. They suggested three levels for grading severity: *nonfunctional*, indicating severe mania or depression; *moderate severity*, indicating some impairment in work or social functioning; and *mild severity*, indicating behavioral or mood alterations but little or no impairment. This charting also should include important life events, behavior and mood changes, and medications or other treatments.

Instruments to Assess the Severity of Bipolar Disorders

In the past decade, a significant advance in the development of reliable and valid mania rating scales has occurred. Newer scales have improved considerably on the design of earlier rating scales. Some of these improvements include:

- Clearer operational definitions of symptoms
- Well-defined anchor points for assessing severity
- More relevant item content (i.e., the inclusion of symptoms consistent with DSM criteria)
- Guidelines for administration, scoring, and interpretation
- Use of more appropriate statistical methods for assessing test–retest reliability (i.e., the intraclass correlation coefficient) and sensitivity/specificity (i.e., receiver operating characteristic [ROC] curve analysis)
- Larger sample sizes
- The inclusion of comparison groups to assess discriminant validity.

These instruments evolved initially from nurses' rating scales in the early 1970s to numerous clinician-rated scales and, more recently, self-rating scales. In addition, scales are now available that assess simultaneously the presence of symptoms for both mania and depression—useful in cases of mixed bipolar disorder.

The profusion of bipolar rating scales has made it necessary to provide meaningful comparisons that can guide researchers and clinicians in their choice of instruments. Space limitations do not permit an exhaustive review and comparison of all the different scales available for bipolar disorder. Indeed, many of the earlier published scales are seldom used today. Furthermore, comprehensive reviews of many of these scales are currently available. The most recent, by Livianos-Aldana and Rojo-Moreno (2001), covers most of the current scales and provides specific recommendations for their use. Poolsup, Li Wan Po, and Oyebode (1999) also provide a recent but less comprehensive review. Moreover, Poolsup et al. exclude self-rating scales from their evaluation, describing them as unreliable.

The following sections provide a discussion and evaluation of some of the most widely used rating scales for bipolar disorders as well as a review of the most recently developed scales, some of which are not included in previous reviews. Because depression rating scales have already enjoyed great acceptance and diffusion among researchers and clinicians, they are not included in this discussion. The purpose here is to provide sufficient information to guide clinicians in their choice of a scale that best satisfies a specific clinical or research need.

In selecting among scales, a number of factors must be considered. For example, will nurses or clinicians administer the scale? Will the scale be used for psychiatric inpatients, outpatients, or for general use in primary care settings? How much time is required to administer the scale? For example, in cases where clinical resources are limited, self-rating scales may be the practical choice. Will the scale be used for screening purposes or to monitor treatment response? Does the scale assess manic symptoms only or mixed symptoms? Finally, it is important to emphasize that, in general, affective rating scales are intended to assess the presence and severity of manic and depressive symptoms, not diagnose bipolar disorders.

The development of a useful rating scale requires two essential psychometric properties: reliability and validity. *Reliability* refers to the consistency of measurement over time. Test–retest reliability ensures that scores from the measurement do not vary significantly with repeated administrations. Reliability also may refer to the internal consistency of the scale or the agreement among individual components of a measure. Internal consistency is higher to the extent that the individual items measure a single dimension. Interrater reliability refers to the agreement among or between raters. With proper training, different raters should produce similar scores or results. *Validity* refers to the extent to which a scale measures what it purports to measure. Thus, scores for patients with bipolar disorder should (1) differ significantly from patients with other disorders, and (2) be similar to the scores of other bipolar patients (discriminant validity). Ideally, a mania scale should correlate highly with other measures of bipolar disorder (e.g., global measures and clinician scales), often referred to as concurrent validity.

General Psychopathological Inventories

A number of personality inventories and checklists (e.g., Minnesota Multiphasic Personality Inventory, Individual Mood and Behavior Checklist, Millon's Multiaxial Clinical Inventory, Comprehensive Psychopathological Rating Scale, Symptom Checklist 90) contain mania and depression subscales as part of an overall battery. These instruments are designed primarily as personality inventories, more useful for diagnostic screening purposes than for assessing severity of mania or response to treatment. As such, they are impractical to use for patients with bipolar disorder because of the time required to complete them. In addition, these inventories often do not assess key symptoms of mania. More recently developed mania rating scales are briefer, more comprehensive, and better suited to assess the presence and severity of acute mania.

Observer-Rated Mania Scales

Manic-State Rating Scale

Observer-rated mania scales were designed to be administered primarily by nursing staff, after long-term observation (i.e., a 6- to 8-hour nursing shift) of the patient, usually on a hospital ward. The first to appear in the literature was the Manic-State Rating Scale (MSRS) by Beigel, Murphy, and Bunney (1971). The MSRS contains 26 items assessing both the frequency (0–5) and intensity (1–5) of various signs and symptoms. The authors report good interrater reliability among nurses for most items and good agreement between scale scores and global ratings of mania. Limitations of the scale include a long observation period, the inclusion of items not specific to mania (e.g., suspiciousness and depressed affect), and the omission of a key manic symptom (i.e., sleep disturbance). In addition, some items on the scale, such as hallucinations and delusions, require more than simple observations to rate reliably.

Manchester Nurse Rating Scale for Mania

A more recent and improved nurses' rating scale is that of Brierley, Szabadi, Rix, and Bradshaw (1988), the Manchester Nurse Rating Scale for Mania (MNRS-M). The MNRS-M, suitable for the daily monitoring of affective states, consists of nine items rated from 0 (not present) to 3 (usually present). Most of the items are modifications of the MSRS (Beigel et al., 1971).

The MNRS-M is completed by nursing staff after observing behavior over a typical shift; it does not require the specialized training that is needed to administer the MSRS. Interrater reliability for the MNRS-M is good (r = .95), as is concurrent validity with global ratings of mania (r = .65) and the Young Mania Rating Scale (YMRS) (Young, Biggs, Ziegler, & Meyer, 1978). Compared to the MSRS, the MNRS-M is compact and easier to complete but still lacks a measure of sleep disturbance. There is also a version to assess depression (MNRS-D), making the combination suitable for evaluating mixed affective states.

Clinician-Rated Mania Scales

Bech–Rafaelson Mania Scale

Bech, Rafaelson, Kramp, and Bolwig (1978) borrowed from the MSRS (Beigel et al., 1971) and the Petterson, Fyro, and Sedvall (1973) mania scale to develop the Bech–Rafaelson Mania Scale (BRMS). The BRMS consists of 11 items, each of which is rated from 0 (normal) to 4 (extreme). Although the BRMS contains items to assess most of the symptoms of mania, four of the 11 items are devoted to activity level alone (e.g., motor, verbal, sexual, work, and interests), and there is no specific item to assess distractibility. Interrater reliability is reportedly high (r =.80–.95). Recently, Bech (2002) has documented the effectiveness of the BRMS as an outcome measure in numerous clinical trials of bipolar disorder over the past 20 years. However, by itself, it cannot be used to assess mixed states.

Young Mania Rating Scale

Currently, the most widely used clinician-administered rating scale for mania is the Young Mania Rating Scale (YMRS; Young et al., 1978). This scale contains 11 items, four of which are scored 0–4, the remaining seven 0–8, based on increasing severity. The rationale for assigning some items twice the weight was to compensate for potentially poor cooperation from severely ill patients. The YMRS is designed to be administered by trained clinicians within a 15- to 30-minute clinical interview. It has been used extensively for assessing treatment response, especially in clinical trial studies, and is considered the gold standard by scale developers, who use it for evaluating concurrent validity with newer scales. The authors report good interrater reliability for both items (r = .66–.92) and total scores (r = .93), and good concurrent validity (r = .71) with the MSRS (Beigel et al., 1971), global ratings (r = .88), and the Petterson et al. (1973) mania scale (r = .89).

The YMRS does have some limitations. In the absence of a factor analysis, the author's decision to double the weight for some items is questionable from both a theoretical and statistical point of view. There are no guidelines or prompt questions to ensure standardized administration. The scale includes some symptoms less central to mania (e.g., appearance and insight), while combining distinct symptoms into one (e.g., decreased need for sleep and insomnia, flight of ideas and distractibility). Because the YMRS was normed on only 20 patients, there is no evidence of discriminant validity. This lack is important in that, not only should a scale demonstrate good sensitivity (correctly identify individuals with a specified trait) but also acceptable specificity (correctly exclude individuals without the trait). Furthermore, there is no report of test–retest reliability. Perhaps the most serious criticism of the YMRS is that it combines symptoms of mania with psychotic symptoms, from which a single overall total score is derived. These symptoms should be assessed separately, inasmuch as they may respond differently to treatment. Similar to the above scales, it is not suitable for evaluating mixed states.

Hypomania Interview Guide–Seasonal Affective Disorder

Comparatively little has been published in the area of rating hypomanic states. However, at least one such scale is available, the Hypomania Interview Guide–Seasonal Affective Disorder (HIGH-SAD; Williams, Link, Rosenthal, & Terman, 1987). The HIGH-SAD is a 12-item interview-based scale. Feldman-Naim et al. (1998) reported a correlation of $r = .77$ with the YMRS (Young et al., 1978).

Clinician-Administered Rating Scale for Mania

Perhaps the most well-validated mania scale is the one developed by Altman, Hedeker, Janicak, Peterson, and Davis (1994), the Clinician-Administered Rating Scale for Mania (CARS-M). Altman and colleagues attempted to address the deficiencies of earlier scales by incorporating a number of methodological improvements in designing the CARS-M. Their scale, derived largely from the SADS (Endicott & Spitzer, 1978), contains 15 items divided into two subscales. Items 1–10 comprise the mania subscale, and items 11–15, the psychosis subscale. All the items except one (i.e., insight) are scored from 0 (absent) to 5 (severe). Items were chosen for inclusion based on DSM-III-R (American Psychiatric Association, 1987) criteria for manic disorder. The authors included items to assess psychotic symptoms (e.g., hallucinations, delusions, thought disorder), insight, and orientation. However, these items are contained in a separate subscale and thus do not confound the assessment of manic symptoms with psychotic symptoms. The CARS-M contains standardized questions to facilitate reliable administration, and guidelines are available from the authors to address severity levels, administration, scoring, and interpretation.

The interview takes approximately 15–30 minutes to administer and allows collateral information (e.g., nursing observations) to be used in scoring. Test–retest reliability was determined on a subsequent sample of 36 patients (16 bipolar, 20 nonbipolar). Discriminant validity was addressed by including patients with schizophrenia, major depression, and schizoaffective disorder. A total of 96 patients were assessed before and after 4–6 weeks of treatment.The YMRS (Young et al., 1978) also was administered to assess concurrent validity. The mean interrater reliability (for five raters) across CARS-M items was $r = .83$ and for total scores $r = .93$. Test–retest reliability for manic patients was significant for the mania subscale ($r = .78$, $p < .01$) and the psychosis subscale ($r = .95$, $p < .01$). Concurrent validity between the CARS-M and the YMRS was very good ($r = .94$). A principal components analysis of all 15 items revealed two prominent factors, accounting for 49% of the total variance. These were identified as "mania" and "psychosis," respectively. Multivariate analysis of covariance clearly demonstrated that scores for manic patients were significantly higher than for the other diagnostic groups on the mania subscale. Results also showed that the CARS-M is sensitive to treatment effects, as scores were significantly lower for both subscales following treatment. Finally, in order to assess the sensitivity and specificity of the CARS-M, Altman et al., following initial publication, performed a receiver operating curve (ROC) analysis. Results showed a sensitivity of .97 and a specificity of .95 at a mania subscale cutoff score of 15 or higher. A limitation of the CARS-M is that it cannot be used to evaluate mixed bipolar states. For this, the authors recommended adding a depression rating scale.

Scale for Manic States

Cassidy, Murry, Forest, and Carroll (1998) attempted to address their principal criticism of current mania scales, namely, that they do not adequately assess mixed states. Their instrument, the Scale for Manic States (SMS), includes items relevant to both mania (15 items) and mixed states (5 items). Items are rated from 0 (not present) to 5 (most severe) and were included in the SMS because of their relevance to mixed states, as demonstrated in statistical studies. The authors reasoned that, if mania scales do not routinely assess dysphoric features, then such features would not be identified as part of the manic syndrome. They argued, perhaps questionably, that mixed bipolar states cannot be studied by simply adding a standard depression rating scale, inasmuch as such scales contain items (e.g., weight loss, insomnia, poor concentration) that are irrelevant to the distinctively mixed state. However, there is no mention of how scores are derived or used to determine severity levels with this scale, especially in the case of mixed states. In addition, psychotic symptoms appear to be included in the assessment of affective symptoms. The authors reported significant correlations between the SMS and the MSRS (Beigel et al., 1971; $r = .84$) and between the SMS and clinical global ratings ($r = .86$). Interrater reliability among three raters was $r = .98$. Their study did not include comparison groups but only patients diagnosed as having either bipolar, manic (n = 273), or mixed (n = 43) disorder. One DSM criterion for mania (i.e., distractibility) is omitted from the SMS and there is no report of the scale's test–retest reliability. Results from their study showed that symptoms of dysphoria, lability, irritability, anxiety, guilt, and suicidality are frequently seen in mania.

Global Mania Scales

Clinical Global Impressions Bipolar Scale

The Clinical Global Impressions scale (CGI; Guy, 1976) is one of the earliest general global rating questionnaires used primarily for psychopharmacology treatment studies. Because it is nonspecific, it has been criticized as being too general and unreliable. However, Spearing, Post, Leverich, Brandt, and Nolen (1997) have revised the CGI specifically for use in bipolar illness. The modified version, the Clinical Global Impressions Bipolar (CGI-BP) scale, contains guidelines clarifying the concepts used and explaining the rating rules. Improvements over the original version include separate scores for depression and mania, symmetrical scores on a 7-point scale, categories to rate symptoms on admission, during an acute episode, and during prophylactic periods, and a separate section to rate medication side effects. Interrater reliabilities included (1) severity of illness r = .91 (2) change from last assessment r = .86, and (3) change from worst phase of illness r = .76.

Mania–Depression Scale

The Mania–Depression Scale (MDS; Mazmanian et al., 1994) is a global clinician-rated severity scale that provides a single score ranging from –5 (depressive stupor), through 0 (euthymic), to +5 (manic delerium). Each severity point has well-defined descriptive behaviors. The authors reported that nursing staff completed the scale at the end of every 12-hour shift. The MDS is easy to administer, allows for the assessment of both manic and depressed states, and is sensitive to diurnal variation and treatment effects. There is also a self- rating patient version of the scale. Interrater reliability is good (r = .84), and the MDS correlates well (r = .59) with the self-rating Beck Depression Inventory (Beck, Ward, Mendelson, Mock, & Erbaugh, 1961), a visual analogue mood scale (r = .71), and the patient version of the MDS (r = .85).

Self-Rating Mania Scales

Unlike the widespread acceptance of self-rating depression scales, the development of self-rating mania scales has been slow and arduous. Only within the last decade has there been credible evidence demonstrating that manic patients can rate their symptoms reliably. Prior to this shift, it was thought that manic patients were generally too uncooperative or lacking in insight to provide valid self-reports. An early study by Platman, Plutchik, Fieve, and Lawlor (1969), which showed a very low correlation between self-reports and staff ratings during manic episodes, may have discouraged subsequent research in this area. Results from this study also showed that the agreement between staff and patient self-ratings improved considerably after patients had recovered from their illness. Many years later, Goodwin and Jamison (1990), in reference to the use of self-rating mania scales, stated that "poor judgment, uncooperativeness, cognitive impairment, distractibility, and denial combine to make meaningful measurement essentially impossible" (p. 320). And more recently, Poolsup et al. (1999) excluded self-rating instruments from their critical appraisal of mania rating scales "because it is now widely recognized that such scales are unreliable in this condition" (p. 434). However, this notion can be supported no longer in view of recent empirical studies (Altman, Hedeker, Peterson, & Davis, 1997; Altman, Hedeker, Peterson, & Davis, 2001).

As Livianos-Aldana and Rojo-Moreno (2001) observed in their comprehensive review of mania rating scales, self-rating scales offer undeniable advantages. They require only a small amount of time from clinicians, they are free from the rater's interpretive and theoretical bias, and they offer a unique perspective from the patient's point of view. However, as is true with observer-rated scales, they also have limitations. Self-rating scales may be more sensitive to fluctuations in patients' mood than those administered by others. They are subjective reports from individuals with varied symptoms, experiences, and cognitive capacities. They may be prone to subjective bias, exaggeration, and underreporting of symptoms. Furthermore, severity of illness may undermine a patient's ability to complete self-ratings. For example, Altman et al. (1997) have shown that self-rating mania scales can be completed reliably by most patients with mild to moderate symptoms, and even by some with severe symptoms. However, as symptoms (or psychoses) increase in severity, self-rating tends to become less reliable and valid. Despite these limitations, advances in diagnostic criteria and methodology have contributed to the development of a number of useful scales.

Instruments to Assess Severity of Symptoms

Internal State Scale. Bauer et al. (1991) applied a visual analogue format to their self-rating scale of bipolar symptoms, the Internal State Scale (ISS). The ISS, designed to measure symptoms of both mania and depression, is a 17-item scale in which each item is rated on a 100-mm visual analogue line. Items were selected primarily to sample self-perceptions (e.g., feeling irritable, feeling great) rather than behavioral patterns (e.g., sleep, weight gain). The time period for rating is the preceding 24 hours. Factorial analysis resulted in four subscales: Depression, Well-Being, Activation, and Perceptual Conflict. The Activation subscale most accurately predicts scores on the YMRS (Young et al., 1978) ($r = .60$). The Depression subscale score correlated with the Hamilton Depression Rating Scale (HAM-D; Hamilton, 1960), as did the Well-Being subscale ($r = .73$). Based on discriminant function analysis and the use of scoring algorithms (i.e., cutoff scores), the ISS correctly classified 96% of depressed patients, 80% of manic patients, and 92% of control participants. Test–retest reliability was assessed on only 12 control participants rather than affective patients. The absence of patient control groups precludes a determination of whether or not the ISS can distinguish between patients with affective disorders and other diagnoses (e.g., schizophrenia and schizoaffective disorder). The authors argued that activation, as opposed to mood state, is a core feature of mania. However, they failed to include some key features of mania, such as decreased need for sleep, pressured speech, and grandiosity. Thus, sensitivity may be less than optimal because of the omission of key manic symptoms from the ISS. Scoring for the ISS is somewhat cumbersome and time consuming. The ISS would be the most appropriate scale to use for individuals who are unable to read.

Bauer, Vojta, Kinosian, Altshuler, and Glick (2000) investigated further the utility of the ISS for mixed states in a multisite, public-sector sample. This study included persons with mania/hypomania ($n = 16$), major depression ($n = 26$), mixed episodes ($n = 14$), and euthymia ($n = 30$). The authors reported replicating the results of the original study that had demonstrated the ability of the ISS to discriminate mood states in patients with bipolar disorder. The one exception was the Depression subscale, which was not significantly lower for depressed patients in this study. They also developed a revised scoring algorithm for the ISS to formally identify mixed states. The overall kappa score ($r = .55$) indicated only moderate agreement between ISS-defined and physician-defined mood state.

Self-Report Manic Inventory. Shugar, Schertzer, Toner, and DiGasbarro (1992) published an alternative self-rating scale, the Self-Report Manic Inventory (SRMI), a 48-item true–false inventory designed primarily to assess DSM-III-R symptoms of mania. The authors intended the instrument to serve as both a diagnostic tool and a measure of severity. However, they failed to include a structured diagnostic interview (e.g., SCID) as part of the study, in order to establish the validity of the SRMI as a diagnostic tool. Thus, it would be inappropriate to use it for diagnostic purposes. They also attempted to evaluate the impact of poor insight on the validity of patient self-report. Unfortunately, their single item assessing insight ("I knew I was getting ill") is suspect without an external measure (e.g., family report, clinician ratings) to compare the validity of patients' self-report. Nevertheless, results indicated no difference in the number of items endorsed by patients with or without insight. A comparison group of mixed psychotic disorders was included to demonstrate discriminant validity. Discriminant function analysis demonstrated that a cutoff score of 14 produced a sensitivity of 80% and a specificity of 33%. Test–retest reliability for manic patients was $r = .93$ and for the whole sample, $r = .73$. However, the interval between testing was too long (45–60 days) to appropriately measure test–retest reliability; ideally, the retest should be administered within a time period of only a few days. The SRMI is easy to administer and score but does not assess symptoms of depression and therefore cannot be used to evaluate mixed states.

In a follow-up study, Bräunig, Shugar, and Krüger (1996) demonstrated that the SRMI is sensitive to change in manic symptoms following treatment, has good test–retest reliability ($r = .86$), and acceptable concurrent validity with the YMRS (Young et al., 1978) at baseline ($r = .63$), posttreatment ($r = .89$), and with change scores ($r = .78$). Again, results showed no difference in scores between patients with and without insight.

Cooke, Krüger, and Shugar (1996) subsequently compared the ISS (Bauer et al., 1991) to the SRMI (Shugar et al., 1992) and the YMRS (Young et al., 1978) in 20 patients with rapid-cycling bipolar disorder. Results showed that both self-report scales correlated well with each other and with the YMRS, but that each covered a different domain of the manic syndrome. The SRMI and the ISS were more sensitive than the YMRS to mood fluctuations in the euthymic to hypomanic range. The authors suggested that the combination of both self-report scales might be more useful than either one alone, especially when assessing mood variations between hypomania and depression. However, results from their study may be compromised because none of the 20 patients ever became manic; rather, most became depressed or hypomanic. As the authors discussed, results from their study may not be applicable to patients with acute or severe mania.

Chinese Polarity Inventory. A rather unique and original scale is the Chinese Polarity Inventory (CPI) by Zheng and Lin (1994). Similar to the ISS, the CPI was designed for the simultaneous measurement of both manic and depressive symptoms. Items were selected from various other instruments, including the MSRS (Beigel et al., 1971), the Petterson et al. (1973) mania scale, the YMRS (Young et al., 1978), and the HAM-D (Hamilton, 1960). Each of the 20 items is comprised of two symmetric subitems, one for depression and one for mania. Items are rated from 0 (none) to 4 (always), and participants are required to rate each item of the CPI in both directions. The authors incorporate cutoff scores to provide levels of severity from normal through severe. Test–retest reliability for the depression subscale is $r = .86$ and for the mania subscale $r = .92$. Concurrent validity for the depression subscale was measured against the HAM-D ($r = .59$), and for the mania subscale, the BRMS (Bech et al., 1978; $r = .53$). The CPI was normed on Chinese patient populations, and thus its validity with Western populations remains to be tested. In addition, as the authors reported, its sensitivity to changes during treatment needs to be established. The CPI does not measure the DSM-IV criterion of distractibility.

Altman Self-Rating Scale for Mania. A more recent and well-validated self-report scale is the Altman Self-Rating Scale for Mania (ASRM; Altman et al., 1997). Because it contains only five items, it is the quickest and easiest to administer and score. Each item is comprised of five statements, scored from 0 (not present) to 4 (present in severe degree). Patients are instructed to select the one statement from each group that best describes their present condition. The scale initially contained 15 items, designed to represent each of the DSM-IV criteria for mania, plus additional items to assess psychotic symptoms. Following principal components analysis, the scale was reduced to five items because of their ability to clearly differentiate between manic and nonmanic participants. Similar to the study by Shugar et al. (1992) on the SRMI, the authors also assessed the impact of both lack of insight and psychosis on self-rating scores.

Concurrent validity was measured by the coadministration of both the CARS-M (Altman et al., 1994) and the YMRS (Young et al., 1978). Comparison groups, rated before and after treatment, included persons with schizophrenia ($n = 22$), schizoaffective disorder ($n = 13$), and major depression ($n = 30$). Test–retest reliability, assessed on 20 patients with depression and 10 with mania on two separate occasions shortly after admission, was very good ($r = .86$). Baseline scores for the manic group were significantly higher than for the other groups. The ASRM proved very sensitive to change; manic patients had significantly decreased posttreatment scores. Concurrent validity was good for both the YMRS ($r = .72$) and the CARS-M ($r = .77$). Sensitivity, determined by receiver operating characteristic (ROC) curve analysis, at a cutoff score of 6 or higher, was 85.5%, and specificity was 87.5%. The authors reported that, for manic patients, the presence or absence of insight (as measured by clinicians with the CARS-M) was unrelated to patients' scores on the ASRM. This result is consistent with the Shugar et al. (1992) study, which also found no differences in scores between patients with or without insight. A limitation of the ASRM is that it does not assess concurrent manic and depressive symptoms and thus would not be useful for evaluating mixed features.

Altman et al. (2001) subsequently compared the ASRM (Altman et al., 1997) to both the ISS (Bauer et al., 1991) and the SRMI (Shugar et al., 1992) in 44 inpatients with acute mania. All three scales were administered together shortly after admission and again after 4–6 weeks of pharmacotherapy. Patients also were rated by clinicians on the CARS-M (Altman et al., 1994). In this study acute mania was defined as a score of 15 or higher on the CARS-M mania subscale, based on a sensitivity rating of 97% and a specificity rating of 95% at this cutoff. Twenty-nine of the 44 patients had mania subscale scores of 15 or higher, 11 had hypomanic symptoms, and four were euthymic. The purpose of this study was to compare the ability of each scale to correctly identify patients with acute symptoms. Accuracy was determined by using the cutoff scores for each scale given by the authors. At baseline, the ISS correctly identified 13 of 29 patients as acutely manic (45% sensitivity), the SRMI 25 of 29 patients (86% sensitivity), and, the ASRM 27 of 29 patients (93% sensitivity). Posttreatment scores were significantly decreased for the ASRM, the SRMI, and the ISS (Activation subscale only). The ASRM and the ISS Well-Being subscale were the only self-rating measures to significantly correlate with the CARS-M Mania subscale at both baseline and posttreatment. Once again, the authors found no significant differences between patients with ($n = 29$) or without ($n = 15$) insight on any of the three measures. However, the presence of psychotic symptoms was associated with significantly higher baseline scores on the ASRM only. Of the three scales, the ASRM was the most sensitive for identifying patients with acute mania, followed by the SRMI. The ISS was not effective for this purpose. The authors attributed the differences among the scales to item content. The ISS omits an important symptom of mania, (i.e., decreased need for sleep), which may have reduced its sensitivity. The SRMI was designed as an outpatient measure, and many of the items pertain to behaviors that are inapplicable to an inpatient setting. Additional research comparing these measures in bipolar outpatients would be useful.

Instruments to Screen for History of Illness or to Identify Individuals at Risk

General Behavior Inventory. Two instruments have been designed specifically to screen for individuals at risk for developing severe affective disorders. The first of these is the General Behavior Inventory (GBI; Depue et al., 1981), designed originally to identify only bipolar affective conditions (on a lifetime or trait basis), and later modified to include both unipolar and bipolar affective conditions ranging from full to subsyndromal intensity (Depue, Krauss, Spoont, & Arbisi, 1989). The GBI is a 73-item self-report inventory in which items are scored from 1 (never/hardly ever) to 4 (very often/almost constantly). It has good test–retest reliability ($r = .71–.75$) and internal consistency ($\alpha = .90–.96$). Research with clinical and nonclinical populations has shown the modified GBI to have good positive predictive power (.87) and negative predictive power (.93) for identifying individuals with chronic intermittent and bipolar conditions, but it is less accurate for individuals with episodic unipolar conditions (Depue & Klein, 1988). The authors suggested that the

GBI be used primarily for research purposes, because its sensitivity in clinical populations is too low. Additional validation studies are needed to further define the limits of the BGI.

Hypomanic Personality Scale. The second instrument designed to identify individuals at risk is the Hypomanic Personality Scale (HYP; Eckblad & Chapman, 1986), a 48-item true–false self-rating inventory. The HYP has high internal consistency (*alpha* = .87) and good test–retest reliability (*r* = .81). Because the HYP does not contain any depression items (unlike the GBI), it does not duplicate the selection of potential bipolar patients with the GBI. In a longitudinal study of the predictive validity of the HYP, Kwapil et al. (2000) have shown that individuals scoring high on this measure not only report more hypomanic episodes at baseline, compared to control participants, but also report more bipolar disorders and depressive episodes at follow-up. While the HYP shows promise as a screening tool, it was normed on predominantly middle-class Caucasian college students. Thus, more research is needed to determine whether these findings would generalize to more ethnically and socially diverse samples. Because most of the participants did not develop manic episodes at follow-up, research does not yet support the use of the HYP for clinical purposes.

Mood Disorder Questionnaire. Hirschfeld et al. (2000) have developed a diagnostic screening instrument for bipolar spectrum disorders, namely, the Mood Disorder Questionnaire (MDQ). The MDQ contains 13 yes/no items that screen for a lifetime history of a manic or hypomanic syndrome. Two additional items are included to assess whether symptoms checked as positive occurred during the same time period, and to what extent they interfered with social, marital, and occupational functioning. The scale was administered to 198 outpatients, most of whom subsequently participated in a telephone diagnostic interview using the SCID. A ROC-derived cutoff score of seven or more items resulted in a sensitivity of 73% and a specificity of 90%. The MDQ is easy to administer and score. However, it does not assess the depressive end of bipolar spectrum disorders and therefore is not appropriate for screening mixed states. Also, because it was designed for screening only, it does not measure severity of symptoms.

SUMMARY AND CONCLUSIONS

This chapter provides a comparative review of psychiatric rating scales currently used to assess, screen, or identify individuals with bipolar disorders. The goal is to provide sufficient information to assist clinicians in their selection of instruments for clinical use, as well as to provide an understanding of

TABLE 3.1. Recommendations for the Selection of Mania Rating Scales

Type of assessment	Scale	Advantages	Limitations
Diagnosis	SCID	• Good reliability and validity • Well-established database • Structured interview format • Several versions available	• Does not assess severity • Some training required for proficiency
Nursing observations	MNRS-M	• Good reliability and validity • No special training required • Depression version available	• Does not assess sleep • Does not assess mixed features
Global severity rating	CGI-BP	• Well-defined severity points • Good reliability and validity • Assesses mixed features	• New scale, lacks database
	MDS	• Good reliability and validity • Brief, easy to administer • Assesses mixed features • Available in nursing and self-rating versions	• New scale, lacks database
Clinician-administered scales	CARS-M	• Extensively validated • Structured format • Effective outcome measure • Good sensitivity and specificity • Good test–retest reliability • Manic and psychotic symptoms assessed separately	• Does not assess mixed features
	YMRS	• Extensive database • Effective outcome measure • Good reliability and validity	• Manic and psychotic symptoms assessed together • Some distinct symptoms combined into one item
Self-rating/ screening measures	ASRM	• Brief, easy to administer • Effective outcome measure • Good sensitivity and specificity • Good reliability and validity	• Does not assess mixed features • Use with outpatients not established
	SRMI	• Good reliability and validity • Easy to administer and score • Effective outcome measure	• Does not assess mixed features • Less effective for inpatients
	MDQ	• Good sensitivity and specificity • Brief and easy to administer • Good reliability and validity • Used for screening history of illness	• Does not assess severity • Does not assess mixed features • New scale, lacks database

how such measures are used in psychiatric research. It is important to empha-size that no single measure should serve as the only method to assess or determine a diagnosis, nor should a single measure be used as the sole basis for clinical decision making. Rather, if used appropriately, these instruments have the potential to provide additional information that may inform the clinical judgment of the researcher or practitioner. The proper interpretation of these measures requires both clinical training and consideration of a vari-ety of factors (e.g., severity of illness, cognitive/intellectual ability, practical issues, etc.). Goodwin and Jamison (1990), after carefully reviewing the strengths and weaknesses of various types of assessment instruments, have recommended that clinicians and researchers use more than one type of measure to obtain a comprehensive assessment (e.g., clinical interview, self-report, nursing observations, etc.). Table 3.1 (on p. 53) summarizes the advantages and limitations of the scales discussed in this chapter.

Bipolar spectrum disorders are likely more prevalent than generally as-sumed. Research findings depend heavily on the definition of the bipolar spectrum, which is still developing and far from settled. New research sug-gests that further subtyping of bipolar spectrum disorders may be neces-sary. In addition, there is still considerable disagreement over how to define mixed bipolar episodes, how to account for brief hypomania (recurrent or sporadic), and how to decide which features constitute the "core" symp-toms of mania. As our concept of what constitutes the syndrome of mania continues to evolve, elaboration and refinement of present methodologies should help improve assessment, diagnosis and, hopefully, treatment of these complex disorders.

REFERENCES

Akiskal, H. S. (1987). The milder spectrum of bipolar disorders: Diagnostic, character-ologic, and pharmacologic aspects. *Psychiatric Annals, 17,* 32–37.

Altman, E. G., Hedeker, D. R., Janicak, P. G., Peterson, J. L., & Davis, J. M. (1994). The Clinician-Administered Rating Scale for Mania (CARS-M): Development, reliability, and validity. *Biological Psychiatry, 36,* 124–134.

Altman, E. G., Hedeker, D., Peterson, J. L., & Davis, J. M. (1997). The Altman Self-Rating Mania Scale. *Biological Psychiatry, 42,* 948–955.

Altman, E., Hedeker, D., Peterson, J. L., & Davis, J. M. (2001). A comparative evaluation of three self-rating scales for acute mania. *Biological Psychiatry, 50,* 468–471.

American Psychiatric Association. (1987). *Diagnostic and statistical manual of mental dis-orders* (3rd ed., rev.). Washington, DC: Author.

American Psychiatric Association. (1994). *Diagnostic and statistical manual of mental Disorders* (4th ed.). Washington, DC: Author.

Angst, J. (1998). The emerging epidemiology of hypomania and bipolar II disorder. *Journal of Affective Disorders, 50,* 143–151.

Bauer, M. S., Crits-Christoph, P., Ball, W. A., Dewees, E., McAllister, T., Alahi, P., Cacciola, J., & Whybrow, P. C. (1991). Independent assessment of manic and depressive symp-toms by self-rating. *Archives of General Psychiatry, 48,* 807–812.

Bauer, M. S., Vojta, C., Kinosian, B., Altshuler, L., & Glick, H. (2000). The Internal State Scale: Replication of its discriminating abilities in a multisite, public sector sample. *Bipolar Disorders, 2,* 340–346.

Bech, P. (2002). The Bech–Rafaelson Mania Scale in clinical trials of therapies for bipolar disorder: A 20-year review of its use as an outcome measure. *CNS Drugs, 16,* 47–63.

Bech, P., Rafaelson, O. J., Kramp, P., & Bolwig, T. G. (1978). The mania rating scale: Scale construction and inter-observer agreement. *Neuropharmacology, 17,* 430–431.

Beck, A. T., Ward, C. H., Mendelson, M., Mock, J., & Erbaugh, J. (1961). An inventory for measuring depression. *Archives of General Psychiatry, 4,* 561–571.

Beigel, A., Murphy, D. L., & Bunney, W. E. (1971). The manic-state rating scale. *Archives of General Psychiatry, 25,* 256–261.

Bräunig, P., Shugar, G., & Krüger, S. (1996). An investigation of the Self-Report Manic Inventory as a diagnostic and severity scale for mania. *Comprehensive Psychiatry, 37,* 52–55.

Brierley, C. E., Szabadi, E., Rix, K. J. B., & Bradshaw, C. M. (1988). The Manchester Nurse Rating Scale for the daily simultaneous assessment of depressive and manic ward behaviors. *Journal of Affective Disorders, 15,* 45–54.

Carpenter, W. T., Jr., Strauss, J. S., & Muleh, S. (1973). Are there pathonomonic symptoms in schizophrenia? An empiric investigation of Schneider's first-rank symptoms. *Archives of General Psychiatry, 28,* 847–852.

Cassidy, F., Murry, E., Forest, K., & Carroll, B. J. (1998). Signs and symptoms of mania in pure and mixed episodes. *Journal of Affective Disorders, 50,* 187–201.

Cooke, R. G., Krüger, S., & Shugar, G. (1996). Comparative evaluation of two self-report mania rating scales. *Biological Psychiatry, 40,* 279–283.

Depue, R. A., & Klein, D. N. (1988). Identification of unipolar and bipolar affective conditions in nonclinical and clinical populations by the General Behavior Inventory. In D. Dunner, E. Gershon, & J. Barrett (Eds.), *Relatives at risk for mental disorder* (pp. 257–282). New York: Raven Press.

Depue, R. A., Krauss, S., Spoont, M. R., & Arbisi, P. (1989). General Behavior Inventory identification of unipolar and bipolar affective conditions in a nonclinical university population. *Journal of Abnormal Psychology, 98,* 117–126.

Depue, R. A., Slater, J. F., Wolfstetter-Kausch, H., Klein, D., Goplerud, E., & Farr, D. (1981). A behavioral paradigm for identifying persons at risk for bipolar depressive disorder: A conceptual framework and five validation studies [Monograph]. *Journal of Abnormal Psychology, 90,* 381–437.

Dunayevich, E., Sax, K. W., Kech, P. E., Jr., McElroy, S. L., Sorter, M. T., McConville, B. J., & Strakowski, S. M. (2000). Twelve-month outcome in bipolar patients with and without personality disorders. *Journal of Clinical Psychiatry, 61,* 134–139.

Eckblad, M., & Chapman, L. J. (1986). Development and validation of a scale for hypomanic personality. *Journal of Abnormal Psychology, 95,* 214–222.

Endicott, J., & Spitzer, R. L. (1978). A diagnostic interview: The Schedule for Affective Disorders and Schizophrenia. *Archives of General Psychiatry, 35,* 837–844.

Feldman-Naim, S., Lowe, C. H., Myers, F. S., Turner, E. H., Weinstock, L. M., & Leibenluft, E. (1998). Validation of the hypomania interview guide: Seasonal affective disorder (HIGH-SAD) version in patients with rapid cycling bipolar disorder. *Depression and Anxiety, 8,* 166–168.

Goodwin, F. K., & Jamison, K. R. (1990). *Manic–depressive illness.* New York: Oxford University Press.

Guy, W. (1976). Clinical global impression. In *ECDEU assessment manual for psychopharmacology* (rev. ed.). Rockville, MD: National Institute of Mental Health.

Hamilton, M. (1960). A rating scale for depression. *Journal of Neurology, Neurosurgery, and Psychiatry, 23,* 56–62.

Hirschfeld, R. M. A., Williams, J. B. W., Spitzer, R. L., Calabrese, J. R., Flynn, L., Keck, P.

E., Lewis, L., McElroy, S. L., Post, R. M., Rapport, D. J., Russell, J. M., Sachs, G. S., & Zajecka, J. (2000). Development and validation of a screening instrument for bipolar spectrum disorder: The Mood Disorder Questionnaire. *American Journal of Psychiatry, 157,* 1873–1875.

Janicak, P. G., Davis, J. M., Preskorn, S. H., & Ayd, F. J., Jr. (2001). *Principles and practice of psychopharmacotherapy* (3rd ed.). Philadelphia: Lippincott, Williams & Wilkins.

Janowsky, D. S., El-Yousef, M., & Davis, J. M. (1974). Interpersonal maneuvers of manic patients. *American Journal of Psychiatry, 131,* 250–254.

Kwapil, T. R., Miller, M. B., Zinser, M. C., Chapman, L. J., Chapman, J., & Eckblad, M. (2000). A longitudinal study of high scorers on the Hypomanic Personality Scale. *Journal of Abnormal Psychology, 109,* 222–226.

Livianos-Aldana, L., & Rojo-Moreno, L. (2001). Rating and quantification of manic syndromes. *Acta Psychiatrica Scandinavica, 104*(Suppl. 409), 1–33.

Mazmanian, D., Sharma, V., Persad, E., Kueneman, K., Burnham, J., Franklin, J., Hemmings, M., & Leiska, G. (1994). Development and validation of a scale for rating mood states of psychiatric inpatients. *Hospital and Community Psychiatry, 45,* 238–241.

Petterson, U., Fyro, B., & Sedvall, G. (1973). A new scale for the longitudinal rating of manic states. *Acta Psychiatrica Scandinavica, 49,* 248–256.

Platman, S., Plutchik, R., Fieve, R., & Lawlor, W. (1969). Emotion profiles associated with mania and depression. *Archives of General Psychiatry, 20,* 210–214.

Poolsup, N., Li Wan Po, A., & Oyebode, F. (1999). Measuring mania and critical appraisal of rating scales. *Journal of Clinical Pharmacy and Therapeutics, 24,* 433–443.

Pope, H., & Lipinski, J. (1978). Differential diagnosis of schizophrenia and manic depressive illness: A reassessment of the specificity of schizophrenia symptoms in the light of current research. *Archives of General Psychiatry, 35,* 811–828.

Post, R. M., Roy-Bryne, P. P., & Uhde, T. W. (1988). Graphic representation of the life course of illness in patients with affective disorder. *American Journal of Psychiatry, 145,* 844–848.

Regier, D. A., Farmer, M. E., Rae, D. S., Locke, B. Z., Keith, S. J., Judd, L. L., & Goodwin, F. K. (1990). Comorbidity of mental disorders with alcohol and other drug abuse. Results from the epidemiologic catchment area (ECA) study. *Journal of the American Medical Association, 264,* 2511–2518.

Robins, L. N., Helzer, J. E., Croughan, J., & Radcliff, K. S. (1981). National Institute of Mental Health Diagnostic Interview Schedule: Its history, characteristics, and validity. *Archives of General Psychiatry, 38,* 381–389.

Rosen, L. N., Rosenthal, N. E., Dunner, D. L., & Fieve, R. R. (1983). Social outcome compared in psychotic and nonpsychotic bipolar I patients. *Journal of Nervous and Mental Diseases, 171,* 272–275.

Shugar, G., Schertzer, S., Toner, B. B., & DiGasbarro, I. (1992). Development, use, and factor analysis of a self-report inventory for mania. *Comprehensive Psychiatry, 33,* 325–331.

Spearing, M. K., Post, R. M., Leverich, G. S., Brandt, D., & Nolen, W. (1997). Modification of the Clinical Global Impressions (CGI) scale for use in bipolar illness (BP): The CGI-BP. *Psychiatric Research, 73,* 159–171.

Spitzer, R. L., & Endicott, J. (1977). *Schedule for Affective Disorders and Schizophrenia–Lifetime version* (SADS-L). New York: New York State Psychiatric Institute.

Spitzer, R. L., & Endicott, J. (1978). *Schedule for Affective Disorders and Schizophrenia–Change version* (3rd ed.). New York: Biometrics Research.

Spitzer, R. L., Endicott, J., & Robins, L. (1979). Use of the Research Diagnostic Criteria and the Schedule for Affective Disorders and Schizophrenia to study affective disorders. *American Journal of Psychiatry, 136,* 52–56.

Spitzer, R. L., Williams, J. B. W., Gibbon, M., & First, M. B. (1992). The Structured Clinical Interview for DSM-III-R. I: History, rationale, and description. *Archives of General Psychiatry, 49,* 624–629.

Taylor, M. A., & Abrams, R. (1973). The phenomenology of mania: A new look at some old patients. *Archives of General Psychiatry, 29,* 520–522.

Williams, J. B. W., Link, M. J., Rosenthal, N. E., & Terman, M. (1987). *Hypomania interview guide (including hyperthymia) for seasonal affective disorder (HIGH-SAD).* New York: New York State Psychiatric Institute.

Young, R. C., Biggs, J. T., Ziegler, V. E., & Meyer, D. A. (1978). A rating scale for mania: Reliability, validity, and sensitivity. *British Journal of Psychiatry, 133,* 429–435.

Zheng, Y. P., & Lin, K. M. (1994). The reliability and validity of the Chinese Polarity Inventory. *Acta Psychiatrica Scandinavica, 89,* 126–131.

CHAPTER FOUR

ASSESSMENT OF BIPOLAR SPECTRUM DISORDERS IN CHILDREN AND ADOLESCENTS

ERIC A. YOUNGSTROM
ROBERT L. FINDLING
NORAH FEENY

The diagnosis of bipolar disorder in children and adolescents is currently generating a great deal of attention and controversy (Kluger & Song, 2002; Papolos, 1999). Much less is known about bipolar disorder in youths than in adults, and most of the assessment tools available were initially developed for use with adults. It is unclear how appropriate these instruments are for assessing bipolar disorder in children or adolescents, due to developmental changes in the presentation of the disorder (Geller & Luby, 1997; Geller et al., 2002) as well as the usual constraints on using self-report information with younger children (Anastasi & Urbina, 1997).

Despite such concerns, the differential diagnosis of bipolar disorder is a high-stakes decision. There are several treatments that appear promising *if* bipolar disorder is diagnosed correctly (McClellan & Werry, 1997). However, the costs of diagnostic errors may be particularly high in the case of juvenile bipolar disorder. False positives—that is, accidentally misdiagnosing a child who does not have bipolar disorder—carries the consequence of unnecessarily medicating the child with lithium or anticonvulsant medication—treatments that risk much more serious side effects than typically are incurred with other first-line pharmacotherapies for juvenile psychiatric disorders (Findling, Feeny, Stansbrey, DelPorto-Bedoya, & Demeter, 2002; Findling, Reed, & Blumer, 1999; Rosenberg, Holttum, &

Gershon, 1994). On the other hand, false negatives—that is, failing to recognize bipolar disorder accurately—are at least equally costly. Untreated bipolar disorder follows a progressive course, with recurrent episodes that become increasingly severe and resistant to treatment (Geller & Luby, 1997; Goodwin & Jamison, 1990). There also is concern that the stimulant and antidepressant medications that are most likely to be prescribed if juvenile bipolar disorder is misdiagnosed may actually be harmful, potentially precipitating or worsening a manic episode (DelBello et al., 2001; Geller, Zimerman, Williams, Bolhofner, & Craney, 2001; Soutullo et al., 2002). Despite the difficulties involved in making an accurate bipolar diagnosis, there is great need for clinicians to become more familiar with the assessment process.

The goals of this chapter are to (1) review what is currently known about the diagnostic presentation of bipolar spectrum disorders (BSD) in children and adolescents, (2) offer practical suggestions for improving the differential diagnosis of BSD in youths, (3) review assessment tools that might help in screening or making differential diagnoses, and (4) provide an overview of potential outcome measures. Because each of these topics can be discussed only briefly in the available space, selected references are indicated that offer more detailed treatment of each topic. It also is important for readers to recognize that the scientific understanding of juvenile BSD is changing extremely rapidly, and significant advances are likely to be made in the next 2 to 5 years. This chapter attempts to alert readers to such potential developments.

DIAGNOSIS OF BIPOLAR DISORDER
IN CHILDREN AND ADOLESCENTS

Prevalence

The scant data available suggest that the prevalence of BSD in adolescents is likely to be similar to adults, and somewhat lower in children. Prevalence estimates range from 0 to 1.2% for bipolar I in youths, 0.1% to 0.6% for bipolar II, and 0.3% for bipolar not otherwise specified (NOS; Costello et al., 1996; Kessler, 1994; Kessler, Avenevoli, & Merikangas, 2001; Lewinsohn, Klein, & Seeley, 1995; Shaffer, Fisher, Greenwald, & Greenberg, 2002; Shaffer, Fisher, Lucas, Dulcan, & Schwab-Stone, 2000; Wittchen, Nelson, & Lachner, 1998).

These studies were well designed and executed. However, there are concerns that the published rates may substantially underestimate the prevalence of BSD. Adult studies may have missed up to 50% of the bipolar I cases, which are diagnostically straightforward compared to bipolar II or bipolar NOS (Kessler, Rubinow, Holmes, Abelson, & Zhao, 1997). Estimates of juvenile prevalence are even more problematic, because all of the studies, to date, have used diagnostic criteria for adult presentations of BSD. No epidemiological study has used an instrument such as the Washington University Kiddie Schedule for Affective Disorders and Schizophrenia (WASH-U KSADS; Geller, Zimerman, Williams, Bolhofner, Craney, Delbello, et al., 2001), which includes increased content and developmentally appropriate anchors. For now, it seems safest to conclude that BSD does occur in children and adolescents, but infrequently, and probably at a rate similar to, or lower than, the rate found in adults.

Three other issues are important to consider here. First, many of the children currently being diagnosed as having a bipolar disorder do not fit the classic symptom pattern of bipolar I or bipolar II, whereas the above prevalence estimates are based on strict DSM-IV or ICD-9 criteria (Carlson & Kelly, 1998; Nottelmann et al., 2001). Manic symptoms that do not fit strict DSM-IV criteria may occur two to six times as often as the classic presentation of bipolar I or II (Carlson et al., 2003; Kashani et al., 1987; Lewinsohn, Seeley, Buckley, & Klein, 2002), much as "soft spectrum" bipolar disorder may be more common than bipolar I in adults (Akiskal, 1996).

The second concern is that epidemiological base rates may bear little resemblance to what clinicians actually see in their practice (Wozniak et al., 1995; Wozniak, Biederman, & Richards, 2001). The actual prevalence rate of juvenile BSD is a complex function of the population base rate, the degree of impairment created by the disorder, public awareness, and treatment accessibility, among other factors. Third, the lack of a known prevalence for juvenile BSD directly impedes efforts at accurate diagnosis. When using the same diagnostic tools (Kraemer, 1992), lower prevalence of BSD at a given site makes it harder to diagnose correctly than in settings where BSD is more common.

Comorbidity

More than half of youths meeting DSM-IV criteria for BSD exhibit at least one other Axis I diagnosis (Findling et al., 2001; Geller & Luby, 1997; Weckerly, 2002). The most commonly co-occurring diagnoses are attention-deficit/hyperactivity disorder (ADHD), conduct disorder, oppositional defiant disorder, anxiety disorders, and substance abuse. It is unclear whether these presentations reflect "true" comorbidity of distinct clinical phenomena, or if they reflect symptom overlap or other artifacts (Caron & Rutter, 1991). The high rate of comorbid ADHD (50–80%) has caused considerable debate about the validity of the comorbid designation, in particular (Biederman et al., 1996; Klein, Pine, & Klein, 1998). From a clinical perspective, it is unfortunate that many of the most commonly co-occurring conditions are also the ones most difficult to differentiate from BSD in youths.

Differential Diagnosis

There are several disorders that can be challenging to disentangle from BSD in youth (Bowring & Kovacs, 1992; Carlson, 2002). If the patient presents with a depressed episode, then it may not be possible to distinguish the depressed phase of a BSD from a *unipolar mood disorder*. Some data suggest that psychotic features, vegetative symptoms (especially psychomotor retardation or sleep disturbance), and family history of bipolar disorder may be predictive of a bipolar, as opposed to a unipolar, depression (Birmaher, Arbelaez, & Brent, 2002; Geller, Zimerman, Williams, Bolhofner, & Craney, 2001).

ADHD, like the manic or hypomanic phase of BSD, involves increased motor activity, disturbed concentration, and is associated with greater aggressiveness and poor impulse control (Klein et al., 1998). Juvenile BSD and severe *oppositional defiant disorder* also present similarly, inasmuch as both involve defiance and resistance to efforts to redirect behavior, and also may include pronounced aggression (Carlson, 2002). *Conduct disorder* is difficult to distinguish from BSD, inasmuch as hypomanic and manic episodes also are associated with increased substance use, sexual disinhibition and promiscuity, disregard for rules, poor impulse control, and aggression (Kovacs & Pollock, 1995). Adding to the diagnostic challenge is the fact that each of these disorders is much more common than BSD, with epidemiological prevalence estimates for conduct disorder ranging from roughly 3% in females and 6–16% in males (Hinshaw & Anderson, 1996); for ADHD, 3–5% (American Psychiatric Association, 2000; Brown et al., 2001), and for oppositional defiant disorder, roughly 12–16% (Nottelmann & Jensen, 1995). Similarly, unipolar depression occurs in between 2 and 8% of children ages 4–18 years, with gender differences in rate becoming pronounced in adolescence (Cyranowski, Frank, Young, & Shear, 2000). The bottom line is that all of these disorders are far more common in the community than is BSD (especially classic bipolar I or II), and these disorders also probably make up a dramatically larger proportion of the referrals to clinical settings. As a result, the majority of those youths for whom it is difficult to make the differential diagnosis are likely *not* to have a BSD, but instead to have one of the more common disorders.

Diagnostic Criteria for Bipolar Disorders

Currently, no adjusted criteria for diagnosing bipolar disorders in children or adolescents versus adults exist (American Psychiatric Association, 2000). Research groups studying juvenile BSD are inconsistent in their agreement with the adult nosology in two major respects. One is about the relative importance of elated mood or grandiosity versus irritability (e.g., Biederman et al., 2000; Geller et al., 2000). The second point of contention concerns the durational criteria and the frequency of cycling (Biederman et al., 1996; Geller & Luby, 1997). Children and adolescents are likely to exhibit rapid cycling much more frequently than adults (50–80% of youths vs. 10–20% of adults; American Psychiatric Association, 2000; Findling et al., 2001; Geller et al., 2000). Some data even suggest that children may show ultradian cycling (changing polarity within the same day; Geller et al., 2000). In contrast, others find that children with bipolar disorder do not show defined boundaries to their mood episodes, but rather show a chronic presentation with mixed mood symptoms, typically with irritability and aggression as significant features (Biederman, Faraone, Chu, & Wozniak, 1999; Wozniak et al., 2001). Yet other data suggest that it is possible to use strict DSM-IV durational criteria to identify juvenile cases of bipolar I (Findling et al., 2001) or cyclothymia (Findling, Kahana, Youngstrom, & Calabrese, 2002), with chronic or ultrarapid cycling classified as bipolar NOS. Additional research is needed to validate the potential benefit of modified durational criteria or a more stringent phenotype (such as Geller and Luby's (1997) Pre-pubescent and Early Adolescent Bipolar [PEA-BP] definition) before these can be used clinically.

Developmental Differences in Presentation

Although the same criteria are applied to children and adolescents in determining if there is a bipolar disorder, there are important developmental differences in presentation that complicate the recognition of mood symptoms. One issue is that depressed mood in youths often involves substantial irritability (American Psychiatric Association, 2000; Kovacs, 1996). This factor clouds the issue of whether irritability is diagnostic of a depressed, manic, or mixed episode in children. Another crucial concern is the presence of developmental constraints on the expression of many manic symptoms (Geller et al., 2002). Children are unlikely to have credit cards with which to charge impulsive and exorbitant purchases, nor can they bounce checks and squander savings on risky investments. Society also provides few and constrained opportunities for children to demonstrate hypersexuality. Bizarre appearance is also difficult to gauge clinically: Parents who are concerned enough to bring their children for assessment also are going to make them appear presentable for the office visit; and contemporary norms for grooming and dress (e.g., body piercing, hair dying, tattoos) make it difficult to separate socially versus psychiatrically motivated changes in appearance. The lack of insight into one's illness that can be characteristic of mania in adults is also difficult to discern from what falls within normal limits for children and adolescents (Youngstrom, Danielson, Findling, Gracious, & Calabrese, 2002).

Clinicians and researchers in the field are beginning to learn more about what features characterize bipolar disorders in children and adolescents (Geller et al., 2002). Commonly described examples of extreme risk-taking behavior include attempting to get out of a moving automobile or jumping off of a garage or house roof (Geller et al., 2002; Weckerly, 2002). *The important point to note is that current approaches involve searching for the same diagnostic symptoms but recognizing that they may interact with developmental factors to produce new forms of expression.* This point is different from a statement that some symptoms are irrelevant for children, or that children show other symptoms that may not be present in adults.

Broad Phenotype

There is a group of children and adolescents that presents with emotional "rages" and aggressive behavior but which does not fit into the classic bipolar categories codified in DSM-IV (Biederman, 1995; Biederman et al., 2000). This group might include cases that would have been labeled as "minimal brain dysfunction" or childhood onset schizophrenia in decades past when the boundaries of those categories were more loosely defined (Carlson, 2002). It is possible that these emotionally explosive and aggressive children might constitute a "broad phenotype" of bipolar disorder (Carlson et al., 2003; Nottelmann, 2002). This pediatric broad phenotype appears to be two to five times more common in clinical settings than does "classic" bipolar I. Whereas research groups can reliably diagnose bipolar I at age 10 (and probably age 5 or 7), there are neither clear diagnostic guidelines nor good prevalence data for the broad phenotype. It also is unknown whether the broad phenotype represents (1) a developmental precursor to classic adult bipolar disorder, (2) a distinct subtype of bipolar disorder, or (3) an unrelated illness. However, the suspicion is that the majority of children diagnosed as bipolar in the community fall into this broad phenotype category (Carlson et al., 2003).

Diagnostic Instruments

A large number of diagnostic instruments is available for use with children and adolescents, and the field has not identified a single tool that should serve as the "gold standard," nor are there clear front-runners. The various KSADS versions probably have been the most widely used semistructured diagnostic interviews in juvenile mood disorder research. At present, most research groups are using some combination of the present and lifetime version (KSADS-PL; Kaufman et al., 1997) and the WASH-U KSADS (see Nottelmann et al., 2001, for review), although epidemiological studies are more likely to use more highly structured interviews, such as the Diagnostic Interview Schedule for Children (DISC; Shaffer et al., 2002) or the Composite International Diagnostic Interview (CIDI; e.g., Wittchen et al.,

1998). Unfortunately, the use of different instruments is likely to contribute to some of the differences in findings across studies.

Though essential in research settings, semistructured and structured interviews are cumbersome and complicated enough to administer that they are impractical for use in most clinical settings. The key strength and limitation of the KSADS family of instruments, as opposed to the more structured interviews, is that the KSADS draws more heavily on clinical judgment. Thus the KSADS instruments require more training and clinical acumen but hold the potential for higher clinical validity, whereas structured interviews such as the C-DISC and CIDI concentrate on improving the interrater reliability of diagnoses.

SUGGESTIONS FOR IMPROVING DIFFERENTIAL DIAGNOSIS

Several clinical strategies, when implemented, can significantly increase the odds of diagnosing BSD correctly. First, taking a comprehensive *family history* provides a highly valuable piece of datum, given the high heritability of bipolar disorder (DelBello & Geller, 2001). If either biological parent has a confirmed bipolar illness, then the odds that the child has BSD increase by a factor of five; if both parents have BSD, then the odds may increase even more (Lapalme, Hodgins, & LaRoche, 1997). The fivefold increase in risk is a very powerful piece of diagnostic information—yet, at the same time, the majority of children with bipolar parents does not manifest bipolar disorder (i.e., only 5% of the offspring with a bipolar parent show bipolar I in community samples; Lapalme et al., 1997).

A second method for improving diagnostic accuracy is to *extend the window of assessment*. Because bipolar illness involves a cycling of mood states, the snapshot of behavior observed during an office visit (or over the first few days of an inpatient admission; Carlson & Youngstrom, 2003), even in a best scenario, represents only a part of the whole pattern of illness. The solution is to gather data about mood functioning over an extended time frame, both retrospectively and prospectively. To gather *retrospective* information involves asking the youth and collateral informants (usually parents and possibly teachers) to describe the youth's mood and behavior over a longer time frame (usually weeks to 6 months on behavior checklists, potentially extending to an informal lifetime "mood history"). Life charting of moods (Denicoff et al., 1997; Meaden, Daniels, & Zajecka, 2000) is valuable if the family is willing and able to provide it. This method requires a family member or the client to diagram the fluctuations in the youth's mood states over a period of months or years. The Depression and Bipolar Support Alliance distributes checkbook-sized life charts, at little or no cost (see *www.dbsalliance.org*). The chief disadvantages to life charting are the considerable investment of time and effort required on the client's or parent's part (Meaden et al., 2000), and the fact that retrospective recall of mood functioning is inaccurate and influenced by current mood states (Coyne, Thompson, & Racioppo, 2001).

Several strategies for extending the window of assessment *prospectively* are available. One would be to use life charting in a prospective fashion, having the adolescent or the family track daily changes in mood state over a period of weeks and then bringing in the chart for review at each office visit. Prospective charting avoids the problems of bias and inaccuracy inherent in retrospective reports. The main disadvantage to prospective charting is that many families have difficulty completing it.

Another strategy for gathering data prospectively is to plan follow-up mood assessments of the course of treatment. Often assessment and diagnosis are perceived as procedures handled during the intake process and seldom revisited during active treatment. A more effective plan might be to label BSD as a "rule out" for cases with risk factors or suggestive symptoms in the intake assessment, and then schedule follow-up mood assessments at weekly or monthly intervals. Some of the assessment tools that are helpful in accomplishing this goal also function well as measures of treatment response (see below). At the same time, treatment response data may provide diagnostically relevant information (Wozniak et al., 2001), although pharmacological challenges with lithium or anticonvulsants are *not* appropriate methods for determining a BSD diagnosis—much as stimulant challenge is not appropriate as a method of diagnosing ADHD. BSD is likely to require continued assessment over the long term in order to maintain treatment gains and prevent relapse (Danielson, Feeny, Findling, & Youngstrom, in press; Newman, Leahy, Beck, Reilly-Harrington, & Gyulai, 2002).

Yet another technique for improving the accuracy of BSD diagnosis is to incorporate psychometric assessment tools, as discussed below. The next few years will see rapid improvements in this area, as several research groups evaluate new measures specific to juvenile BSD (e.g., Axelson, 2002; Gracious, Youngstrom, Findling, & Calabrese, 2002; Pavuluri, 2002; Youngstrom, Findling, Danielson, & Calabrese, 2001), and information also is gathered about how well measures crossvalidate in independent samples (Woldorf, Youngstrom, Danielson, Findling, & Calabrese, 2002).

It is generally recommended that evaluations of children and adolescents integrate information from multiple informants about the youth's functioning. The use of collateral sources of information becomes especially important in BSD, where a lack of insight into illness is a common feature of manic and hypomanic states (Sachs, Guille, & McMurrich, 2002). Interestingly, data suggest that parents are probably the best informants to differentiate bipolar from nonbipolar illness in youths, including teenagers (Findling, Youngstrom, Danielson, et al., 2002; Youngstrom, Gracious, Danielson, Findling, & Calabrese, in press). Parent report has significantly outperformed youth self-report on at least two different instruments (i.e., the Achenbach checklists and the General Behavior Inventory—see below; Youngstrom, Findling, Calabrese, et al., 2003). Furthermore, parent report is substantially more sensitive and specific to BSD than is teacher report (Geller, Warner, Williams, & Zimerman, 1998; Hazell, Lewin, & Carr, 1999; Kahana, Youngstrom, Findling, & Calabrese, in press). The relative diagnostic value of parent versus teacher report is not surprising: Teachers are sensitive to disruptive behavior but not to internalizing symptoms, and teachers tend to interpret most externalizing behaviors as symptoms of ADHD (Abikoff, Courtney, Pelham, & Koplewicz, 1993). However, the fact that parents' reports outperform youth self-report as predictors of BSD contradicts the popular clinical perception that self-report is the most valid source of information about mood disorders (Loeber, Green, & Lahey, 1990). Based on the available data, it is clearly important to gather information from parents about the youth's mood functioning whenever possible, even with adolescents.

An important tactic when marshalling all of this assessment data is to *concentrate on the cardinal symptoms* of BSD (Geller, Williams et al., 1998). Because symptoms such as distractibility and aggression are likely to be highly impairing, they are major motivators for seeking treatment and thus important targets for treatment (Wozniak et al., 2001). However, they also are not specific to any single disorder. Irritability in youths is analogous to fever—it is indicative that there is something wrong and its degree can provide some gauge of the seriousness of the problem, but it is not pathognomonic of any particular disorder (Aman, De Smedt, Derivan, Lyons, & Findling, 2002). Elated mood and inflated self-esteem or grandiosity, on the other hand, have accumulated substantial support as being relatively specific to BSD, particularly when assessment data suggest a change from the individual's baseline (Findling et al., 2001; Geller, Williams et al., 1998). Pressured speech, racing thoughts, and hypersexuality also are likely to be somewhat more specific to BSD. However, these symptoms also are likely to be complex to evaluate, especially in young children, where it becomes difficult to differentiate these symptoms from expressive language disabilities (Carlson, 2002; see also Gracious et al., 2002, for discussion of parent report about hypersexuality).

Finally, it is crucial to *look for evidence of cycling*. Since Kraepelin initially formulated the diagnosis of manic depression, it has been considered a cycling illness (Goodwin & Jamison, 1990). In spite of the controversy about the rate of cycling in children, the majority of research groups agrees that youths with bipolar I or II *do* cycle (Carlson et al., 2003; Findling et al., 2001; Geller & Luby, 1997). Evaluators need to be aware that families might report certain behavior problems as being chronic in spite of the presence of mood cycling. Irritability is a case in point: Youths are frequently irritable in both manic and depressed phases of illness, often remaining irritable between mood episodes as well if there are comorbid psychiatric conditions. However, the *ecology* of the irritability changes. During a manic episode, the youth wants to pursue pleasurable goal-directed activity and responds with irritability to attempts to limit or redirect that behavior. During a depressive phase, the youth will present as more sullen, not wanting to do anything, and responding with irritability to efforts to engage or motivate him or her (Findling et al., 2001). In our experience, most families quickly comprehend the difference in these situations and can provide useful reports about the presence or absence of mood cycling, even in the context of chronic irritability. In contrast, reliance on a questionnaire or structured interview that simply asks about irritability is likely to miss the changes in ecology and mood context.

PSYCHOMETRIC TOOLS AS ADJUNCTS TO DIAGNOSIS

This section briefly discusses two "families" of broad assessment tools that measure several dimensions of functioning, as well as more specialized measures that concentrate specifically on mood symptoms (see Youngstrom, Findling, Carlson, & Ferziger, in press, for a more detailed review). Although there is a variety of broad behavior checklists available, we are only aware of published BSD studies using the Achenbach System of Empirically Based Assessments (ASEBA; Achenbach & Rescorla, 2001) and the Gadow and Sprafkin Symptom Inventories (Gadow & Sprafkin, 1994, 1997, 1999). Additional areas of functioning are important to evaluate in order to gain a comprehensive picture of an individual's status: for example, measures of psychotic features, depressive symptoms, and aggressive behavior (focusing more specifically on the impulsive vs. provocative or reactive vs. instrumental distinction; Weisbrot & Ettinger, 2002; see Youngstrom, Findling et al., in press for elaboration).

The Achenbach System of Empirically Based Assessments

The Achenbach scales are among the most widely researched instruments that assess juvenile bipolar disorder. Six different research groups have published data using the Child Behavior Checklist (CBCL; Biederman et al., 1995; Carlson, Loney, Salisbury, & Volpe, 1998; Dienes, Chang, Blasey, Adleman, & Steiner, 2002; Geller, Warner et al., 1998; Hazell et al., 1999; Kahana et al., in press). Youths with BSD can be statistically discriminated from nonbipolar youths by the scores from a combination of scales on the CBCL (typically, higher scores on the aggressive, delinquent behavior, attention problems, and anxious/depressed scales), whereas teacher report provides fewer and smaller differences, and youth report shows the fewest and smallest differences (i.e., relative elevations on delinquent behavior, which were only statistically significant in the Kahana et al., in press, study). The ASEBA instruments primarily appear to capture a higher level of externalizing problems in youths with BSD (Carlson et al., 1998). After controlling for the externalizing problem score, no other clinical syndrome scales of the ASEBA instruments provide meaningful predictive value in distinguishing BSD from other diagnoses (Kahana et al., in press).

The ASEBA instruments were not designed to measure manic or hypomanic symptoms, per se, and they do not include the cardinal symptoms of mania (i.e., elated mood or grandiosity, pressured speech); nor do they assess cycling or duration of mood states. The ASEBA checklists appear to provide a good measure of general impairment associated with BSD. However, the ASEBA scales do not perform as well as some of the more specialized instruments discussed below in differentiating BSD from other diagnoses (Youngstrom, Findling, Calabrese, et al., 2003). Probably the greatest value of the ASEBA instruments is that their usage may help calibrate different research groups' descriptions of juvenile BSD (Nottelmann et al., 2001).

Symptom Inventories

Currently, the Gadow and Sprafkin Symptom Inventories (Gadow & Sprafkin, 1994, 1997, 1999) are the other broad-spectrum assessment devices used in published studies on BSD. These checklists, which list DSM symptom criteria for most major juvenile Axis I disorders, are completed by parents, teachers, and adolescents. The inventories may provide an inexpensive way of gathering diagnostically relevant information from multiple sources. Relatively simple algorithms—such as requiring manic symptoms to be endorsed by any two out of three informants—could lead to a fairly specific way of identifying juvenile BSD (i.e., by correctly labeling the majority of people *without BSD*; Thuppal, Carlson, Sprafkin, & Gadow, 2002). Replication by other research groups will help establish the degree of diagnostic efficiency provided by the symptom inventories.

Specialized Rating Scales of Mania

Currently, the Young Mania Rating Scale (YMRS; Young, Biggs, Ziegler, & Meyer, 1978) is the most widely used clinician rating scale of manic symptoms in child, adolescent, and adult populations. No published mania rating scales developed specifically for use with children are presently in use (although Axelson's KSADS-MRS is currently under investigation), and only the YMRS has gained widespread usage in child and adolescent populations. The adoption of the YMRS as a clinical rating scale for children involves several changes from the context in which the YMRS was originally validated. These changes include all of the usual concerns when applying an adult measure to a juvenile population: the possibility of developmental changes in the manifestation of manic symptoms and the presence of developmental constraints on the expression of symptoms. Additionally, the YMRS was originally developed to be completed by health care professionals in an inpatient setting, where raters would have the opportunity to observe behavior over an 8-hour shift. However, when applied to children and adolescents, the YMRS is typically used with *outpatients*. Thus, the clinician no longer directly observes behavior over an extended period of time. Instead, self-report and parent report about behavior during the past week or 2 constitute the major sources of information.

Fortunately, published psychometric data on the YMRS in child and adolescent samples are available. Early investigations of the YMRS indicated that it was internally consistent and discriminated between groups of youths with bipolar disorder versus ADHD (Fristad, Weller, & Weller, 1992; Fristad, Weller, & Weller, 1995). More recent studies with larger samples indicate that the YMRS measures a single factor of general mania (Youngstrom, Findling, Sachs, et al., 2003; Youngstrom et al., 2002). Youths with ADHD showed moderate elevations on several YMRS items, but scores were significantly lower than for the BSD group (Fristad et al., 1995; Youngstrom et al., 2002).

The YMRS demonstrates fair to excellent internal consistency (average $\alpha = .75$, ranging from .62 to .91). The weakest items appear to be *bizarre appearance* and *lack of insight*, both of which show the lowest mean scores, standard deviations, and corrected item-total correlations. The multisite study also provides some information about 1-week retest stability of the YMRS in cohorts of bipolar youths beginning treatment: stability appears to be in the vicinity of $r = .55$ ($n = 122$) or $r = .67$ ($n = 27$). Because the youths in both of these groups had begun treatment, it is likely that stability in an untreated cohort should be comparable or higher. Pooling these estimates suggests that the YMRS has a standard error of the difference of approximately 7 points, meaning that changes of 11.5 points, or larger, are 95% likely to reflect improvement (one-tailed; see Jacobsen & Truax, 1991, for calculations).

When used with prepubescent outpatients, raters have included a parent interview as part of the evaluation on which item scores are based. The rating period under consideration also appears to have been extended to the past week. Based on the data described above, the YMRS appears to be a reasonably reliable and valid measure of mania in youths ages 5–17, even with these procedural modifications. However, there also are significant ways in which the YMRS could be improved, such as the revision or elimination of the bizarre appearance, lack of insight, and hypersexuality items, or the addition of new items that assess mania-related symptoms not previously reflected in the YMRS or DSM criteria (e.g., Geller et al., 2002). Currently, efforts are underway to develop an adolescent mania rating scale that contains more detailed and developmentally appropriate anchors in order to standardize scoring and increase interrater reliability. Until a revised version or an alternate mania rating scale with clearly superior properties becomes available, the YMRS remains the first choice for clinician ratings of manic symptoms in juveniles.

Data also are becoming available on more specialized mood rating scales that can be completed by parents and adolescents, such as an adaptation of the YMRS as a questionnaire, for completion by a parent to describe child functioning (Gracious et al., 2002). The Parent-YMRS has shown good internal consistency and excellent diagnostic efficiency, discriminating youths with diagnoses of bipolar spectrum disorders from those with unipolar depression, ADHD or disruptive behavior disorders, or other psychiatric diagnoses. Advantages of the P-YMRS include its brevity (11 items) and the shared content with the clinician-rated YMRS, which is the most widely used mania rating scale in juvenile samples. The P-YMRS also appears to be sensitive to treatment effects (Youngstrom, Gracious, & Findling, unpublished data, Case Western Reserve University), and its concise format lends itself to repeated assessment of outcomes.

The General Behavior Inventory (GBI; Depue, Krauss, Spoont, & Arbisi, 1989) is another instrument with considerable potential. The GBI is a 73-item tool designed to assess symptoms of depression, hypomania, mania, and mixed states. Slightly different versions of the GBI ask about different time frames, including the past week (e.g., Mallon, Klein, Bornstein, & Slater, 1986), past year, and lifetime (e.g., Depue, 1987) history. The GBI provides very thorough content coverage of mood-related symptoms, incorporating many behaviors that appear associated with mood states, even though these are not included in the formal diagnostic criteria. The GBI was originally developed as a way of screening for subsyndromal presentations of mood disorders in college samples, and it appears to be a highly specific instrument in that capacity (Depue et al., 1989). Subsequent research has found that the GBI performs well as a self-report measure in adult samples (Klein & Depue, 1984; Klein, Depue, & Slater, 1985), and the "past week" versions also appear sensitive to treatment effects (Mallon et al., 1986). Recently published data indicate that the GBI can be used as a self-report measure in youths as young as 10 while still retaining high levels of internal consistency ($\alpha = .95$ and $.97$ for the hypomanic/biphasic and depressed scales, respectively) and good diagnostic efficiency (Danielson, Youngstrom, Findling, & Calabrese, 2003). GBI scores also appear to be the best predictor of future onset of BSD (Lewinsohn, Seeley, & Klein, 2002).

The GBI also works well when adapted for use as a parent-report measure of child mood symptoms in youths ages 5–17 years. With minimal modifications to instructions and item wording, the Parent-GBI yields excellent reliability ($\alpha = .97$ and $.96$) and diagnostic efficiency (Findling, Youngstrom, Danielson, et al., 2002; Youngstrom et al., 2001). Based on a sample of 196 youths (30 with bipolar I, 40 with other bipolar spectrum disorders, 31 with unipolar depression, and 64 with ADHD or disruptive behavior disorders without comorbid mood disorder), parent report on the P-GBI hypomanic/biphasic scale successfully discriminated youths with BSD from youths with unipolar depression (AUC = .87, 86% classification) as well as ADHD or disruptive behavior disorders (AUC = .84, 81% classification) (Youngstrom et al., 2001). These results have recently been replicated in an independent sample of more than 300 youths evaluated at the same specialty clinic (Woldorf et al., 2002). Both the adolescent and parent-report versions of the GBI appear to be sensitive to treatment effects, based on an open-label study of more than 90 youths receiving Depakote and lithium combination therapy (Findling, McNamara, et al., in press).

Although the GBI and P-GBI demonstrate impressive reliability, diagnostic efficiency, and probably good sensitivity to treatment effects, their length is an obstacle for use in outcome assessment. Paradoxically, the GBI forms might be most useful in working with individual cases, where the high reliability translates into more precise estimation of an individual's true scores and response to treatment. The P-YMRS appears to be the leading candidate for a collateral source of information about manic symptoms; it offers a compelling combination of conciseness, linked content to the clinician YMRS, and sensitivity to treatment effects. The P-YMRS leaves room for improvement, but it appears appropriate to use the P-YMRS at least until more information becomes available about alternatives.

OUTCOME MEASUREMENT

BSD creates serious challenges in terms of measuring outcomes. The cycling nature of the illness leads to substantial variability in mood ratings from week to week, accounting for much of the variance in psychometric ratings of outcome. Because of this variance, the adult BSD literature has moved toward augmenting symptom ratings such as the YMRS (often the primary outcome measure for acute treatment studies) with more global clinical ratings as supplemental outcome measures, such as the Global Assessment of Functioning (GAF, or Axis V of the DSM), the Children's Global Assessment Scale (CGAS; Shaffer et al., 1983) or the Clinical Global Impressions of Bipolar response to treatment (CGI-BP). Global functioning ratings implicitly combine different aspects of symptomatology and functioning, and they may "smooth" some of the transient fluctuations in psychometric symptom ratings. Variants of survival analysis and Cox regression are presently the dominant methods for evaluating long-term maintenance clinical trials, where the dependent variable becomes the length of time to a clinically meaningful outcome, such as recurrence of a mood episode, termination of treatment due to mood symptoms or medication side effects, or discontinuation for any reason (e.g., Findling, Youngstrom, & Calabrese, 2002a, 2002b; Frank & Spanier, 1995; Miklowitz, Frank, & George, 1996). Although these global measures of outcome are coarse, they translate directly into clinical practice, where outcomes are often defined globally by the clinician and family.

There are at least three other models of outcome assessment worth considering. One is the approach that quantifies percentage of symptom reduction from baseline. This method has several shortcomings, including the fact that much of the variance in outcome ratings depends on the state of cycling, and the psychometric criticisms of percent-change approaches (Jacobson & Truax, 1991). However, the percent-change model is straightforward to interpret and, for now, is the most common model presented in the acute treatment literature for juvenile BSD (e.g., Frazier et al., 2001; Kafantaris, 1995; Kowatch et al., 2000; Wagner et al., 2002).

The second is effect-size estimation, such as reporting Cohen's d as a standardized estimate of the difference in treatment response on an outcome measure applied to two treatment groups (e.g., Carlson & Youngstrom, 2003). Effect-size estimation has advantages as a format for presenting group data, but it does not speak to individual clinical change.

The third model is the "clinically significant change" model, articulated by Jacobson and colleagues (Jacobson & Truax, 1991) and developed by Speer and others (Kendall, Marrs-Garcia, Nath, & Sheldrick, 1999; Speer, 1998). The Jacobson clinical significance model emphasizes two components: (1) reliable change, whereby an individual's change in scores is larger than could be attributed to measurement error in the given tool, and (2) passing an objective functional benchmark, based on normative distributions of scores for clinical and nonclinical populations. The advantages of the clinically significant change approach are that it focuses on individual change in the same way that practicing clinicians must, and it capitalizes on the psychometric information about the precision of scores and how they compare to meaningful reference groups. The main drawback of the Jacobson model is that it requires more information than typically is available for most measures. Few manuals or articles report the standard error of the difference score, for example, which is used in estimating reliable change. Similarly, estimation of two out of the three benchmarks suggested by Jacobson requires a nonclinical reference sample (Kendall et al., 1999). However, the most widely used clinical rating scales, such as the Young Mania Rating Scale (YMRS; Young et al., 1978) and the Child Depression Rating Scale—Revised (CDRS-R; Poznanski, Miller, Salguero, & Kelsh, 1984), have published data available on clinical samples but not a nonclinical standardization sample. Still, the clinically significant change model is gaining popularity, and it is likely to develop rapidly in the area of juvenile BSD (see Youngstrom, Findling, et al., in press, for elaboration, including details about using the available instruments within this framework).

In summary, the cyclical nature of BSD creates special challenges for evaluating outcomes, both in the context of clinical trials as well as individual practice. Sophisticated methods are available for modeling and documenting change, but each approach has strengths and limitations. Best practices in outcome assessment involve blending symptom ratings (such as the YMRS) and global functioning.

SUMMARY AND CLINICAL EXAMPLE

The literature reviewed in this chapter supports several conclusions. One is that BSD does occur in children and adolescents, though at a frequency lower than in adults but still much higher than previously believed. In order to rule the diagnosis of a BSD in or out, with some degree of accuracy, clinicians may need to modify their information gathering in several ways. In research settings, the use of a semistructured diagnostic interview is probably requisite to conducting informative studies. The WASH-U KSADS provides the most comprehensive assessment of BSD and ancillary features, but it also imposes the greatest burden on participants and requires the most training to administer.

In most clinical settings, structured and semistructured clinical interviews remain prohibitively expensive in terms of training costs and patient time. Clinical assessment in applied settings ideally emphasizes (1) gathering a family history of mood and related symptoms, (2) collecting report data from collateral sources (such as parents and teachers) about mood functioning, (3) concentrating on evidence of mood cycling and cardinal symptoms (such as periods of elevated mood or grandiosity), and (4) extending the window of assessment both retrospectively (by collecting mood data using psychometric instruments or life charting) and prospectively (via life charting and repeated scheduled mood assessments over the course of treatment). Several psychometric tools appear promising in terms of aiding differential diagnosis, and several more instruments that could make significant contributions are under investigation.

For evaluating outcomes and response to treatment, we recommend the use of an array of instruments, including global assessments of functioning (e.g., CGI-BP and CGAS) as well as more targeted measures of mood functioning (e.g., YMRS, CDRS-R, C-BPRS [Child—Brief Psychiatric Rating Scale; Hughes, Rintelmann, Emslie, Lopez, & MacCabe, 2001], P-GBI, GBI, etc.) and measures of quality of life (e.g., the Pediatric Quality of Life Scale; Varni, Seid, & Rode, 1999, and the KINDL; Ravens-Sieberer & Bullinger, 1998). As the relevant information becomes available, clinicians and policy-makers might be interested in employing the clinical-significance framework developed by Jacobson and Traux (1991) (although this model has proved to be a rigorous standard against which to measure clinical outcomes).

Finally, in terms of making differential diagnoses of BSD in children and adolescents, we must stress the benefit of actuarial approaches to decision making (Sackett, Straus, Richardson, Rosenberg, & Haynes, 2000). BSD is an exceptionally difficult condition to recognize correctly in youths, and cognitive heuristics are making it even more difficult for clinicians. The recent coverage in the popular press (Kluger & Song, 2002), for example, has drastically increased the number of parents who are bringing their children for evaluation because "they might have bipolar disorder." However, it is not intuitively obvious how best to combine the different pieces of available information (Grove, Zald, Lebow, Snitz, & Nelson, 2000). Actuarial approaches to diagnostic decision making offer the best vehicle for translating research findings into clinical practice (Sackett et al., 2000, provide detailed instructions).

As an example, imagine a 10-year-old male referred because of concerns about distractibility and aggressive behavior. His father has been diagnosed with bipolar I, and the son scores in the top 10% on the parent version of the GBI (51+ using the 0–3 Likert scoring; compared to benchmarks contained in Youngstrom, Findling, Calabrese, et al., 2003). The boy also obtained an externalizing problems t-score of 78 on the Achenbach Teacher Rating Form (TRF) from the teacher with whom he has the most contact. Assuming that the clinical setting does not see an unusual number of youths with bipolar disorder, then the probability that this youth has a bipolar disorder, based on a strictly statistical combination of the available information, could easily range from 27% (assuming a base rate of 1% for BSD, comparable to the community epidemiological estimates) to 70% (assuming a base rate of 6% for BSD—1% for bipolar I, and five times as much prevalence for other bipolar spectrum disorders).

This example illustrates how information that is readily available can inform diagnostic decisions *and* how much uncertainty remains. The scenario presents a relatively strong case for BSD, with family history and reports from two collateral sources all supportive of a BSD diagnosis. Even so, in order to feel confident enough to begin a treatment for BSD, yet more information would need to be gathered. The above clinical data would only suggest a 90% posterior probability of BSD in settings where the prevalence of BSD was 20% or higher. Careful attention to cardinal symptoms of BSD and to spontaneous fluctuations in mood over time would likely provide the decisive pieces of information in determining whether or not this specific youth had a BSD.

We have learned a great deal about BSD in children and adolescents over the last 5 years. We also have a great deal about which to be humble: The public health need certainly outstrips what we know about the diagnosis of this pernicious disorder. The good news is that a considerable amount of research is in progress that will inform how we diagnose and monitor BSD in children and adolescents in the near future. This chapter attempts to provide a broad but concise overview of the field, while simultaneously referring readers to more detailed sources and to relevant work in progress. Even with the partial information and unsettled debates that characterize the current literature, there is much that clinicians can already employ to help make this high-stakes diagnosis more accurately.

ACKNOWLEDGMENTS

A Bipolar Disorder Clinical Research Center Grant from the Stanley Foundation supported this research. We would like to thank Denise Delporto Bedoya, MA, Christine Demeter, BA, Deanne Pastva, BS, and Resa Whipkey, BS, for their assistance. We also thank Sheri Johnson and Jennifer Kogos Youngstrom for their helpful feedback. Special thanks are given to participating youths and their families.

REFERENCES

Abikoff, H., Courtney, M., Pelham, W. E., & Koplewicz, H. S. (1993). Teachers' ratings of disruptive behaviors: The influence of halo effects. *Journal of Abnormal Child Psychology, 21,* 519–533.

Achenbach, T. M., & Rescorla, L. A. (2001). *Manual for the ASEBA School-Age Forms and Profiles.* Burlington, VT: University of Vermont, Research Center for Children, Youth, and Families.

Akiskal, H. S. (1996). The prevalent clinical spectrum of bipolar disorders: Beyond DSM-IV. *Journal of Clinical Psychopharmacology, 16,* 4S–14S.

Aman, M. G., De Smedt, G., Derivan, A., Lyons, B., & Findling, R. L. (2002). Double-blind, placebo-controlled study of risperidone for the treatment of disruptive behaviors in children with subaverage intelligence. *American Journal of Psychiatry, 159,* 1337–1346.

American Psychiatric Association. (2000). *Diagnostic and statistical manual of mental disorders* (4th ed., text rev.). Washington, DC: Author.

Anastasi, A., & Urbina, S. (1997). *Psychological testing* (7th ed.). New York: MacMillan.

Axelson, D. (2002). *KSADS Mania Rating Scale.* Pittsburgh: University of Pittsburgh Medical Center.

Biederman, J. (1995). Developmental subtypes of juvenile bipolar disorder. *Harvard Review of Psychiatry, 3,* 227–230.

Biederman, J., Faraone, S. V., Chu, M. P., & Wozniak, J. (1999). Further evidence of a bidirectional overlap between juvenile mania and conduct disorder in children. *Journal of the American Academy of Child and Adolescent Psychiatry, 38,* 468–476.

Biederman, J., Faraone, S., Mick, E., Wozniak, J., Chen, L., Ouellette, C., Marrs, A., Moore, P., Garcia, J., Mennin, D., & Lelon, E. (1996). Attention-deficit hyperactivity disorder and juvenile mania: An overlooked comorbidity? *Journal of the American Academy of Child and Adolescent Psychiatry, 35,* 997–1008.

Biederman, J., Mick, E., Faraone, S. V., Spencer, T., Wilens, T. E., & Wozniak, J. (2000). Pediatric mania: A developmental subtype of bipolar disorder? *Biological Psychiatry, 48,* 458–466.

Biederman, J., Wozniak, J., Kiely, K., Ablon, S., Faraone, S., Mick, E., Mundy, E., & Kraus, I. (1995). CBCL clinical scales discriminate prepubertal children with structured interview-derived diagnosis of mania from those with ADHD. *Journal of the American Academy of Child and Adolescent Psychiatry, 34,* 464–471.

Birmaher, B., Arbelaez, C., & Brent, D. (2002). Course and outcome of child and adolescent major depressive disorder. *Child and Adolescent Psychiatric Clinics of North America, 11,* 619–638.

Bowring, M. A., & Kovacs, M. (1992). Difficulties in diagnosing manic disorders among children and adolescents. *Journal of the American Academy of Child and Adolescent Psychiatry, 31,* 611–614.

Brown, R. T., Freeman, W. S., Perrin, J. M., Stein, M. T., Amler, R. W., Feldman, H. M., Pierce, K., & Wolraich, M. L. (2001). Prevalence and assessment of attention-deficit/hyperactivity disorder in primary care settings. *Pediatrics, 107,* E43.

Carlson, G. A. (2002). Bipolar disorder in children and adolescents: A critical review. In D. Shaffer & B. Waslick (Eds.), *The many faces of depression in children and adolescents* (Vol. 21, pp. 105–128). Washington, DC: APPI Press.

Carlson, G. A., Jensen, P. S., Findling, R. L., Meyer, R. E., Calabrese, J. R., delBello, M., Emslie, G., Flynn, L., Goodwin, F., Hellander, M., Kowatch, R., Kusumakar, V., Laughren, T., Leibenluft, E., McCracken, J., Nottelmann, E., Pine, D., Sachs, G., Shaffer, D., Simar, R., Strober, M., Weller, E., Wozniak, J., & Youngstrom, E. A. (2003). Methodological issues and controversies in clinical trials with child and adolescent patients with bipolar disorder: Report of a consensus conference. *Journal of Child and Adolescent Psychopharmacology, 13,* 1–15.

Carlson, G. A., & Kelly, K. L. (1998). Manic symptoms in psychiatrically hospitalized children: What do they mean? *Journal of Affective Disorders, 51,* 123–135.

Carlson, G. A., Loney, J., Salisbury, H., & Volpe, R. J. (1998). Young referred boys with DICA-P manic symptoms vs. two comparison groups. *Journal of Affective Disorders, 121,* 113–121.

Carlson, G. A., & Youngstrom, E. A. (2003). Clinical implications of pervasive manic symptoms in children. *Biological Psychiatry, 53,* 1050–1058.

Caron, C., & Rutter, M. (1991). Comorbidity in child psychopathology: Concepts, issues and research strategies. *Journal of Child Psychology and Psychiatry and Allied Disciplines, 32,* 1063–1080.

Costello, E. J., Angold, A., Burns, B. J., Stangl, D. K., Tweed, D. L., Erkanli, A., & Worthman, C. M. (1996). The Great Smoky Mountains Study of youth: Goals, design, methods, and the prevalence of DSM-III-R disorders. *Archives of General Psychiatry, 53,* 1129–1136.

Coyne, J. C., Thompson, R., & Racioppo, M. W. (2001). Validity and efficiency of screening for history of depression by self-report. *Psychological Assessment, 13,* 163–170.

Cyranowski, J. M., Frank, E., Young, E., & Shear, K. (2000). Adolescent onset of the gender difference in lifetime rates of major depression. *Archives of General Psychiatry, 57,* 21–27.

Danielson, C. K., Feeny, N. C., Findling, R. L., & Youngstrom, E. A. (in press). Psychosocial treatment of bipolar disorder in adolescents: A proposed cognitive-behavioral intervention. *Cognitive and Behavioral Practice.*

Danielson, C. K., Youngstrom, E. A., Findling, R. L., & Calabrese, J. R. (2003). Discriminative validity of the General Behavior Inventory using youth report. *Journal of Abnormal Child Psychology, 31,* 29–39.

DelBello, M. P., & Geller, B. (2001). Review of studies of child and adolescent offspring of bipolar parents. *Bipolar Disorders, 3,* 325–334.

DelBello, M. P., Soutullo, C. A., Hendricks, W., Niemeier, R. T., McElroy, S. L., & Strakowski, S. M. (2001). Prior stimulant treatment in adolescents with bipolar disorder: Association with age at onset. *Bipolar Disorders, 3,* 53–57.

Denicoff, K. D., Smith-Jackson, E. E., Disney, E. R., Suddath, R. L., Leverich, G. S., & Post, R. M. (1997). Preliminary evidence of the reliability and validity of the prospective life-chart methodology (LCM-P). *Journal of Psychiatric Research, 31,* 593–603.

Depue, R. A., Krauss, S., Spoont, M. R., & Arbisi, P. (1989). General Behavior Inventory identification of unipolar and bipolar affective conditions in a nonclinical university population. *Journal of Abnormal Psychology, 98,* 117–126.

Dienes, K. A., Chang, K. D., Blasey, C. M., Adleman, N., & Steiner, H. (2002). Characterization of children of bipolar parents by parent report CBCL. *Journal of Psychiatric Research, 36,* 337–345.

Findling, R. L., Feeny, N. C., Stansbrey, R. J., DelPorto-Bedoya, D., & Demeter, C. (2002). Somatic treatment for depressive illnesses in children and adolescents. *Child and Adolescent Psychiatric Clinics of North America, 11,* 555–578.

Findling, R. L., Gracious, B. L., McNamara, N. K., Youngstrom, E. A., Demeter, C., & Calabrese, J. R. (2001). Rapid, continuous cycling and psychiatric co-morbidity in pediatric bipolar I disorder. *Bipolar Disorders, 3,* 202–210.

Findling, R. L., Kahana, S. Y., Youngstrom, E. A., & Calabrese, J. R. (2002). *Cyclotaxia: Subsyndromal symptoms of mania and depression in offspring with a bipolar parent.* Manuscript submitted for publication.

Findling, R. L., McNamara, N. K., Gracious, B. L., Youngstrom, E. A., Stansbrey, R. J., Reed, M. D., Demeter, C., Branicky, L. A., Resler, R. M., Fisher, K. E., & Calabrese, J. R. (in press). Combination lithium and divalproex in pediatric bipolarity. *Journal of the American Academy of Child and Adolescent Psychiatry.*

Findling, R. L., Reed, M. D., & Blumer, J. L. (1999). Pharmacological treatment of depression in children and adolescents. *Paediatric Drugs, 1,* 161–182.

Findling, R. L., Youngstrom, E. A., & Calabrese, J. R. (2002a, December). *Divalproex sodium versus lithium as maintenance pharmacotherapy in pediatric bipolarity.* Paper presented at the American College of Neuropsychopharmacology, Puerto Rico.

Findling, R. L., Youngstrom, E. A., & Calabrese, J. R. (2002b, December). *Evolving maintenance trial designs in pediatric bipolarity.* Paper presented at the American College of Neuropsychopharmacology, Puerto Rico.

Findling, R. L., Youngstrom, E. A., Danielson, C. K., DelPorto, D., Papish David, R., Townsend, L., & Calabrese, J. (2002). Clinical decision-making using the General Behavior Inventory in juvenile bipolarity. *Bipolar Disorders, 4,* 34–42.

Frank, E., & Spanier, C. (1995). Interpersonal psychotherapy for depression: Overview, clinical efficacy, and future directions. *Clinical Psychology: Science and Practice, 2,* 349–369.

Frazier, J. A., Biederman, J., Tohen, M., Feldman, P. D., Jacobs, T. G., Toma, V., Rater, M. A., Tarazi, R. A., Kim, G. S., Garfield, S. B., Sohma, M., Gonzalez-Heydrich, J., Risser, R. C., & Nowlin, Z. M. (2001). A prospective open-label treatment trial of olanzapine monotherapy in children and adolescents with bipolar disorder. *Journal of Child and Adolescent Psychopharmacology, 11,* 239–250.

Fristad, M. A., Weller, E. B., & Weller, R. A. (1992). The Mania Rating Scale (MRS): Can it be used with children? A preliminary report. *Journal of the American Academy of Child and Adolescent Psychiatry, 31,* 252–257.

Fristad, M. A., Weller, R. A., & Weller, E. B. (1995). The Mania Rating Scale (MRS): Further reliability and validity studies with children. *Annals of Clinical Psychiatry, 7,* 127–132.

Gadow, K. D., & Sprafkin, J. (1994). *Child Symptom Inventories Manual*. Stonybrook, NY: Checkmate Plus.

Gadow, K. D., & Sprafkin, J. (1997). *Adolescent Symptom Inventory: Screening manual*. Stonybrook, NY: Checkmate Plus.

Gadow, K. D., & Sprafkin, J. (1999). *Youth's Inventory–4 Manual*. Stonybrook, NY: Checkmate Plus.

Geller, B., & Luby, J. (1997). Child and adolescent bipolar disorder: A review of the past 10 years. *Journal of the American Academy of Child and Adolescent Psychiatry, 36,* 1168–1176.

Geller, B., Warner, K., Williams, M., & Zimerman, B. (1998). Prepubertal and young adolescent bipolarity versus ADHD: Assessment and validity using the WASH-U KSADS, CBCL and TRF. *Journal of Affective Disorders, 51,* 93–100.

Geller, B., Williams, M., Zimerman, B., Frazier, J., Beringer, L., & Warner, K. L. (1998). Prepubertal and early adolescent bipolarity differentiate from ADHD by manic symptoms, grandiose delusions, ultra-rapid or ultradian cycling. *Journal of Affective Disorders, 51,* 81–91.

Geller, B., Zimerman, B., Williams, M., Bolhofner, K., & Craney, J. L. (2001). Bipolar disorder at prospective follow-up of adults who had prepubertal major depressive disorder. *American Journal of Psychiatry, 158,* 125–127.

Geller, B., Zimerman, B., Williams, M., Bolhofner, K., Craney, J. L., DelBello, M. P., & Soutullo, C. A. (2000). Diagnostic characteristics of 93 cases of prepubertal and early adolescent bipolar disorder phenotype by gender, puberty and comorbid attention deficit hyperactivity disorder. *Journal of Child and Adolescent Psychopharmacology, 10,* 157–164.

Geller, B., Zimerman, B., Williams, M., Bolhofner, K., Craney, J. L., DelBello, M. P., & Soutullo, C. (2001). Reliability of the Washington University in St. Louis Kiddie Schedule for Affective Disorders and Schizophrenia (WASH-U KSADS) mania and rapid cycling sections. *Journal of the American Academy of Child and Adolescent Psychiatry, 40,* 450–455.

Geller, B., Zimerman, B., Williams, M., DelBello, M. P., Frazier, J., & Beringer, L. (2002). Phenomenology of prepubertal and early adolescent bipolar disorder: Examples of elated mood, grandiose behaviors, decreased need for sleep, racing thoughts and hypersexuality. *Journal of Child and Adolescent Psychopharmacology, 12,* 3–9.

Goodwin, F. K., & Jamison, K. R. (1990). *Manic–depressive illness*. New York: Oxford University Press.

Gracious, B. L., Youngstrom, E. A., Findling, R. L., & Calabrese, J. R. (2002). Discriminative validity of a parent version of the Young Mania Rating Scale. *Journal of the American Academy of Child and Adolescent Psychiatry, 41,* 1350–1359.

Grove, W. M., Zald, D. H., Lebow, B. S., Snitz, B. E., & Nelson, C. (2000). Clinical versus mechanical prediction: A meta-analysis. *Psychological Assessment, 12,* 19–30.

Hazell, P. L., Lewin, T. J., & Carr, V. J. (1999). Confirmation that Child Behavior Checklist clinical scales discriminate juvenile mania from attention deficit hyperactivity disorder. *Journal of Paediatrics and Child Health, 35,* 199–203.

Hinshaw, S. P., & Anderson, C. A. (1996). Conduct and oppositional defiant disorders. In E. J. Mash & R. A. Barkley (Eds.), *Child psychopathology* (pp. 113–149). New York: Guilford Press.

Hughes, C. W., Rintelmann, J., Emslie, G. J., Lopez, M., & MacCabe, N. (2001). A revised anchored version of the BPRS-C for childhood psychiatric disorders. *Journal of Child and Adolescent Psychopharmacology, 11,* 77–93.

Jacobson, N. S., & Truax, P. (1991). Clinical significance: A statistical approach to defining meaningful change in psychotherapy research. *Journal of Consulting and Clinical Psychology, 59,* 12–19.

Kafantaris, V. (1995). Treatment of bipolar disorder in children and adolescents. *Journal of the American Academy of Child and Adolescent Psychiatry, 34,* 732–741.

Kahana, S. Y., Youngstrom, E. A., Findling, R. L., & Calabrese, J. R. (in press). Using Achenbach's System of Empirically Based Assessment to differentiate between ADHD and bipolar spectrum disorders. *Journal of Child and Adolescent Psychopharmacology.*

Kashani, J. H., Beck, N. C., Hoeper, E. W., Fallahi, C., Corcoran, C. M., McAllister, J. A., Rosenberg, T. K., & Reid, J. C. (1987). Psychiatric disorders in a community sample of adolescents. *American Journal of Psychiatry, 144,* 584–589.

Kaufman, J., Birmaher, B., Brent, D., Rao, U., Flynn, C., Moreci, P., Williamson, D., & Ryan, N. (1997). Schedule for Affective Disorders and Schizophrenia for School-Age Children—Present and Lifetime version (K-SADS-PL): Initial reliability and validity data. *Journal of the American Academy of Child and Adolescent Psychiatry, 36,* 980–988.

Kendall, P. C., Marrs-Garcia, A., Nath, S. R., & Sheldrick, R. C. (1999). Normative comparisons for the evaluation of clinical significance. *Journal of Consulting and Clinical Psychology, 67,* 285–299.

Kessler, R. C. (1994). The National Comorbidity Survey of the United States. *International Review of Psychiatry, 6,* 365–376.

Kessler, R. C., Avenevoli, S., & Merikangas, K. R. (2001). Mood disorders in children and adolescents: An epidemiologic perspective. *Biological Psychiatry, 49,* 1002–1014.

Kessler, R. C., Rubinow, D. R., Holmes, C., Abelson, J. M., & Zhao, S. (1997). The epidemiology of DSM-III-R bipolar I disorder in a general population survey. *Psychological Medicine, 27,* 1079–1089.

Klein, D. N., & Depue, R. A. (1984). Continued impairment in persons at risk for bipolar affective disorder: Results of a 19-month follow-up study. *Journal of Abnormal Psychology, 93,* 345–347.

Klein, D. N., Depue, R. A., & Slater, J. F. (1985). Cyclothymia in the adolescent offspring of parents with bipolar affective disorder. *Journal of Abnormal Psychology, 94,* 115–127.

Klein, R. G., Pine, D. S., & Klein, D. F. (1998). Resolved: Mania is mistaken for ADHD in prepubertal children. *Journal of the American Academy of Child and Adolescent Psychiatry, 37,* 1093–1096.

Kluger, J., & Song, S. (2002). Young and bipolar. *Time, 51,* pp. 39–47.

Kovacs, M. (1996). Presentation and course of major depressive disorder during childhood and later years of the life span. *Journal of the American Academy of Child and Adolescent Psychiatry, 35,* 705–715.

Kovacs, M., & Pollock, M. (1995). Bipolar disorder and comorbid conduct disorder in childhood and adolescence. *Journal of the American Academy of Child and Adolescent Psychiatry, 34,* 715–723.

Kowatch, R. A., Suppes, T., Carmody, T. J., Bucci, J. P., Hume, J. H., Kromelis, M., Emslie, G. J., Weinberg, W. A., & Rush, A. J. (2000). Effect size of lithium, divalproex sodium, and carbamazepine in children and adolescents with bipolar disorder. *Journal of the American Academy of Child and Adolescent Psychiatry, 39,* 713–720.

Kraemer, H. C. (1992). *Evaluating medical tests: Objective and quantitative guidelines.* Newbury Park, CA: Sage.

Lapalme, M., Hodgins, S., & LaRoche, C. (1997). Children of parents with bipolar disorder: A meta-analysis of risk for mental disorders. *Canadian Journal of Psychiatry, 42,* 623–631.

Lewinsohn, P. M., Klein, D. N., & Seeley, J. R. (1995). Bipolar disorders in a community sample of older adolescents: Prevalence, phenomenology, comorbidity, and course. *Journal of the American Academy of Child and Adolescent Psychiatry, 34,* 454–463.

Lewinsohn, P. M., Seeley, J. R., Buckley, M. E., & Klein, D. N. (2002). Bipolar disorder in adolescence and young adulthood. *Child and Adolescent Psychiatric Clinics of North America, 11,* 461–476.

Lewinsohn, P. M., Seeley, J. R., & Klein, D. N. (2002, September). *Longitudinal course of bipolar disorder from adolescence to age 30 in the community.* Paper presented at the Society for Research in Psychopathology, San Francisco.

Loeber, R., Green, S. M., & Lahey, B. B. (1990). Mental health professionals' perception of the utility of children, mothers, and teachers as informants on childhood psychopathology. *Journal of Clinical Child Psychology, 19,* 136–143.

Mallon, J. C., Klein, D. N., Bornstein, R. F., & Slater, J. F. (1986). Discriminant validity of the General Behavior Inventory: An outpatient study. *Journal of Personality Assessment, 50,* 568–577.

McClellan, J., & Werry, J. (1997). Practice parameters for the assessment and treatment of children and adolescents with bipolar disorder: American Academy of Child and Adolescent Psychiatry. *Journal of the American Academy of Child and Adolescent Psychiatry, 36,* 157S–176S.

Meaden, P. M., Daniels, R. E., & Zajecka, J. (2000). Construct validity of life chart functioning scales for use in naturalistic studies of bipolar disorder. *Journal of Psychiatric Research, 34,* 187–192.

Miklowitz, D. J., Frank, E., & George, E. L. (1996). Clinical trials: Bipolar disorder. *Psychopharmacology Bulletin, 32,* 613–621.

Newman, C. F., Leahy, R. L., Beck, A. T., Reilly-Harrington, N. A., & Gyulai, L. (2002). *Bipolar disorder: A cognitive therapy approach.* Washington, DC: American Psychological Association.

Nottelmann, E. (2002). *Prepubertal bipolar disorder—not otherwise specified.* Paper presented at the National Institute of Mental Health Research Roundtable, Washington, DC.

Nottelmann, E., Biederman, J., Birmaher, B., Carlson, G. A., Chang, K. D., Fenton, W. S., Geller, B., Hoagwood, K. E., Hyman, S. E., Kendler, K. S., Koretz, D. S., Kowatch, R. A., Kupfer, D. J., Leibenluft, E., Nakamura, R. K., Nottelmann, E. D., Stover, E., Vitiello, B., Weiblinger, G., & Weller, E. (2001). National Institute of Mental Health research roundtable on prepubertal bipolar disorder. *Journal of the American Academy of Child and Adolescent Psychiatry, 40,* 871–878.

Nottelmann, E. D., & Jensen, P. S. (1995). Comorbidity of disorders in children and adolescents: Developmental perspectives. In T. H. Ollendick & R. J. Prinz (Eds.), *Advances in clinical child psychology* (Vol. 17, pp. 109–155). New York: Plenum Press.

Papolos, D. F. (1999). *The bipolar child: The definitive and reassuring guide to childhood's most misunderstood disorder.* New York: Broadway Books.

Pavuluri, M. (2002, September). *Prospective treatment study: Reliability and validity of the Child Bipolar Rating Scale—Parent/Teacher version (CBRS-P/T).* Paper presented at the NIMH roundtable on the Broad Phenotype of Juvenile Bipolar Disorder, Bethesda, MD.

Poznanski, E. O., Miller, E., Salguero, C., & Kelsh, R. C. (1984). Preliminary studies of the reliability and validity of the Children's Depression Rating Scale. *Journal of the American Academy of Child Psychiatry, 23,* 191–197.

Ravens-Sieberer, U., & Bullinger, M. (1998). Assessing health-related quality of life in chronically ill children with the German KINDL: First psychometric and content analytic results. *Quality of Life Research: An International Journal of Quality of Life Aspects of Treatment, Care and Rehabilitation, 7,* 399–407.

Rosenberg, D. R., Holttum, J., & Gershon, S. (1994). *Textbook of pharmacotherapy for child and adolescent psychiatric disorders.* New York: Brunner/Mazel.

Sachs, G. S., Guille, C., & McMurrich, S. L. (2002). A clinical monitoring form for mood disorders. *Bipolar Disorders, 4,* 323–327.

Sackett, D. L., Straus, S. E., Richardson, W. S., Rosenberg, W., & Haynes, R. B. (2000).

Evidence-based medicine: How to practice and teach EBM (2nd ed.). New York: Livingstone.

Shaffer, D., Fisher, P., Greenwald, S., & Greenberg, T. (2002, June). *Child and adolescent bipolar disorder: Measurement.* Paper presented at the American Academy of Child and Adolescent Psychiatry and Best Practices Conference, Current Controversies and Methodological Challenges Regarding Clinical Trials in Juvenile Bipolar Disorder, Washington, DC.

Shaffer, D., Fisher, P., Lucas, C. P., Dulcan, M. K., & Schwab-Stone, M. E. (2000). NIMH Diagnostic Interview Schedule for Children Version IV (NIMH DISC-IV): Description, differences from previous versions, and reliability of some common diagnoses. *Journal of the American Academy of Child and Adolescent Psychiatry, 39,* 28–38.

Shaffer, D., Gould, M. S., Brasic, J., Ambrosini, P., Fisher, P., Bird, H., & Aluwahlia, S. (1983). A children's global assessment scale (CGAS). *Archives of General Psychiatry, 40,* 1228–1231.

Soutullo, C. A., DelBello, M. P., Ochsner, J. E., McElroy, S. L., Taylor, S. A., Strakowski, S. M., & Keck, P. E., Jr. (2002). Severity of bipolarity in hospitalized manic adolescents with history of stimulant or antidepressant treatment. *Journal of Affective Disorders, 70,* 323–327.

Speer, D. C. (1998). *Mental health outcome evaluation.* San Diego, CA: Academic Press.

Thuppal, M., Carlson, G. A., Sprafkin, J., & Gadow, K. D. (2002). Correspondence between adolescent report, parent report, and teacher report of manic symptoms. *Journal of Child and Adolescent Psychopharmacology, 12,* 27–35.

Varni, J. W., Seid, M., & Rode, C. A. (1999). The PedsQL: Measurement model for the pediatric quality of life inventory. *Medical Care, 37,* 126–139.

Wagner, K. D., Weller, E. B., Carlson, G. A., Sachs, G., Biederman, J., Frazier, J. A., Wozniak, P., Tracy, K., Weller, R. A., & Bowden, C. (2002). An open-label trial of divalproex in children and adolescents with bipolar disorder. *Journal of the American Academy of Child and Adolescent Psychiatry, 41,* 1224–1230.

Weckerly, J. (2002). Pediatric bipolar mood disorder. *Journal of Developmental and Behavioral Pediatrics, 23,* 42–56.

Weisbrot, D. M., & Ettinger, A. B. (2002). Aggression and violence in mood disorders. *Child and Adolescent Psychiatric Clinics of North America, 11,* 649–671.

Wittchen, H.-U., Nelson, C. B., & Lachner, G. (1998). Prevalence of mental disorders and psychosocial impairments in adolescents and young adults. *Psychological Medicine, 28,* 109–126.

Woldorf, G. M., Youngstrom, E. A., Danielson, C. K., Findling, R. L., & Calabrese, J. R. (2002, August). *Discriminant validity of the Parent General Behavior Inventory: A replication.* Paper presented at the Annual Meeting of the American Psychological Association, Chicago.

Wozniak, J., Biederman, J., Kiely, K., Ablon, J. S., Faraone, S., Mundy, E., & Mennin, D. (1995). Mania-like symptoms suggestive of childhood-onset bipolar disorder in clinically referred children. *Journal of the American Academy of Child and Adolescent Psychiatry, 34,* 867–876.

Wozniak, J., Biederman, J., & Richards, J. A. (2001). Diagnostic and therapeutic dilemmas in the management of pediatric-onset bipolar disorder. *Journal of Clinical Psychiatry, 62*(Suppl. 14), 10–15.

Young, R. C., Biggs, J. T., Ziegler, V. E., & Meyer, D. A. (1978). A rating scale for mania: Reliability, validity, and sensitivity. *British Journal of Psychiatry, 133,* 429–435.

Youngstrom, E. A., Danielson, C. K., Findling, R. L., Gracious, B. L., & Calabrese, J. R. (2002). Factor structure of the Young Mania Rating Scale for use with youths aged 5 to 17 years. *Journal of Clinical Child and Adolescent Psychology, 31,* 567–572.

Youngstrom, E. A., Findling, R. L., Calabrese, J. R., Demeter, C., Delporto Bedoya, D., & Price, M. E. (2003). *Diagnostic accuracy of six potential screening instruments for bipolar disorder in youths aged 5 to 17 years.* Manuscript submitted for publication.

Youngstrom, E. A., Findling, R. L., Carlson, G. A., & Ferziger, R. (in press). Screening and outcome measures for child and adolescent bipolar disorder. *Journal of Child and Adolescent Psychopharmacology.*

Youngstrom, E. A., Findling, R. L., Danielson, C. K., & Calabrese, J. R. (2001). Discriminative validity of parent report of hypomanic and depressive symptoms on the General Behavior Inventory. *Psychological Assessment, 13,* 267–276.

Youngstrom, E. A., Findling, R. L., Sachs, G., Carlson, G. A., Wozniak, J., Fristad, M., Kafantaris, V., Frazier, J., DelBello, M., Chang, K., Scheffer, R., & Leibenluft, E. (2003, March). *Manic symptoms in bipolar and nonbipolar youths across eleven research groups using the Young Mania Rating Scale.* Paper presented at the NIMH Pediatric Bipolar Disorder Conference, Washington, DC.

Youngstrom, E. A., Gracious, B. L., Danielson, C. K., Findling, R. L., & Calabrese, J. R. (in press). Toward an integration of parent and clinician report on the Young Mania Rating Scale. *Journal of Affective Disorders.*

CHAPTER FIVE

PSYCHOSOCIAL PREDICTORS OF SYMPTOMS

SHERI L. JOHNSON
BJÖRN MEYER

As discussed in the first chapters of this volume, bipolar disorder has severe consequences for affected individuals, family members, and society. Even with the best of current medical treatments, many individuals continue to experience frequent relapses and chronic subsyndromal symptoms (Judd et al., 2002). Given the wide variability in course across individuals, as well as over time within individuals, there is a need to understand the variables that predict symptoms.

Although heritability is well established as the central variable explaining vulnerability to this disorder, biological variables do not fully explain individual differences in severity or changes in course over time. As widely demonstrated by the field of psychoimmunology, social and psychological variables have a clear and direct impact on neurotransmitter levels, peptides, and cytokines, as well as a broad range of disease processes (Glaser & Kiecolt-Glaser, 1994). Given this impact, it is natural to investigate the influence of psychosocial variables on the expression of vulnerability to this essentially biological disorder. Indeed, in recent years, the influence of psychosocial variables on the course of bipolar disorder has become increasingly well substantiated.

In an attempt to describe the lives and characteristics of individuals with bipolar disorder, the vast majority of research has been cross-sectional.

Much of this research has focused on ascertaining whether individuals with bipolar disorder experience difficult social environments and poor resources for coping with these environments. We would expect that the experience of repeated symptoms and hospitalizations would create difficulties for friendships and intimate relationships, work, and self-esteem—and, indeed, it does appear that bipolar disorder is associated with social and psychological problems, including marital conflict and family burden (McKnight, Nelson-Gray, Gullick, 1989; Perlick et al., 1999), fewer resourceful coping strategies (Meyer, 2001), and lower self-esteem (Serretti et al., 1999). There also is evidence that bipolar disorder may be associated with specific neuropsychological deficits in sustained attention, even after controlling for subsyndromal symptoms (Clark, Iversen, & Goodwin, 2002) and the cognitive side effects of mood-stabilizing medication (Judd, 1979; Squire, Judd, Janowsky, & Huey, 1980). Deficits in long-delay verbal recall have been noted among family members of individuals with bipolar disorder as well (Gourovitch et al., 1999; Keri, Kelemen, Benedek, & Janka, 2001). In sum, many troubling correlates of bipolar disorder have been established.

In this chapter, we focus our attention on the predictors of symptom course. Psychosocial variables also may influence social and occupational functioning, treatment adherence, and suicidality. The predictors of functioning are discussed by Hammen (Chapter 3, this volume). Aside from such issues, the question that seems most central in guiding psychotherapeutic interventions is: Which variables predict when—and for whom—severe symptoms will occur? Hence, we turn toward longitudinal studies designed to assess the triggers for symptom changes. In reviewing these areas, we first note variables that seem to predict poorer outcomes, without attention to the specific types of symptoms that are predicted. We discuss social–environmental triggers, followed by psychological variables. Recent literature has begun to identify patterns that may be distinct for the prediction of depression compared to mania. Thus, after discussing variables that predict symptoms more generally, we turn toward predictors of depression and mania specifically.

PREDICTORS OF POOR OUTCOME

Expressed Emotion

Expressed emotion (EE), defined as emotionally intrusive or hostile comments from family members toward individuals with the disorder, was one of the first environmental variables shown to influence the course of bipolar disorder (Miklowitz, Goldstein, Nuechterlein, Snyder, & Mintz, 1988; Priebe, Wildgrube, & Mueller-Oerlinghausen, 1989). Traditionally, EE is measured by conducting the Camberwell interview, in which family members are asked a series of questions regarding the patient and his or her illness. Family members who make more than six hostile or overly intrusive comments within the interview period are labeled as high EE. Considerable evidence supports the validity of the Camberwell interview. For example, families that display high EE levels during the interview also display more negativity during problem-solving interactions (Simoneau, Miklowicz, & Saleem, 1998).

Although EE has been shown to influence the course of a broad range of disorders, the effect size appears to be substantially larger for individuals with mood disorders than for those with schizophrenia (Butzlaff & Hooley, 1998). The deleterious effects of EE appear to be particularly important when received from parents, compared to marital partners (Miklowitz et al., 2000). Although less research addressing adolescent bipolar disorder is available, low maternal warmth does seem to predict a relapse (Geller et al., 2002).

Many individuals have wondered whether EE is a reaction to the patient's particular symptoms. That is, do patients with certain symptoms or personality features elicit more criticism or overinvolvement? A series of studies have suggested that EE seems to hold predictive power even after accounting for subsyndromal symptoms and personality traits (Hooley, Rosen, & Richters, 1995).

This finding raises the question of how EE operates. A current theory is that EE is influenced by the family's attributions for illness. That is, family members who see symptoms as under the patient's control, rather than uncontrollable and biologically driven, may be more prone to blame the person and to feel angry (Hooley, 1998; Hooley & Licht, 1997). In this light, psychoeducation for family members and patients appears particularly critical.

Social Support

Although family members are often central sources of support for many patients, many individuals with bipolar disorder experience such estrangement from their family members that other individuals become the source of their social support. Hence, it is important to integrate an understanding of specific family processes with information about other interpersonal resources. Several studies suggest that individuals with bipolar disorder experience less social support than those without mental disorders, and that social support is lower for people with a history of more manic episodes (Romans & McPherson, 1992). Within bipolar disorder, however, individuals vary considerably in the number and closeness of friendships they sustain. At times, hypomanic symptoms and related traits may promote increased social and sexual engagement (Greenhouse, 2002). An absence of emotional support has been related to a poorer course of the disorder, including more frequent relapse and less successful lithium treatment

(Johnson, Meyer, Winett, & Small, 2000; Stefos, Bauwens, Staner, Pardoen, & Mendlewicz, 1996).

Negative Life Events

Numerous studies investigating life events and bipolar disorder have been conducted, but the methodological quality has varied substantially, with concomitant differences in results. Life-events research is vulnerable to a broad range of confounding variables, including poor reporting, as well as the tricky issue of quantifying stressful consequences of the illness (Hammen, 2000). Life-stress interviews intended to address these issues have been developed, and the findings using these interview measures have consistently supported links between life events and increases in symptoms (Johnson & Roberts, 1995). These findings seem to hold even after excluding life events that are provoked by symptoms or poor coping. For example, independent negative life events have been found to be associated with a 4.5-fold increase in the risk of relapse (Ellicott, Hammen, Gitlin, Brown, & Jamison, 1990; Hunt, Bruce-Jones, & Silverstone, 1992) and a slower time to recovery from episodes (Johnson & Miller, 1997).

As has been found in research with people who have schizophrenia and major depression (Brown & Harris, 1989), not all life events are equally likely to provoke symptom changes. Severe events, such as the loss of a family member or core friend seem to be particularly important in provoking symptoms, whereas smaller events, such as fender-benders or minor altercations, have not been found to substantially increase the risk of symptoms (Johnson et al., 1997). Similarly, there is some evidence that interpersonal events are particularly influential (Hammen, Ellicott, & Gitlin, 1992). Hence, within the life-stress domain, the best predictors of course appear to be major negative life events, particularly those that involve loss.

Personality

During an episode, maladaptive personality traits appear elevated (cf. Solomon, Shea, Leon, & Mueller, 1996). Therefore, the likelihood of obtaining an Axis II diagnosis is lower if an individual is assessed after recovery. Even during euthymic periods, however, individuals with bipolar disorder, like those with remitted unipolar depression, appear to endorse neuroticism (Bagby et al., 1996) as well as Cluster B (dramatic, emotionally erratic) and Custer C (fearful, avoidant) personality disorders (George, Miklowitz, Richards, Simoneau, & Taylor, 2002).

Cross-sectional attempts to assess the levels of personality disturbance associated with bipolar disorder, however, have been criticized for failing to attend to the possibility that some personality features may reflect the psychological aftermath of the illness as well as chronic subsyndromal symptoms (cf. Hirschfeld et al., 1983). For example, although studies have found higher levels of neuroticism among individuals with bipolar disorder (see Klein, Durbin, Shankman, & Santiago, 2002), it is unclear whether these higher levels reflect chronic subsyndromal depression. Ideal designs would involve studying (1) individuals before the onset of mood symptoms, or (2) family members of affected individuals. In the only available study of personality features preceding onset (Clayton, Ernst, & Angst, 1994), the personality traits studied did not differentiate the 36 individuals who did develop mania from those who did not (n = 2,894). To date, then, personality correlates of bipolar disorder have varied widely depending on the methodological approaches used, but neuroticism and different facets of extroversion have received attention.

A key question is whether personality variables predict symptoms over time. Cross-sectional studies suggest that individuals with comorbid personality disorders appear more likely to experience chronic subsyndromal symptoms between episodes (George et al., 2002), and they appear to spend more time in the hospital (Barbato & Hafner, 1998). Prospectively, one study found that sociotropy—that is, a personality trait involving excessive need for reassurance and sensitivity to interpersonal life events—predicted increases in symptom severity over time in persons with bipolar disorder (Hammen et al., 1992). These few studies, then, suggest that personality disorders and maladaptive traits contribute to poor outcomes.

Summary

Individuals who are able to maintain noncritical family relationships, strong social support networks, and lower rates of major life events are likely to experience fewer symptoms of their disorder over time. Beyond the social environment, a better course of disorder may be possible for people with fewer negative interpretations of themselves and their life events, those who are less neurotic, and those who are less dependent on others' opinions of them. Sadly, some of the cross-sectional evidence suggests that bipolar disorder may come hand in hand with difficulties in these areas. Hence, psychotherapeutic interventions may be needed to help individuals develop more supportive social environments, positive self-evaluations, and adaptive cognitions regarding stress. Maladaptive personality traits that persist beyond the recovery period may suggest the need for more intensive therapeutic interventions as well.

POLARITY-SPECIFIC FINDINGS

Bipolar disorder includes a broad range of symptom expressions, including subsyndromal chronic symptoms, acute episodes, and ongoing hopelessness and motivational deficits. The most striking distinction, of course, is between symptoms of depression and mania. Which of these symptom types can we predict from psychosocial variables? In recent years, our team has begun to examine whether psychosocial variables operate differently in the prediction of depression versus mania, and, to some extent, evidence has substantiated the existence of polarity-specific effects.

Before examining the predictors of mania and depression separately, it is important to note that not all individuals with mania experience depression. Moreover, evidence documents that depressive and manic symptoms appear to follow separate, distinguishable courses. For example, depression and mania are not correlated across time within individuals (Johnson & Darcy, 2003). Hence, it appears important to distinguish between these two symptom types.

Predictors of Depression within Bipolar Disorder

Severe life events are one of the most robustly documented predictors of depression in persons with unipolar disorder (Brown & Harris, 1989). Individuals with bipolar disorder and those with unipolar disorder have been found to report comparable rates of severe, independent life events before an episode of depression (Perris, 1984; Hammen, 1995). In the Hammen study, which is notable for use of a prospective design and interview-based measures of life events, individuals with unipolar disorder appeared to generate more events that could be attributed to the disorder than individuals with bipolar disorder. Nonetheless, rates of severe, independent life events appear comparable preceding episodes of unipolar and bipolar depression.

Isometsa, Heikinen, Henriksson, Aro, and Lonnquist (1995) compared the prevalence of life events preceding completed suicides of individuals with bipolar and unipolar disorder. Next of kin completed the Recent Life Change survey regarding stressors experienced by the deceased person before his or her death. Negative life events appeared to be equally common precipitants to suicide, in that 64% of individuals with bipolar disorder and 66% of individuals with unipolar depression had experienced at least one severe life event shortly before their death.

Given the parallel role of negative life events in people with bipolar and unipolar depression, we might expect that a related psychosocial variable—social support—also would play a role in persons with bipolar depression. Indeed, we found that poor social support predicted increases in depression, but not mania, over time (Johnson, Meyer, et al., 2000). Conceptually, it is easy to understand how a lack of social resources might trigger depressive inactivity and dysphoria, but it would be more difficult to explain why the absence of social contact should lead to manic symptoms.

Beyond the role of environmental factors such as life events and social support, a few studies have examined personality traits as predictors of bipolar depression. Neuroticism has been defined as the tendency to experience dysphoric affect, and so it is not surprising that this trait has been a focus of much of the work on vulnerability to depression. Neuroticism has predicted intensification in depressive but not manic symptoms (Heerlein, Richter, Gonzalez, & Santander, 1998; Lozano & Johnson, 2001).

These findings are consistent with several studies supporting the view that neuroticism predicts unipolar depression (Gunderson, Triebwasser, Phillips, & Sullivan, 1999), and that there is genetic overlap between neuroticism and unipolar depression (e.g., Roberts & Kendler, 1999). Indeed, bipolar and unipolar disorder appear to be associated with comparable neuroticism levels (Bagby et al., 1996). Similarly, family members of individuals with depression, regardless of the presence of mania, have been found to display negative affective personality traits (Hecht, van Culker, Berger, & von Zerssen, 1998). In sum, neuroticism appears to be related to bipolar well as unipolar depression.

Beyond studying personality, research has also begun to examine how problematic cognitive styles, which are known to play an important role in unipolar depression (e.g., Alloy et al., 2000), relate to symptom course in bipolar disorder. For example, among undergraduates with a lifetime diagnosis of either hypomanic or depressive symptoms, one study found that dysfunctional attitudes, negative attributional styles, and self-referential encoding of negative information each interacted with negative events to predict increases in depressive symptoms across a 1-month period (Reilly-Harrington, Alloy, Fresco, & Whitehouse, 1999). Unfortunately, separate analyses were not reported for individuals with bipolar spectrum versus unipolar disorders, but the results appeared consistent with the idea that bipolar depression, like unipolar depression, can be predicted from dysfunctional cognitive processes. Consistent with this idea, Johnson, Meyer, et al. (2000) found that low self-esteem predicted greater increases in depression (but not mania) over time. To the extent that low self-esteem reflects negative cognitive appraisals of the self, this study also supported the notion that problematic cognitions place bipolar individuals at risk for intensification of depression over time.

Whereas only a few studies with prospective designs have examined cognition as a predictor of bipolar symptoms, more evidence is available from cross-sectional studies. Similar to those with unipolar depression, for instance, individuals with bipolar disorder tend to endorse a range of negative cognitive styles during their depressive episodes, including elevated scores on the Attributional Style Questionnaire (Seligman et al., 1979), the Automatic Thoughts Questionnaire (Hill, Oei, & Hill, 1989; Hollon, Kendall, & Lumry, 1986), the Dysfunctional Attitudes Scale (Hollon et al., 1986), and lower scores on self-esteem measures (Ashworth, Blackburn, & McPherson, 1982; Roy, 1991). Furthermore, within both bipolar and unipolar disorders, attributions regarding failure have been found to correlate with depression severity (Seligman et al., 1988). In sum, these studies suggest that bipolar as well as unipolar depression may reflect (or be the result of) negative cognitive styles.

If negative cognitive styles function as an enduring risk factor for bipolar depression, then one would expect these cognitions to be present even during remission. However, research on this issue has yielded mixed results—although some studies have documented more negative cognitive styles during remission (Scott, Stanton, Garland, & Ferrier, 2000), many of the negative cognitive facets evident during bipolar depression appear to diminish with recovery. During remission, individuals with bipolar disorder scored within the normal range on the Automatic Thoughts Questionnaire (Hollon et al., 1986). Similarly, they reported actual versus ideal self-discrepancies, self-esteem levels, and attributions for negative events that were similar to those in the normal control group (Bentall & Thompson, 1990; Lyon, Startup, & Bentall, 1999; Winters & Neale, 1985). In some studies of remitted individuals, those with bipolar disorder made less stable attributions for negative events and reported higher self-esteem than individuals with unipolar depression (Ashworth et al., 1982; Tracy et al., 1992; Winters & Neale, 1985). Hence, findings regarding depressive cognitive styles during remission are inconsistent. The difficulty in identifying negative cognitive styles during remission, however, may be explained by a set of methodological issues.

First, it may be important to assess cognitive processes, rather than self-report of cognition, in persons with bipolar disorder (Lyon et al., 1999). One common example of an information-processing measure is the Emotion Stroop Test. In this task, words are displayed in different colors. Individuals are asked to state the color while ignoring the word. Because sad, happy, and neutral content words are included, the task provides a measure of how distracting words referring to positive and negative emotion are while a person attempts to state colors. One study of individuals with bipolar I disorder (Lyon et al., 1999) and two studies of undergraduates have found that a history of hypomanic symptoms was related to interference for depressive words on an Emotion Stroop task (Bentall & Thompson, 1990), even after controlling for anxiety levels (French, Richards, & Scholfield, 1996). Not all studies of attention to negative stimuli, however, have identified negative information-processing patterns in individuals with bipolar I disorder (David, 1993).

Second, research on cognitive processes in persons with unipolar depression has substantiated the need to activate schemas to adequately test underlying cognitive vulnerability. For example, differences between nondisturbed subjects in the control group and individuals with remitted depression can be documented when the latter individuals are in a negative mood state (cf., Gotlib & Neubauer, 2000; Hedlund & Rude, 1995). In the only study we are aware of that included a schema-activation manipulation, patients with remitted bipolar disorder demonstrated decreased latency to both sad and happy word sets on an emotion stroop task, as well as significantly elevated Dysfunctional Attitudes Scale (DAS) scores compared to normal controls (Lex, 2000).

Third, some of the inconsistency in findings may reflect a need to ascertain whether the individuals studied actually have a history of depression. Alloy, Reilly-Harrington, Fresco, Whitehouse, and Zechmeister (1999) found that among undergraduates with lifetime hypomanic symptoms, participants with no history of depression appeared similar to the normal control group in their cognitive styles; in contrast, those with a history of depression endorsed more negative cognitive styles than did those in the control group. Unfortunately, most examinations of cognitive vulnerability and bipolar disorder have not considered depression history.

In short, it seems clear that during an episode of depression, many individuals with bipolar disorder experience negative cognitions about themselves and their experiences. Studies of negative cognitive styles in persons during euthymic periods have produced more inconsistent findings, but the methods employed in many of these studies may have compromised the ability to detect subtle or latent cognitive vulnerabilities. A few recent studies that have considered schema-activation procedures suggest that depressogenic cognition can be demonstrated even after recovery among individuals with bipolar disorder, particularly among those with a lifetime history of depression.

In summary, several preliminary conclusions emerge from the research on psychosocial predictors of depression in persons with bipolar disorder. First, negative life events, low social support, neuroticism, and poor self-esteem appear tied to increases in depression over time. Negative cognitive styles also appear to be correlated with bipolar depression. Although replications are needed, these findings are remarkably parallel with the findings regarding unipolar depression. Drawing on psychosocial as well as neurobiological comparisons of bipolar and unipolar disorder, we have argued that unipolar and bipolar depression are the same in terms of symptom patterns as well as the predictors of course (Kizer, Johnson, & Winters, 2003).

Unique Predictors of Mania

If the predictors of bipolar and unipolar depression are parallel, the question arises of whether the same predictors also influence the course of manic symptoms. Some theorists have suggested that life events may provoke both depressive and manic episodes through dysregulation of underlying neurobiological systems. At the same time, some evidence suggests that the predictors of mania may be somewhat unique. First we describe evidence for relatively unique predictors of mania, including sleep deprivation and heightened activity in the behavioral activation system. Then, we turn toward a model of parallels between depression and mania, and we review some evidence. Our discussion integrates this complicated set of patterns.

Sleep Deprivation

Both depression and mania are correlated with disturbances in sleep (e.g., Thase et al., 1997; Wehr, Sack, & Rosenthal, 1987). Intriguingly, sleep deprivation may help relieve depressive symptoms temporarily (Wu & Bunney, 1990). Case reports (Wehr, Goodwin, Wirz-Justice, Breitmaier, & Craig, 1982) and naturalistic studies (Barbini, Bertelli, Colombo, & Smeraldi, 1996; Leibenluft, Albert, Rosenthal, & Wehr, 1996) suggest that manic episodes also may follow sleep loss. As many as 10% of patients with bipolar disorder developed hypomanic or manic symptoms after induced sleep deprivation (Colombo, Benedetti, Barbini, Campori, & Smeraldi, 1999). Interestingly, Frank and Swartz (Chapter 8, this volume) propose that life events may operate at least partially through disrupting sleep patterns. More specifically, they suggest that environmental events and poor social networks may influence bipolar symptoms via the mediating pathway of disrupting circadian rhythms. That is, environmental events may interfere with the regular provision of social zeitgebers ("time givers"). Individuals with bipolar disorder report a greater number of schedule-disrupting life events before mania than before depression (Malkoff-Schwartz et al., 1998, 2000). Although there is evidence that negative life events also can operate through channels independent of sleep disruption (Winett, 2000), sleep regulation appears vital in maintaining health in individuals with bipolar disorder. As described in Chapter 8, Interpersonal and Social Rhythm Therapy provides specific strategies for helping individuals with bipolar disorder monitor and regulate their sleep patterns. Recent case studies have suggested that increasing sleep regulation in individuals with bipolar disorder may have important effects in reducing symptoms (Wehr et al., 1998).

Behavioral Activation

In a line of investigation largely separate from sleep research, several investigators over the past 20 years have proposed that manic symptoms are tied to excessive activity in the behavioral facilitation system/behavioral activation system/behavioral approach system (BAS; Depue & Zald, 1993; Depue & Iacono, 1989; Gray, 1982, 1990; Fowles, 2001). This biobehavioral system is believed to facilitate a broad range of motivational and cognitive processes in support of goal-directed behavior. Heightened BAS activity is expected to result in positive affect (Watson & Tellegen, 1985), sociability, incentive–reward motivation, goal-directed behavior, search for excitement, and motor activity (Depue & Zald, 1993). Scores on a self-report measure of BAS sensitivity (Carver & White, 1994) have been associated with learning and affect in response to cues of incentive (Zinbarg & Mohlman, 1998; Carver & White, 1994). The BAS outputs correspond closely to the manic symptoms of mood change, inflated self-esteem, increased talkativeness, flight of ideas, increased goal-directed activity, and excessive involvement in pleasurable activities. Based on this overlap, Depue has hypothesized that mania may be the outcome of excessively high BAS activity (Depue & Iacono, 1989). More specifically, a series of authors has noted that bipolar disorder may reflect dysregulation of the ventral tegmental dopamine-secreting neurons, which have been hypothesized to be a central tract involved in BAS (Depue & Zald, 1993; Hestenes, 1992).

Decreased BAS sensitivity (i.e., lower reward sensitivity) has been theorized to relate to depression. Support for this model has been obtained in behavioral (Henriques & Davidson, 1990) as well as neurotransmitter research (Naranjo, Tremblay, & Busto, 2001). Self-report studies of BAS sensitivity have suggested lower BAS sensitivity associated with depression in undergraduate (Beevers & Meyer, 2002; Meyer, Johnson, & Carver, 1999) but not community (Johnson, Turner, & Iwata, 2003) or bipolar (Meyer, Johnson, & Winters, 2001) samples. Nonetheless, links between BAS sensitivity and depression remain a focus of current inquiry.

Many authors have hypothesized that mania is linked to heightened BAS sensitivity. That is, individuals with bipolar disorder are expected to show more reactivity to cues of incentive. We have found that BAS sensitivity, using the Carver and White (1994) self-report measure, is associated with vulnerability to manic symptoms among undergraduates identified as at-risk for bipolar spectrum disorders (Meyer et al., 1999; Johnson, Ruggero, & Carver, 2003).

In another study (Meyer et al., 2001), we administered BAS scales to 59 participants with bipolar I disorder after they achieved recovery for 2 full months. BAS reward-responsiveness scores predicted mania severity over the next 6 months, even after controlling for subsyndromal symptoms.

This study also addressed the question of whether BAS sensitivity is better viewed as a stable indicator of risk or whether it shows state-dependent variability. That is, although BAS output levels would be expected to vary depending on the number of opportunities or cues of incentive that are present, we were interested in whether self-reported BAS *sensitivity* levels would vary with fluctuations in mania. For this purpose, we followed these 59 individuals for an average of 20 months and examined whether BAS scores covaried with mania symptom scores. Mixed-effects regression models showed that reward-responsiveness scores remained constant as mania scores varied. These findings were consistent with the hypothesis that reward responsiveness functions as a symptom-independent, stable characteristic in individuals with bipolar disorder.

Other studies examining the behavioral activation system have used EEG measures of anterior cortical asymmetry as an index of BAS activity. Anterior cortical asymmetry has been found to correlate with the relative BAS and behavioral inhibition sensitivity (BIS) (Sutton & Davidson, 1997; Harmon-Jones & Allen, 1997), and approach systems are generally hypothesized to be lateralized in the left anterior cerebral cortex (Davidson, 1998). In one study, four women with a history of hypomania displayed relatively reduced left frontal activity (Allen, Iacono, Depue, & Arbisi, 1993). Evidence also suggests excessive left frontal activity among undergraduates vulnerable to manic symptoms. For example, Harmon-Jones et al. (2002) reported that lifetime vulnerability to mania was related to increases in left frontal activity in response to an anger-evoking event.

In sum, BAS sensitivity, as measured by self-report and psychophysiological indices, appears to play an important role in bipolar disorder. Recent research suggests that BAS sensitivity tends to be higher among bipolar than comparison samples, and that relatively higher BAS sensitivity appear to predict greater risk of mania over time.

If heightened BAS sensitivity in bipolar disorder causes exaggerated responsiveness to cues of incentive and thus plays a role in triggering mania, then we would expect that these intense incentive responses also could be demonstrated directly. Based on this reasoning, manic symptoms should increase when cues of incentive are present; for example, we would expect manic symptoms to increase following life events that involve goal attainment. This hypothesis was supported within a sample of 43 individuals with bipolar disorder (Johnson, Sandrow, et al., 2000). In this prospective study, we selected the life event with the highest score on the Brown and Harris goal attainment scale (Leenstra, Ormel, & Giel, 1995); typically, these events involved a new job, new schooling, or new relationships. Only events that were rated as independent of symptoms were included. After controlling for manic symptoms before the event, the intensity of the goal attainment event predicted an increase in manic symptoms over the next 2 months, but did not predict depression. In comparison, more general positive events did not predict increases in mania, supporting the expected specificity of the effect to events that involved personal striving and motivation (Johnson, Sandrow, et al., 2000).

In summary, BAS sensitivity is related to a lifetime risk of hypomanic symptoms in samples of undergraduates, and predicted the course of mania in samples of people with bipolar disorder. BAS elevations in people with bipolar disorder have been documented using both self-report and psychophysiological measures, and goal-attainment life events appear to trigger mania.

Intriguingly, evidence from personality and cognitive domains also appears congruent with the BAS model of manic symptoms. For example, Adler and other psychodynamic authors hypothesized that individuals with a lifetime history of mania have excessively high expectations (Peven & Shulman, 1983). Bipolar disorder has been described as characterized by drive, work motivation, and stimulus-seeking behavior (Akiskal, Hirshfeld, & Yerevanian, 1983). First-degree relatives of individuals with bipolar disorder describe elevated achievements compared to nondisturbed individuals (Coryell et al., 1989). Similarly, achievement-striving items (e.g., high goal investment and newly established goals), measured 6 months after an index episode, predicted increases in manic symptoms over the next 4 months, controlling for baseline mania (Lozano & Johnson, 2001). Broader personality traits related to positive affect have been found to be associated with bipolar disorder (Bagby et al., 1996; Goodwin & Jamison, 1990), to predict the duration of initial episodes of mania (Strakowski, Stoll, Tohen, Faedda, & Goodwin, 1993), and to be correlated with more lifetime episodes of mania than depression (Hecht et al., 1998; von Zerssen, 2002).

Other work has focused on cognitions regarding incentive. One model suggests that the course of mania will be predicted by cognitions regarding reward (Leahy, 1999). We also observed elevated positive cognitions regarding reward among 464 college students who endorsed hypomanic symptoms (Meyer, Beevers, & Johnson, 2002). Specifically, using Little's (1989) Personal Projects Task to assess goal appraisals, we observed that current hypomanic symptoms correlated with the tendency to construe one's goals as attainable.

An initial success may have important implications for goal appraisals by individuals with a history of hypomania. Stern and Berrenberg (1979) examined expectancies concerning success in individuals with a history of hypomanic symptoms. After sham success feedback, undergraduates with a history of hypomanic symptoms were more likely to attribute their success to internal factors and to expect success on the next task than they were in the absence of success feedback; control subjects did not show these effects. After failure or neutral feedback, individuals with a history of hypomania did not differ from others on any cognitive measures. Recently, we replicated and extended these findings (Johnson et al., 2003); among undergraduates, hypomanic symptoms were associated with increased success expectancies, but only after an initial success. Hence, hypomania appears to be associated with an increased confidence, or success expectancy, particularly after an initial success. Once individuals begin to experience hypomanic symptoms, cognitive changes emerge such as increased confidence, increased recall of previous personal successes (Eich, Macaulay, & Lam, 1997; Weingartner, Miller, & Murphy, 1977), and increased attentional bias for positive stimuli (cf. Lyon et al., 1999). Current hypomanic symptoms, then, appear to be associated with increased confidence in the ability to achieve goals, particularly after a success.

As with bipolar depression, less research is available concerning cognitive correlates of bipolar disorder during euthymic periods. Are there cognitive features of mania that can be detected outside of mood episodes? Recently, in a study of undergraduates, we found that vulnerability to lifetime hypomanic symptoms was associated with setting higher goals (Johnson et al., 2003). Students with a history of hypomanic symptoms chose more difficult goals, even after controlling for mood and current symptoms. Bipolar disorder also has been related to higher standards for goal attainment compared to normal control subjects (Lam, Wright, & Smith, 2002).

Taken together, a series of studies suggests that individuals with bipolar disorder and their family members may demonstrate increased goal striving and sensitivity to rewards. Increases in confidence during hypomanic periods may make individuals particularly likely to behave overly actively after a success. These difficulties in goal regulation and reward responsiveness may be expressed in symptoms of mania following life events involving goal attainment. A separate line of research suggests that manic symptoms may be likely to follow sleep deprivation. Interestingly, both elevated BAS (Depue & Iacono, 1989) and sleep deprivation (Ebert & Berger, 1998) have been tied to dysregulation of the dopamine system. A growing body of multidisciplinary research suggests that BAS and other variables influencing dopamine regulation may be important to consider in understanding mania.

Variables That May Predict Both Depression and Mania

Our research has suggested that social support and negative life events predict depression, but in our findings, these variables have not been substantial predictors of mania. Rather, variables related to behavioral activation and sleep deprivation seem to predict greater risk for mania. Other researchers, however, have found that negative life events in interaction with negative cognitive styles, as measured by self-report scales, do predict increases in hypomanic symptoms among an undergraduate sample (Reilly-Harrington et al., 1999). Similarly, there are several published case reports of mania occurring at funerals (Johnson & Roberts, 1995). Individuals who are hospitalized for mania report lower levels of life events than individuals with depression but higher levels than control participants (Johnson & Roberts, 1995), and in one recent retrospective study, the rates of life events were similar before manic and depressive episodes (Malkoff-Schwartz et al., 2000). It remains possible that this correlation reflects a general tendency toward stressful lives rather than a specific trigger of mania. There is also some evidence that increases in mania following negative events may be particularly likely if mild hypomanic symptoms are already present (Johnson, Kizer, Ruggero, & Miller, 2003). Notwithstanding the need for more research, one model is available that integrates the evidence that mania could follow both goal-relevant and failure-relevant triggers.

One way to integrate these findings is to take into account early psychodynamic models of the "manic defense."

Beyond emphasizing high levels of goal striving, Adler and other psychodynamic authors also suggested that individuals with bipolar disorder use success to ward off an underlying feelings of insecurity, a process labeled the "manic defense" (Peven & Shulman, 1983). That is, they theorized that individuals with bipolar disorder might experience greater emotional responses to failures, and then cope with this experience through increased pursuit of goals as well as cognitive defensiveness manifested in overly high self-esteem (Lyon et al., 1999). Clinicians should be aware that some individuals with bipolar disorder find simplistic statements of this theory to be pejorative, as the theory seems to dismiss the biological basis of mania. It is worth being aware that any individual who experiences the loss and depression that are common to bipolar disorder would be likely to find him- or herself fighting against failure, and that an impulse to ward off depression is commendable, even if the approaches taken include some risks. This hypothesized need for success to ward off failure, whatever its source, may be expressed in greater goal pursuit, which may lead to sleep disruption and excessive involvement in goal pursuit, which in turn may intensify hypomanic symptoms.

Despite 100 years of clinical reports and theory, there are relatively few direct tests of this model. At a simple level, there is no evidence, using standard personality measures, that individuals with bipolar disorder or bipolar spectrum symptoms are more defensive than individuals with no mood disorder (Hirschfeld, Klerman, Keller, Andreasen, & Clayton, 1986; Bentall & Thompson, 1990). On the other hand, there is evidence that overt measures of self-esteem are less correlated with measures of attention and recall of negative material in persons with bipolar disorder (Lyon et al., 1999; Winters & Neale, 1985).

In short, the nature of cognitive vulnerability to mania remains a bit puzzling. There is some debate about whether mania reflects a response to goal pursuit, with excessive belief in the ability to achieve success, or whether mania reflects a defensive reaction to failure—or both. Others might see mania as a more purely biological phenomenon, with less psychosocial influence. It remains possible that different individuals will evidence different patterns of risk factors for mania.

SUMMARY OF PSYCHOSOCIAL RISK VARIABLES AND THE COURSE OF BIPOLAR DISORDER

In this chapter, we have provided an overview of several different predictors of symptom course in people with bipolar disorder. Many variables are associated with increases in symptoms over time, including expressed emotion, negative life events, poor social support, negative cognitive styles, and personality difficulties. Many of these variables seem to exert a stronger influence on depression than mania, and it seems that many of the psychosocial variables that predict unipolar depression may influence the course of bipolar depression. Mania appears specifically influenced by sleep deprivation and increased activity within the behavioral activation system. Although the evidence is not as robust, writers over the past 100 years have suggested that manic symptoms can occasionally reflect a reaction to negative life events and cognitions. Such a reaction could reflect biological instability or a more psychological process—namely, that manic activity may be triggered as a defense against overwhelming feelings of loss or failure. It may be that some individuals use the inborn goal orientation to ward off impending depression. Much more research is needed about each of these basic ideas; once we get away from the general predictions of poorer outcome, the landscape becomes fuzzier. The next generation of research will need to carefully assess the differential pathways into mania and depression, and the extent to which they overlap.

In sum, psychosocial variables appear to play an important role in the exacerbation of symptoms in bipolar disorder, and positive social environments and psychological traits may help reduce the toll of this disorder. Beyond the research regarding direct effects on symptoms, an exciting set of studies has begun to explore how psychosocial variables influence social functioning and treatment adherence. A model emerges of bipolar disorder as a genetic condition that may be substantially shaped by a person's environmental and psychological resources.

This research suggests the importance of psychosocial treatments as adjuncts to medication management. As covered in the chapters in this book, empirically guided treatment manuals are now available for addressing family concerns, psychosocial impairment, interpersonal stressors, sleep regulation, increased peer support, and acceptance of disorder. Some of these draw fairly directly on the decades of work on unipolar depression and are supported by the strong parallels between bipolar and unipolar depression. Other techniques, such as sleep regulation strategies, are based more specifically on risk factors that are robustly associated with the course of mania (see Chapter 8, this volume). The broad range of interpersonal, family, and cognitive techniques dovetails well with the literature suggesting that many different psychosocial variables are important influences on the course of bipolar disorder.

Despite the hope and knowledge embodied in this relatively young field, many questions that are important for guiding interventions remain unanswered. For example, as more predictors are documented, there is a need for help in setting priorities—which variables are the most important starting points for intervention? Furthermore, little is known about the mechanisms through which such variables operate. Basic research on the influences of social support and stress on biological mechanisms may help us understand the process through which psychosocial variables become translated into symptoms. To date, the environmental and biological research literatures have remained fairly separate.

Nonetheless, this body of research illuminates important targets for assessment and treatment within bipolar disorder. Fortunately, many treatment techniques are available to address these targets.

REFERENCES

Akiskal, H. S., Hirschfeld, R. M. A., & Yerevanian, B. I. (1983). The relationship of personality to affective disorders. *Archives of General Psychiatry, 40,* 801–810.

Allen, J. J., Iacono, W. G., Depue, R. A., & Arbisi, P. (1993). Regional electroencephalographic asymmetries in bipolar seasonal affective disorder before and after exposure to bright light. *Biological Psychiatry, 33,* 642–646.

Alloy, L. B., Abramson, L. Y., Hogan, M. E., Whitehouse, W. G., Rose, D. T., Robinson, M. S., Kim, R. S., & Lapkin, J. B. (2000). The Temple–Wisconsin Cognitive Vulnerability to Depression Project: Lifetime history of Axis I psychopathology in individuals at high and low cognitive risk for depression. *Journal of Abnormal Psychology, 109,* 403–418.

Alloy, L. B., Reilly-Harrington, N., Fresco, D. M., Whitehouse, W. G., & Zechmeister, J. S. (1999). Cognitive styles and life events in subsyndromal unipolar and bipolar disorders: Stability and prospective prediction of depressive and hypomanic mood swings. *Journal of Cognitive Psychotherapy, 13,* 21–40.

Ashworth, C. M., Blackburn, I. M., & McPherson, F. M. (1982). The performance of depressed and manic patients on some repertory grid measures: A cross-sectional study. *British Journal of Medical Psychology, 55,* 247–255.

Bagby, R. M., Young, L. T., Schuller, D. R., Bindseil, K. D, Cooke, R. G., Dickens, S. E., Levitt, A. J., & Joffe, R. T. (1996). Bipolar disorder, unipolar depression and the Five-Factor Model of Personality. *Journal of Affective Disorders, 41,* 25–32.

Barbato, N., & Hafner, R. J. (1998). Comorbidity of bipolar and personality disorder. *Australia and New Zealand Journal of Psychiatry, 32,* 276–280.

Barbini, B., Bertelli, S., Colombo, C., & Smeraldi, E. (1996). Sleep loss, a possible factor in augmenting manic episode. *Psychiatry Research, 65,* 121–125.

Beevers, C. G., & Meyer, B. (2002). Lack of positive experiences and positive expectancies mediate the relationship between BAS responsiveness and depression. *Cognition and Emotion, 16,* 549–564.

Bentall, R. P., & Thompson, M. (1990). Emotional stroop performance and the manic defence. *British Journal of Clinical Psychology, 29,* 235–237.

Brown, G. W., & Harris, T. O. (Eds.) (1989). *Life events and illness.* New York: Guilford Press.

Butzlaff, R. L., & Hooley, J. M. (1998). Expressed emotion and psychiatric relapse: A meta-analysis. *Archives of General Psychiatry, 55,* 547–552.

Carver, C. S., & White, T. L. (1994). Behavioral inhibition, behavioral activation, and affective responses to impending reward and punishment: The BIS/BAS scales. *Journal of Personality and Social Psychology, 67,* 319–333.

Clark, L., Iversen, S. D., & Goodwin, G. M. (2002). Sustained attention deficit in bipolar disorder. *British Journal of Psychiatry, 180,* 313–319.

Clayton, P. J., Ernst, C., & Angst, J. (1994). Premorbid personality traits of men who develop unipolar or bipolar disorders. *European Archives of Psychiatry and Clinical Neuroscience, 243,* 340–346.

Colombo, C., Benedetti, F., Barbini, B., Campori, E., & Smeraldi, E. (1999). Rate of switch from depression into mania after therapeutic sleep deprivation in bipolar depression. *Psychiatry Research, 86,* 267–270.

Coryell, W., Endicott, J., Keller, M., Andreasen, N., Grove, W., Hirschfeld, R.M.A., & Scheftner, L. W. (1989). Bipolar affective disorder and high achievement: A familial association. *American Journal of Psychiatry, 146,* 983–988.

David, A. S. (1993). Spatial and selective attention in the cerebral hemispheres in depression, mania, and schizophrenia. *Brain and Cognition, 23,* 166–180.

Davidson, R. J. (1998). Affective style and affective disorders: Perspectives from affective neuroscience. *Cognition and Emotion, 12,* 307–330.

Depue, R. A., & Iacono, W. G. (1989). Neurobehavioral aspects of affective disorders. *Annual Review of Psychology, 40,* 457–492.

Depue, R. A., & Zald, D. H. (1993). Biological and environmental processes in nonpsychotic psychopathology: A neurobiological perspective. In C. G. Costello (Ed.), *Basic issues in psychopathology* (pp. 127–237). New York: Guilford Press.

Ebert, D., & Berger, M. (1998). Neurobiological similarities in antidepressant sleep deprivation and psychostimulant use: A psychostimulant theory of antidepressant sleep deprivation. *Psychopharmacology, 140,* 1–10.

Eich, E., Macaulay, D., & Lam, R. W. (1997). Mania, depression, and mood dependent memory. *Cognition and Emotion, 11,* 607–618.

Ellicott, A., Hammen, C., Gitlin, M., Brown, G., & Jamison, K. (1990). Life events and the course of bipolar disorder. *American Journal of Psychiatry, 147,* 1194–1198.

Fowles, D. C. (2001). Biological variables in psychopathology: A psychobiological perspective. In H. E. Adams & P. B. Sutker (Eds.), *Comprehensive handbook of psychopathology* (3rd ed., pp. 85–104). New York: Kluwer.

French, C. C., Richards, A., & Scholfield, E. J. C. (1996). Hypomania, anxiety and the emotional stroop. *British Journal of Clinical Psychology, 35,* 617–626.

Geller, B., Craney, J. L., Bolhofner, K., Nickelsburg, M. J., Williams, M., & Zimerman, B. (2002). Two-year prospective follow-up of children with a prepubertal and early adolescent bipolar disorder phenotype. *American Journal of Psychiatry, 159,* 927–933.

George, E. L., Miklowitz, D. J., Richards, J. A., Simoneau, T. L. & Taylor, E. O. (2002). *The comorbidity of bipolar disorder and Axis II personality disorders: Prevalence and clinical correlates.* Manuscript submitted for publication.

Glaser, R., & Kiecolt-Glaser, J. (Eds.). (1994). *Handbook of human stress and immunity.* San Diego, CA: Academic Press.

Goodwin, F. K., & Jamison, K. R. (1990). *Manic–depressive illness.* Oxford, UK: Oxford University Press.

Gotlib, I. H., & Neubauer, D. L., (2000). Information-processing approaches to the study of cognitive biases in depression. In S. L. Johnson, A. M. Hayes, T. Field, P. McCabe, & N. Schneiderman, (Eds.), *Stress, coping, and depression: Proceedings of the Fifteenth Annual Stress and Coping Conference* (pp. 117–144). Mahwah, NJ: Erlbaum.

Gourovitch, M. L., Torrey, E. F., Gold, J. M., Randolph, C., Weinberger, D. R., & Goldberg, T. E. (1999). Neuropsychological performance of monozygotic twins discordant for bipolar disorder. *Biological Psychiatry, 45,* 639–646.

Gray, J. A. (1982). *The neuropsychology of anxiety: An enquiry into the functions of the septo-hippocampal system.* New York: Oxford University Press.

Gray, J. A. (1990). Brain systems that mediate both emotion and cognition. *Cognition and Emotion, 4,* 269–288.

Greenhouse, W. J. (2002). *Predictors of occupational and social functioning in mania: A symptom-regulation model.* Unpublished doctoral dissertation, University of Miami.

Gunderson, J. G., Triebwasser, J., Phillips, K. A., & Sullivan, C. N. (1999). Personality and vulnerability to affective disorders. In C. R. Cloninger (Ed.), *Personality and psychopathology* (pp. 3–32). Washington, DC: American Psychiatric Association.

Hammen, C. L. (1995). Stress and the course of unipolar and bipolar disorders. In C.M. Mazure (Ed.), *Does stress cause psychiatric illness?*(Progress in Psychiatry, No. 46, pp. 87–110). Washington, DC: American Psychiatric Press.

Hammen, C. L. (2000). Interpersonal factors in an emerging developmental model of depression. In S. L. Johnson, A. M. Hayes, T. Field, P. McCabe, & N. Schneiderman (Eds.), *Stress, coping, and depression: Proceedings of the Fifteenth Annual Stress and Coping Conference* (pp. 71–88). Mahwah, NJ: Erlbaum.

Hammen, C., Ellicott, A., & Gitlin, M. J. (1992). Stressors and sociotropy/autonomy: A longitudinal study of their relationship to the course of bipolar disorder. *Cognitive Therapy and Research, 16,* 409–418.

Harmon-Jones, E., Abramson, L. Y., Sigelman, J., Bohlig, A., Hogan, M. E., & Harmon-Jones, C. (2002). Proneness to hypomania/mania symptoms or depression symptoms and asymmetrical frontal cortical responses to an anger-evoking event. *Journal of Personality and Social Psychology, 82,* 610–618.

Harmon-Jones, E., & Allen, J. J. B. (1997). Behavioral activation sensitivity and resting frontal EEG asymmetry: Covariation of putative indicators related to risk for mood disorders. *Journal of Abnormal Psychology, 106,* 159–163.

Hecht, H., van Calker, D., Berger, M., & von Zerssen, D. (1998). Personality in patients with affective disorders and their relatives. *Journal of Affective Disorders, 51,* 33–43.

Hedlund, S., & Rude, S. S. (1995). Evidence of latent depressive schemas in formerly depressed individuals. *Journal of Abnormal Psychology, 104,* 517–525.

Heerlein, A., Richter, P., Gonzalez, M., & Santander, J. (1998). Personality patterns and outcome in depressive and bipolar disorders.*Psychopathology, 31,* 15–22.

Henriques, J. B., & Davidson, R. J. (1990). Regional brain electrical asymmetries discriminate between previously depressed and healthy control subjects. *Journal of Abnormal Psychology, 99,* 22–31.

Hestenes, D. (1992). A neural network theory of manic–depressive illness. In D. S. Levine & S. J. Leven (Eds.), *Motivation, emotion, and goal direction in neural networks* (pp. 209–257). Hillsdale, NJ: Erlbaum.

Hill, C. V., Oei, T. P., & Hill, M. A. (1989). An empirical investigation of the specificity and sensitivity of the Automatic Thoughts Questionnaire and Dysfunctional Attitudes Scale. *Journal of Psychopathology and Behavior Assessment, 11,* 291–311.

Hirschfeld, R. M., Klerman, G. L., Clayton, P.J., Keller, M. B., McDonald-Scott, P., & Larkin, B. H. (1983). Assessing personality: Effects of the depressive state on trait measurement. *American Journal of Psychiatry, 140,* 695–699.

Hirschfeld, R. M., Klerman, G. L., Keller, M. B., Andreasen, N. C., & Clayton, P. J. (1986). Personality of recovered patients with bipolar affective disorder. *Journal of Affective Disorders, 11,* 81–89.

Hollon, S. D., Kendall, P. C., & Lumry, A. (1986). Specificity of depressotypic cognitions in clinical depression. *Journal of Abnormal Psychology, 95,* 52–59.

Hooley, J. M. (1998). Expressed emotion and locus of control. *Journal of Nervous and Mental Disease, 186,* 374–378.

Hooley, J. M., & Licht, D. M. (1997). Expressed emotion and causal attributions in the spouses of depressed patients. *Journal of Abnormal Psychology, 106,* 298–306.

Hooley, J. M., Rosen, L. R., & Richters, J. E. (1995). Expressed emotion: Toward clarification of a critical construct. In G. Miller (Ed.), *The behavioral high-risk paradigm in psychopathology* (pp. 88–120). New York: Springer.

Hunt, N., Bruce-Jones, W. D., & Silverstone, T. (1992). Life events and relapse in bipolar affective disorder. *Journal of Affective Disorders, 25,* 13–20.

Hyman, S. E. (2000). Goals for research on bipolar disorder: The view from NIMH. *Biological Psychiatry, 48,* 436–441.

Isometsa, E., Heikinen, M., Henriksson, M., Aro, H., & Lonnquist, J. (1995). Recent life events and completed suicide in bipolar affective disorder: A comparison with major depressive suicides. *Journal of Affective Disorders, 33,* 99–106.

Johnson, S. L., & Darcy, K. (2003). *Depression and mania: Two poles or two dimensions?* Manuscript submitted for publication.

Johnson, S. L., Fingerhut, R., Miller, I., III, Keitner, G., Ryan, C., & Solomon, D. (1997, October). *Do minor life events impact the course of bipolar disorder?* Poster presentation at the Society for Research on Psychopathology, Palm Springs, CA.

Johnson, S., Meyer, B., Winett, C., & Small, J. (2000). Social support and self-esteem predict changes in bipolar depression but not mania. *Journal of Affective Disorders, 58,* 79–86.

Johnson, S. L., & Miller, I. (1997). Negative life events and time to recovery from episodes of bipolar disorder. *Journal of Abnormal Psychology 106,* 449–457.

Johnson, S.L., Kizer, A., Ruggero, C., & Miller, I. (2003). *Negative and goal attainment life events: Predicting the course of mania and depression in bipolar disorder.* Manuscript in preparation.

Johnson, S. L., & Roberts, J. R. (1995). Life events and bipolar disorder: Implications from biological theories. *Psychological Bulletin, 117,* 434–449.

Johnson, S. L., Ruggero, C., & Carver, C. (2003). *Cognitive, behavioral, and affective responses to reward: Links with hypomanic symptoms.* Manuscript submitted for publication.

Johnson, S. L., Sandrow, D., Meyer, B., & Winters, R., Miller, I., Keitner, G., & Solomon, D. (2000). Life events involving goal-attainment and the emergence of manic symptoms. *Journal of Abnormal Psychology, 109,* 721–727.

Johnson, S. L., Turner, R. J., & Iwata, N. (2003). BIS/BAS levels and psychiatric disorder: An epidemiological study. *Journal of Psychopathology and Behavioral Assessment, 25,* 25–36.

Judd, L. L. (1979). Effect of lithium on mood, cognition, and personality function in normal subjects. *Archives of General Psychiatry, 36,* 860–865.

Judd, L. L., Akiskal, H. S., Schetteler, P. J., Endicott, J., Maser, J., Solomon, D. A., Leon, A. C., Rice, J. A., & Keller, M. B. (2002). The long-term natural history of the weekly symptomatic status of bipolar I disorder. *Archives of General Psychiatry, 59,* 530–537.

Keri, S., Kelemen, O., Benedek, G., & Janka, Z. (2001). Different trait markers for schizophrenia and bipolar disorder: A neurocognitive approach. *Psychological Medicine, 31,* 915–922.

Kizer, A., Johnson, S. L., & Winters, R. (2003). *Distinctions between unipolar and bipolar depression: A review of the evidence.* Manuscript submitted for review.

Klein, D. N., Durbin, C. E., Shankman, S. A., & Santiago, N. J. (2002). Depression and personality. In I. H. Gotlib & C. L. Hammen (Eds.), *Handbook of depression* (pp.115–140). New York: Guilford Press.

Lam, D., Wright, K., & Smith, N. (2002). *Dysfunctional assumptions in bipolar disorder.* Unpublished manuscript.

Lara, M. E., Leader, J., & Klein, D. N. (1997). The association between social support and course of depression: Is it confounded with personality? *Journal of Abnormal Psychology, 106,* 478–482.

Leahy, R. L. (1999). Decision-making and mania. *Journal of Cognitive Psychotherapy, 13,* 83–105.

Leenstra, A. S., Ormel, J., & Giel, R. (1995). Positive life change and recovery from depression and anxiety: A three-stage longitudinal study of primary care attenders. *British Journal of Psychiatry, 166,* 333–343.

Leibenluft, E., Albert, P. S., Rosenthal, N. E., & Wehr, T. A. (1996). Relationship between sleep and mood in patients with rapid-cycling bipolar disorder. *Psychiatry Research, 63,* 161–168.

Lex, C. (2000). *Kognitive Verarbeitung bei Bipolarer Depression* [Cognitive processing in bipolar depression]. Unpublished master's thesis, University of Vienna, Vienna, Austria.

Little, B. R. (1989). Personal Projects Analysis: Trivial pursuits, magnificent obsessions, and the search for coherence. In D. M. Buss & N. Cantor (Eds.), *Personality psychology: Recent trends and emerging directions* (pp. 15–31). New York: Springer Verlag.

Lozano, B. E., & Johnson, S. L. (2001). Can personality traits predict increases in manic and depressive symptoms? *Journal of Affective Disorders, 63,* 103–111.

Lyon, H. M., Startup, M., & Bentall, R. P. (1999). Social cognition and the manic defense: Attributions, selective attention, and self-schema in bipolar affective disorder. *Journal of Abnormal Psychology, 108,* 273–282.

Malkoff-Schwartz, S., Frank, E., Anderson, B., Sherrill, J. T., Siegel, L., Patterson, D., & Kupfer, D. J. (1998). Stressful life events and social rhythm disruption in the onset of manic and depressive bipolar episodes. *Archives of General Psychiatry, 55,* 702–707.

Malkoff-Schwartz, S., Frank, E., Anderson, B. P., Hlastala, S. A., Luther, J. F., Sherrill, J. T., Houck, P. R., & Kupfer, D. J. (2000). Social rhythm disruption and stressful life events in the onset of bipolar and unipolar episodes. *Psychological Medicine, 30,* 1005–1016.

McKnight, D.L., Nelson-Gray, R. O., & Gullick, E. (1989). Interactional patterns of bipolar patients and their spouses. *Journal of Psychopathology and Behavior Assessment, 11,* 269–289.

Meyer, B. (2001). Coping with severe mental illness: Relations of the Brief COPE with symptoms, functioning, and well-being. *Journal of Psychopathology and Behavior Assessment, 23,* 265–277.

Meyer, B., Beevers, C. G., & Johnson, S. L. (2002). *Goal appraisals and vulnerability to bipolar disorder: A personal projects analysis.* Manuscript submitted for publication.

Meyer, B., Johnson, S. L., & Carver, C. S. (1999). Exploring behavioral activation and inhibition sensitivities among college students at risk for bipolar-spectrum symptomatology. *Journal of Psychopathology and Behavior Assessment, 21,* 275–292.

Meyer, B., Johnson, S. L., & Winters, R. (2001). Responsiveness to threat and incentive in bipolar disorder: Relations of the BIS/BAS scales with symptoms. *Journal of Psychopathology and Behavior Assessment, 23,* 133–143.

Miklowitz, D. J., Goldstein, M. J., Nuechterlein, K. H., Snyder, K. S., & Mintz, J. (1988). Family factors and the course of bipolar affective disorder. *Archives of General Psychiatry, 45,* 225–231.

Miklowitz, D. J., Simoneau, T. L., George, E. A., Richards, J. A., Kalbag, A., Sachs-Ericsson, N., & Suddath, R. (2000). *Family-focused treatment of bipolar disorder: One-year effects of a psychoeducational program in conjunction with pharmacotherapy.* Manuscript submitted for publication.

Naranjo, C. A., Tremblay, L. K., & Busto, U. E. (2001). The role of the brain reward system in depression. *Progress in Neuro-Psychopharmacology and Biological Psychiatry, 25,* 781–823.

Perlick, D., Clarkin, J. F., Sirey, J., Raue, P., Greenfield, S., Struening, E., & Rosenheck, R.(1999). Burden experienced by care-givers of persons with bipolar affective disorder. *British Journal of Psychiatry, 175,* 56–62.

Perris, H. (1984). Life events and depression: Part 2. Results in diagnostic subgroups and in relation to the recurrence of depression. *Journal of Affective Disorders, 7,* 25–36.

Peven, D. E., & Shulman, B. H. (1983). The psychodynamics of bipolar affective disorder: Some empirical findings and their implications for cognitive theory. *Individual Psychology: Journal of Adlerian Theory, Research and Practice, 39,* 2–16.

Priebe, S., Wildgrube, C., & Mueller-Oerlinghausen, B. (1989). Lithium prophylaxis and expressed emotion. *British Journal of Psychiatry, 154,* 396–399.

Reilly-Harrington, N. A., Alloy, L. B., Fresco, D. M., & Whitehouse, W. G. (1999). Cognitive styles and life events interact to predict bipolar and unipolar symptomatology. *Journal of Abnormal Psychology, 108,* 567–578.

Roberts, S. B., & Kendler, K. S. (1999). Neuroticism and self-esteem as indices of the vulnerability to major depression in women. *Psychological Medicine, 29,* 1101–1109.

Romans, S. E., & McPherson, H. M. (1992). The social networks of bipolar affective disorder patients. *Journal of Affective Disorders, 25,* 221–228.

Roy, A. (1991). Personality variables in depressed patients and normal controls. *Neuropsychobiology, 23,* 119–123.

Scott, J., Stanton, B., Garland, A., & Ferrier, I. N. (2000). Cognitive vulnerability in patients with bipolar disorder. *Psychological Medicine, 30,* 467–472.

Seligman, M. E. P., Abramson, L. Y., Semmel, A., & von Baeyer, C. (1979). Depressive attributional style. *Journal of Abnormal Psychology, 88,* 242–247.

Seligman, M. E., Castellon, C., Cacciola, J., Schulman, P., Luborsky, L., Ollove, M., & Downing, R. (1988). Explanatory style change during cognitive therapy for unipolar depression. *Journal of Abnormal Psychology, 97,* 13–18.

Serretti, A., Cavallini, M. C., Macciardi, F., Namia, C., Franchini, L., Souery, D., Lipp, O., Bauwens, F., Smeraldi, E., & Mendlewicz, J. (1999). Social adjustment and self-esteem in remitted patients with mood disorders. *European Psychiatry, 14,* 137–142.

Simoneau, T. L., Miklowitz, D. J., & Saleem, R. (1998). Expressed emotion and interactional patterns in the families of bipolar patients. *Journal of Abnormal Psychology, 107,* 497–507.

Solomon, D. A., Shea, M. T., Leon, A. C., & Mueller, T. I. (1996). Personality traits in subjects with bipolar I disorder in remission. *Journal of Affective Disorders, 40,* 41–48.

Squire, L. R., Judd, L. L., Janowsky, D. S., & Huey, L. Y. (1980). Effects of lithium carbonate on memory and other cognitive functions. *American Journal of Psychiatry, 137,* 1042–1046.

Stefos, G., Bauwens, F., Staner, L., Pardoen, D., & Mendlewicz, J. (1996). Psychosocial predictors of major affective recurrences in bipolar disorder: A 4-year longitudinal study of patients on prophylactic treatment. *Acta Psychiatrica Scandinavica, 93,* 420–426.

Stern, G. S., & Berrenberg, J. L. (1979). Skill-set, success outcome, and mania as determinants of the illusion of control. *Journal of Research in Personality, 13,* 206–220.

Strakowski, S. M., Stoll, A. L., Tohen, M., Faedda, G. L., & Goodwin, D. C. (1993). The tridimensional personality questionnaire as a predictor of six-month outcome in first episode mania. *Psychiatry Research, 48,* 1–8.

Sutton, S. K., & Davidson, R. J. (1997). Prefrontal brain asymmetry: A biological substrate of the behavioral approach and inhibition systems. *Psychological Science, 8,* 204–210.

Thase, M. E., Kupfer, D. J., Fasiczka, A. J., Buysse, D. J., Simmons, A. D., & Frank, E. (1997). Identifying an abnormal electroencephalographic sleep profile to characterize major depressive disorder. *Biological Psychiatry, 41,* 964–973.

Tracy, A., Bauwens, F., Martin, F., Pardoen, D., & Mendlowicz, J. (1992). Attributional style and depression: A controlled comparison of remitted unipolar and bipolar patients. *British Journal of Clinical Psychology, 31,* 83–84.

von Zerssen, D. (2002). Development of an integrated model of personality, personality disorders and severe axis I disorders, with special reference to major affective disorders. *Journal of Affective Disorders, 69,* 143–158.

Watson, D., & Tellegen, A. (1985). Towards a consensual structure of mood. *Psychological Bulletin, 98,* 219–235.

Wehr, T. A, Goodwin, F. K., Wirz-Justice, A., Breitmaier, J., & Craig, C. (1982). 48-hour sleep-wake cycles in manic–depressive illness: Naturalistic observations and sleep deprivation experiments. *Archives of General Psychiatry, 39,* 559–565.

Wehr, T. A., Sack, D. A., & Rosenthal, N. E. (1987). Sleep reduction as a final common pathway in the genesis of mania. *American Journal of Psychiatry, 144,* 201–204.

Wehr, T. A., Turner, E. H., Shimada, J. M., Lowe, C. H., Barker, C., & Leibenluft, E. (1998).

Treatment of a rapidly cycling bipolar patient by using extended bed rest and darkness to stabilize the timing and duration of sleep. *Biological Psychiatry, 43,* 822–828.

Weingartner, H., Miller, H., & Murphy, D. L. (1977). Mood-state-dependent retrieval of verbal associations. *Journal of Abnormal Psychology, 86,* 276–284.

Winett, C. A. (2000). *The mediating role of insomnia in the relation between life events and depression and mania.* Unpublished dissertation, University of Miami.

Winters, K. C., & Neale, J. M. (1985). Mania and low self-esteem. *Journal of Abnormal Psychology, 94,* 282–290.

Wu, J. C., & Bunney, W. E. (1990). The biological basis of an antidepressant response to sleep deprivation and relapse: Review and hypothesis. *American Journal of Psychiatry, 147,* 14–21.

Zinbarg, R. E., & Mohlman, J. (1998). Individual differences in the acquisition of affectively valenced associations. *Journal of Personality and Social Psychology, 74,* 1024–1040.

PART II

THERAPY AND TREATMENT ISSUES

CHAPTER SIX

THE CHANGING LANDSCAPE OF PSYCHOPHARMACOLOGY

JOSEPH F. GOLDBERG

In the past decade, the pharmacotherapy of bipolar disorder has changed dramatically. Whereas lithium, conventional antipsychotics, monoamine oxidase inhibitors (MAOIs), and tricyclic antidepressants represented the mainstays of treatment from the 1970s through the 1980s, the range of standard pharmacotherapies has broadened extensively. Fundamental treatment strategies have changed also, raising many critical, unresolved questions. This chapter provides a review of the evidence concerning the following questions.

- Which medications should be considered cornerstone treatments for bipolar illness?
- Which medications fit the definition of a mood stabilizer?
- What are the proposed mechanisms of action for these medications?
- Is long-term pharmacotherapy necessary for all patients with bipolar illness?
- When is lithium an optimal medication for bipolar illness?
- What is the role of divalproex, carbamazepine, and other anticonvulsant drugs in treating bipolar illness?
- Do atypical antipsychotics possess antimanic or antidepressant efficacy?
- To what extent do antidepressants induce rapid cycling or mania? Which medications possess the strongest antidepressant efficacy and the lowest risk of inducing rapid cycling or mania?
- When are combinations of medications the best treatment approach for bipolar disorder?
- What medications are appropriate for special populations, such as children, pregnant women, or medically ill patients?

WHAT IS A MOOD STABILIZER?

At present, only five medications are approved by the United States Food and Drug Administration (FDA) for the treatment of bipolar disorder: lithium (Lithobid, Eskalith, Lithonate; approved in 1970), chlorpromazine (Thorazine; approved in 1973), divalproex (Depakote, Depakene, Depakon; approved in 1995), olanzapine (Zyprexa; approved in 2000), and lamotrigine (Lamictal; approved in 2003). Among these, only lithium and lamotrigine are approved for long-term use, although long-term data now exist for many other medications (such as divalproex and olanzapine). It is important to note that, at present, FDA approval for medications to acutely treat bipolar disorder focuses on efficacy in acute mania; that is, the FDA has not yet approved any medication for acute bipolar depression. The landmark 2003 FDA approval of lamotrigine as a maintenance treatment for bipolar I disorder represents the first long-term therapy approved for bipolar illness in three decades. While lamotrigine was approved to delay recurrences of any illness phase, the data on which the indication was based showed more robust efficacy to prevent depressive episodes than manic episodes. As such, it has been conceptualized as an agent that may stabilize mood "from below" the baseline mood state (Ketter & Calabrese, 2002).

The FDA does not approve drugs for bipolar disorder as "mood stabilizers." Many practitioners use this term to describe medications expected to reduce mood lability, impulsivity, or aggression. Stricter definitions propose that mood stabilizers are agents that treat or prevent distinct manic or depressive episodes, without triggering either (Keck et al., 2002). In this sense, antidepressants would not constitute mood stabilizers insofar as their efficacy for depression is countered by their liability to induce or worsen mania (Wehr & Goodwin, 1987; Goldberg & Whiteside, 2002). Similarly, conventional antipsychotic drugs such as haloperidol appear effective in mania but may induce depression in some patients (Van Putten & May, 1978). In the case of anticonvulsant drugs, some agents (e.g., divalproex and carbamazepine) demonstrate more robust antimanic than antidepressant effects, whereas others (e.g., lamotrigine) appear more efficacious in bipolar depression than mania (Ernst & Goldberg, 2003). No antipsychotics or anticonvulsants have been shown to induce manias over time, and all have some demonstrated efficacy in sustaining long-term euthymia after resolving an initial manic or depressive episode (Ernst & Goldberg, 2003).

CURRENT PHARMACOTHERAPIES: RATIONALE AND MECHANISMS

The medications currently used most often for bipolar disorder, apart from antidepressants—notably, lithium, anticonvulsants, and atypical antipsy-

TABLE 6.1. Psychotropic Drugs Commonly Used in the Treatment of Bipolar Disorder

Medication	Indications	Usual dosage	Common side effects[a]	Comments
lithium (Lithobid, Eskalith)	FDA-approved for acute mania or bipolar prophylaxis	Initially 600–900 mg/day; adjust to reach serum lithium level of 0.8–1.2 mEq/liter	Tremor, thirst, urinary frequency, constipation, blurry vision, sedation, acne	Particular benefit in euphoric mania, initial episodes, bipolar family history; no rapid cycling, no substance abuse; likely intrinsic antisuicide effects; must monitor renal and thyroid function
Anticonvulsants				
divalproex (Depakote)	FDA-approved for acute mania	Initially 750 mg/day; adjust to reach serum valproate level between 50–125 μ/ml; can be orally loaded (20–30 mg/kg) for off-label use in acute mania	Nausea, somnolence, dizziness, vomiting, asthenia, abdominal pain, dyspepsia, rash[b]; other common side effects include tremor, weight gain	Beneficial in pure or mixed manias, rapid cycling, comorbid substance abuse; must monitor hepatic function; concern for toxicity-related thrombocytopenia; possible pancreatitis, polycystic ovarian syndrome; pregnancy exposure may cause spina bifida
carbamazepine (Tegretol)	Used off label in mania or bipolar prophylaxis	Initially 400 mg/day; adjust upward to 1,000–1,600 mg/day; value of serum levels for efficacy in mood is debated	Dizziness, drowsiness, unsteadiness, nausea, vomiting	Beneficial in pure or mixed manias; must monitor for leukopenia and hepatic dysfunction; pregnancy exposure may cause spina bifida
oxcarbazepine (Trileptal)	Used off label in acute mania; no long-term bipolar data	Initially 300 mg/day; adjust upward to 600–2,400 mg/day; no serum levels established for therapeutic efficacy	Fatigue, nausea, vomiting, abdominal pain, dizziness, somnolence, ataxia, double vision[c]	Must monitor serum sodium levels; can render oral contraceptives less effective by metabolizing ethinyl estradiol
lamotrigine (Lamictal)	FDA-approved to prevent recurrent mood episodes in bipolar I disorder; used off label in bipolar depression or bipolar rapid cycling; little data for efficacy in mania	Initially 25 mg/day for 2 weeks, then 50 mg/day for 2 weeks, thereafter increase by 50–100 mg/day to target of 200 mg/day, maximum of 500 mg/day. Dose half as quickly and maximally if combined with valproate; twice as fast if combined with carbamazepine; no established therapeutic serum levels	Headache, nausea, dizziness, skin rash (benign rash in 10%, significant rash in 0.01%)	Skin rashes most often occur in weeks 2–8 of treatment; serious rashes involve blistering, burn-like lesions on face, oropharynx, conjunctivae, or palms and soles, usually with systemic involvement

(continued)

111

TABLE 6.1. (*continued*)

Medication	Indications	Usual dosage	Common side effects	Comments
gabapentin (Neurontin)	Negative data in placebo-controlled trials for mania; main role is for anxiolysis	Target dose of 900–1,800 mg/day; no established therapeutic serum levels	Dizziness, somnolence, edema, nausea, gait unsteadiness, tremor	900 mg is maximal dose absorbed at one time
topiramate (Topamax)	Negative data in placebo-controlled trials for mania; main role is for appetite suppression, possible antidepressant and anti-alcoholism effects	Typically begins at 25–50 mg/day, with gradual upward dosing (usual: 100–200 mg/day), to maximal 1,600 mg/day); no established therapeutic levels	Sedation, word-finding difficulties, renal calculi, secondary narrow-angle glaucoma, paresthesias	Cognitive side effects are likely dose-dependent
Atypical antipsychotics				
olanzapine (Zyprexa)	FDA-approved for acute mania as monotherapy or as add-on therapy to lithium or divalproex	Typically begins at 15 mg/day, increases to 20 mg/day; used experimentally at higher doses (40 mg/day) for rapid symptom control	Asthenia, dry mouth, weight gain, constipation, dyspepsia, increased appetite, somnolence, dizziness, tremor[b]; controversial risk for precipitating Type II diabetes	
clozapine (Clozaril)	Used off label in refractory mood disorders, especially with psychosis or rapid cycling	Typically begins at 25 mg/day, increasing by 25–50 mg/day every few days to 300–600 mg/day (maximum 900 mg/day), as extrapolated from schizophrenia studies	Sedation, dizziness, tachycardia, constipation, hypersalivation occurs in > 10% of subjects; controversial risk for precipitating Type II diabetes	Must monitor white blood cell count weekly or biweekly throughout treatment; may have antisuicide properties

Medication	Status	Dosing	Side effects[a],[b]	Comments
risperidone (Risperdal)	Used off label in acute mania	Typically begins at 1 mg twice a day and increases to target of 4–6 mg/day	Anxiety, somnolence, extrapyramidal symptoms, dizziness, constipation, nausea, dyspepsia, rhinitis, tachycardia, rash	Higher potential for prolactin elevation than other atypical antipsychotics
quetiapine (Seroquel)	Used off label in acute mania	Typically begins at 50 mg twice a day with increases of 100 mg/day to a target dose of 500–600 mg/day (maximum 800 mg/day); higher doses considered experimental	Dizziness, orthostatic hypotension, dry mouth, dyspepsia, weight gain	
ziprasidone (Geodon)	Used off label in acute mania	Typically, 20 mg twice daily to start, increasing up to 80 mg twice a day	Somnolence, extrapyramidal symptoms, respiratory problems	May be associated with prolongation of QTc interval on EKG; may be weight neutral
aripiprazole (Abilify)	Used off label in acute mania	15–30 mg/day initially in acute mania	Anxiety, insomnia, nausea, vomiting, lightheadedness, akathisia	May be weight neutral

Note. Brand names of medications are given in parentheses.

[a]Based on package insert data.

[b]All reported in > 5% of patients during placebo-controlled trials for acute mania.

[c]All reported as more common with drug than placebo in controlled trials for epilepsy.

chotics—are summarized in Table 6.1 (on pp. 111–113). In terms of mechanisms of action, there is presently little direct evidence to link any particular pharmacological activity with observable clinical antimanic or antidepressant effects. Unlike treatments for many other medical conditions, drugs used for bipolar disorder do not ameliorate mood swings via distinctly known physiological effects. Nevertheless, a number of preclinical observations may provide a provisional framework for categorizing drugs with known mood-stabilizing properties. These may be summarized categorically as follows.

Lithium

Convergent lines of evidence suggest that the major physiological targets for lithium involve signaling pathways within nerve cells (Manji & Potter, 1995), leading to neuroprotective effects that could prevent cell death. Specifically, lithium is believed to exert its effects via so-called second messengers involved in transmitting signals from membrane-bound receptor proteins to intracellular targets. Lithium has been shown to inhibit one such messenger, protein kinase C (PKC), in a manner similar to that seen with divalproex, omega-3 fatty acids, and the calcium channel blocker verapamil.

Anticonvulsants

In the 1980s, Robert Post and colleagues advanced the hypothesis that recurrent episodes of mania or depression constitute a form of recurrent brain activity that is loosely analogous to the type of recurrent paroxysmal brain excitation seen in epilepsy (Post et al., 1986; Post & Weiss, 1989). The phenomenon that occurs in recurrent seizures, in which poorly controlled initial episodes hasten further relapses, has been described as kindling—that is, as the development and expression of spontaneous epilepsy. The parallel concept of behavioral sensitization has been used to describe recurrent affective episodes that arise with increasing automaticity.

Anticonvulsant drugs are thought to exert antikindling effects largely by diminishing excitation and enhancing inhibition in brain areas thought to regulate affect (e.g., the limbic system). Some compounds, such as lamotrigine or carbamazepine, primarily exert antiexcitation effects by reducing the outflow or postsynaptic uptake of excitatory amino acids, such as glutamate or aspartic acid (Ernst & Goldberg, 2003). This effect may be accomplished by blocking presynaptic low-voltage sodium channels (in turn, reducing the presynaptic release of glutamate), or by blocking the uptake of glutamate postsynaptically, as occurs with the anticonvulsant topiramate.

Other anticonvulsants, such as divalproex or gabapentin (Neurontin), predominantly increase presynaptic levels of the inhibitory neurotransmitter gamma-aminobutyric acid (GABA). It has been suggested, although not empirically proven, that drugs which predominantly diminish excitatory amino acid (e.g., glutamate) transmission may possess greater antidepressant than antimanic efficacy, whereas those that principally increase levels of GABA may hold greater utility for reducing agitation and excitation, such as that seen in mania or mixed states (Ernst & Goldberg, 2003).

Antipsychotics

Clinicians have long recognized the value of most conventional antipsychotics, including chlorpromazine, for the short-term treatment of psychosis and agitation associated with mania. Atypical antipsychotics represent a major advance with regard to their unique mechanism of action, better side-effect profile, and possibly broader spectrum of psychotropic activity apart from treating psychosis. In addition to olanzapine (Zyprexa), evidence has begun to suggest that other newer generation antipsychotic drugs may possess mood-stabilizing effects, particularly antimanic properties. To varying degrees, each of these agents exerts pharmacological effects at multiple receptor targets that involve not only the dopamine system (as classically linked with antipsychotic efficacy) but also the serotonin, norepinephrine, and cholinergic systems, among others. These receptor-mediated effects are thought to foster possible mood-stabilizing properties and demarcate a major difference in mode of action between newer generation (atypical) and older generation (conventional) antipsychotics.

Antidepressants

Generally, existing antidepressants are thought to influence symptoms largely via serotonergic, noradrenergic, and/or dopaminergic effects, although other neurotransmitter systems (e.g., glucocorticoids) likely play key roles that have yet to be elucidated.

CURRENT PRACTICE GUIDELINES

A growing number of treatment practice guidelines has been advanced for bipolar disorder. Among the most recent include the 2002 revision of the American Psychiatric Association (APA) practice guidelines for the treatment of bipolar disorder (American Psychiatric Association, 2002) as well as the Texas Medication Algorithm Project (TMAP; Suppes et al., 2001). Both sets of recommendations identify lithium, divalproex, or olanzapine as appropriate first-line medications for acute mania. In the case of severe mania, the APA guidelines advise combination therapy, at the outset, with lithium or divalproex plus an antipsychotic drug, preferably an atypical antipsychotic.

Long-term, open-ended pharmacotherapy with an effective antimanic drug generally is advised after a single severe manic episode, especially when a family history of bipolar illness is present. After resolution of the acute phase, efforts often are made to reduce or eliminate medications that may have been adjunctive (e.g., benzodiazepines or antipsychotic drugs), unless they are deemed necessary to treat ongoing symptoms (e.g., psychosis) or to aid in relapse prevention (American Psychiatric Association, 2002). Often it is unknowable whether a medication is playing a primary or secondary role in sustaining a remission, and hence decisions about when and how to discontinue medications can become a trial-and-error endeavor. Because recent data suggest that long-term combination therapy may reduce relapse rates more substantially than monotherapies (Tohen, Suppes, et al., 2002), this issue remains controversial and in need of further investigation.

When and how to discontinue adjunctive medications remain a matter of debate. After stabilizing on lithium or divalproex plus olanzapine, abrupt cessation of olanzapine led to rapid relapse in about half of patients with remitted bipolar disorder for over 3 months (Tohen, Suppes, et al., 2002). It is also unclear whether maintenance doses of medications (other than lithium) can be reduced without compromising efficacy. Most practitioners therefore advocate changing only one medication at a time, and doing so gradually to minimize untoward effects. The spectrum of activity for medications commonly used for bipolar illness is described in Table 6.5 (at the end of the chapter).

CURRENT PHARMACOTHERAPIES: EVIDENCE FOR ANTIMANIC EFFICACY

Lithium

After more than 50 years of experience, lithium remains a cornerstone drug for both the short- and long-term treatment of bipolar disorder. It remains the most extensively studied agent for relapse prevention in bipolar disorder. An emerging database suggests that lithium may possess intrinsic properties that reduce suicide risk (Tondo & Baldessarini, 2000). A distinct bipolar clinical subtype has been recognized for which lithium response may be most favorable (Goldberg, Harrow, & Sands, 1996), as summarized in Table 6.1, along with common side effects.

Anticonvulsant Drugs

Divalproex

Initially developed as an anticonvulsant and later as a remedy for migraine, the psychotropic properties of divalproex emerged primarily in the 1980s and 1990s with regard to bipolar mania (Pope et al., 1991; Bowden et al., 1994), other psychopathological states related to impulsivity/aggression (Swann, 1999), and borderline personality disorder (Hollander et al., 2001). The FDA has not established psychotropic indications for divalproex apart from bipolar mania. Efforts to demonstrate its superiority to placebo during long-term relapse prevention have been unsuccessful thus far (Bowden et al., 2000).

In acute mania, rapid dosing strategies via oral loading can produce therapeutic serum valproate levels faster than usual dosing (Hirschfeld et al., 1999). A therapeutic blood range has been established in acute mania (Bowden et al., 1996; see Table 6.1). Efficacy in acute mania appears comparable to that seen with olanzapine, with possibly less weight gain (Zajecka et al., 2002), although the efficacy of each drug may depend strongly on how rapidly it is dosed initially (Tohen, Baker, et al., 2002). Illness features such as mixed states (Swann et al., 1997) or comorbid substance abuse (Goldberg et al., 1999) may herald a better antimanic response to divalproex than lithium. Augmentation of divalproex (or lithium) with an atypical antipsychotic such as olanzapine (Tohen, Suppes, et al., 2002), risperidone (Sachs, Grossman, et al., 2002), or quetiapine (DelBello et al., 2002; Sachs, Mullen, et al., 2002) may enhance acute antimanic efficacy. Common side effects of divalproex are described in Table 6.1.

Carbamazepine

First described by Okuma, Inanaga, et al. (1979) in Japan and Post et al. (1986) in the United States, carbamazepine has demonstrated efficacy in acute mania but more modest antidepressant and prophylactic efficacy (see Ernst & Goldberg, 2003). It may show added benefit when combined with lithium in rapid-cycling patients (Denicoff et al., 1997). Although carbamazepine is not presently approved by the FDA for the treatment of bipolar disorder, both it and oxcarbazepine are considered by the APA Practice Guidelines for the Treatment of Bipolar Disorder (American Psychiatric Association, 2002) as reasonable alternatives to more first-line antimanic treatments such as lithium or divalproex. Enthusiasm for its use has been limited, in part, because of possible neurotoxicity as well as hepatic enzyme induction and white blood-cell depression. Dosing and side effect information is presented in Table 6.1.

Oxcarbazepine

A derivative form of carbamazepine, oxcarbazepine does not form the epoxide metabolite of carbamazepine responsible for many of that drug's side effects. Regarded by many prescribers as a "cleaner" form of carbamazepine, its use in bipolar disorder has been limited by only a small number of short-term trials in acute mania, although the available trials suggest comparability to lithium or haloperidol (Emrich, 1990). Additionally, its monohydroxy-derivative (MHD) metabolite is currently under study for possible psychotropic effects.

Lamotrigine

Although found to have minimal acute antimanic efficacy (Ichim, Berk, & Brook, 2000), lamotrigine demonstrates better relapse prevention than placebo among bipolar II rapid-cycling outpatients (Calabrese et al., 2000). Initial observations of serious skin rashes, such as Stevens–Johnson syndrome and toxic epidermal necrolysis, led to revised slow-dose escalation recommendations (see Table 6.1) that considerably reduce the risk for serious skin rash.

Gabapentin

Following optimism from initial open trials, gabapentin was found to have no advantage compared to placebo for the treatment of acute mania (Pande, Crockatt, et al., 2000) or severe forms of bipolar disorder (Frye et al., 2000). It has demonstrated modest anxiolytic efficacy for social anxiety disorder (Pande et al., 1999) and panic disorder (Pande, Pollack, et al., 2000), as well as neuropathic pain syndromes, prompting some clinicians to advocate its use as an adjunct for those conditions, as distinct from mania or depression. The relatively benign side-effect profile and ease of administration (see Table 6.1) may account for its popularity among prescribers, despite the negative results in controlled studies.

Topiramate

Interest in this novel anticonvulsant has been spurred, in part, by its demonstrated utility for reducing appetite and possibly reversing weight gain caused by other psychotropic drugs. It has not shown antimanic efficacy better than placebo. A recent randomized controlled trial suggests an advantage for topiramate over placebo in patients with primary alcohol dependence (Johnson et al., 2003). Dosing and side-effect information, as described in Table 6.1, are especially notable for the potential dose-dependent cognitive side effects. Table 6.2 summarizes research on the use of anticonvulsants in bipolar disorder.

Other Anticonvulsants

Little systematic information is available on other anticonvulsants, such as tiagabine, levetiracetam, zonisamide, or pregabalin. Based on antikindling mechanisms associated with anticonvulsants, current research efforts are examining possible mood-stabilizing, anxiolytic, or other psychotropic

TABLE 6.2. Randomized, Double-Blind, Controlled Trials of Anticonvulsants in Bipolar Disorder

Compound	Authors	Design	n	Mean peak dose	Outcome	Comment
Divalproex	Bowden et al. (1994)	3-week comparison of DVP, Li+, or PBO in acute mania	187 DVP 91 Li+ 94 PBO	Day 8 mean VPA = 77 µg/ml; Li+ = 1.0 mEq/liter	DVP = Li+ > PBO	
	Pope et al. (1991)	3-week comparison of DVP or PBO in acute mania	17 DVP 19 PBO	DVP dosed to reach serum; VPA = 50–100 µg/ml	DVP > PBO	
	Bowden et al. (2000)	12-month comparison of DVP, Li+, or PBO for bipolar relapse prevention	69 DVP 36 Li+ 74 PBO	Day 30 median VPA = 83.9 µg/ml; Li+ = 0.9 mEq/liter	Li+ = DVP = PBO	High placebo response rate limits study interpretations
	Lambert & Venaud (1992)	18-month comparison of VAL or Li+ for bipolar relapse prevention	78 VAL 72 Li+	VAL 1,200 mg/day; Li+ not reported	VAL: 0.51 attacks/subject; 83% reduction from prestudy; Li+: 0.61 attacks/subject; 80% reduction from prestudy	Bipolar and unipolar subjects intermixed, not differentiated by treatment arm
	Freeman et al. (1992)	3-week randomized comparison of DVP or Li+	14 DVP 13 Li+	[valproate] 98 µg/ml; Li+ 0.8–1.4 mEq/liter	64% DVP response; 92% Li+ response	
Carbamazepine[a]	Okuma et al. (1979)	3–5 week comparison of CBZ or CPZ in acute mania	30 CBZ 30 CPZ	Not reported	CBZ = CPZ	
	Post et al. (1984)	11–56 day comparison of CBZ or PBO	19	CBZ 600–2,000 mg/day	63% improved	On-off-on design
	Lerer et al. (1987)	4-week comparison of CBZ or Li+	14 CBZ 14 Li+	Median CBZ dose = 1,400 mg/day (serum CBZ = 8.8 µg/ml); median Li+ dose = 2,100 mg/day (serum Li+ = 0.87 mEq/liter)	Trend for better Li+ than CBZ response	

(continued)

TABLE 6.2. (*continued*)

Compound	Authors	Design	n	Mean peak dose	Outcome	Comment
Oxcarbazepine	Emrich (1990)	2-week double-blind comparison of OXCBZ or Li⁺ in acute mania	28 OXCBZ 24 Li⁺	1,400 mg/day 1,100 mg/day	OXCBZ = Li⁺	Short-term study, no placebo
	Emrich (1990)	2-week double-blind comparison of OXCBZ or HAL in acute mania	17 OXCBZ 20 HAL	2,400 mg/day 42 mg/day	OXCBZ = HAL	Short-term study, no placebo
Lamotrigine	Ichim et al. (2000)	4-week double-blind comparison of LTG or Li⁺ in acute mania	15 LTG 15 Li⁺	100 mg/day 800 mg/day	LTG = Li⁺	LTG dosed at 25, then 50, then 100 mg by 3 weeks; rapid escalation raises risk for skin rash
	Calabrese et al. (1999)	7-week double-blind comparison of LTG or PBO in acute depression	66 LTG 50 mg/ day; 63 LTG 200 mg/day; 66 PBO	50 mg/day; 200 mg/day	MADRS: 49% LTG (50 mg) 55% LTG (200 mg) 29% PBO	Separation from PBO by week 3
	Frye et al. (2000)	6-week double-blind comparison of LTG, GPN, or PBO in refractory mood disorders	38 (crossover design)	Mean LTG dose = 274 mg/ day	CGI-BP: 52% LTG; 26% GPN; 23% PBO	
	Calabrese et al. (2000)	6-month double-blind comparison of LTG (50 or 200 mg/day) or PBO for relapse prevention in rapidly cycling bipolar disorder	92 LTG 88 PBO	Mean LTG dose = 288 mg/ day	LTG > PBO for BP II (*not* BP I)	

Drug	Study	Design	N	Dose	Results	Comments
	Bowden et al. (2003)	76-week double-blind comparison of LTG, Li+, or PBO for relapse prevention after a manic episode	58 LTG 44 Li+ 69 PBO	LTG 100–400 mg/day; Li+ dosed to achieve serum level of 0.8–1.1 mEq/liter	LTG > PBO for depression relapse but not mania relapse	
Gabapentin	Pande et al. (2000)	12-week double-blind comparison of GPN or PBO added to lithium or DVP in acute mania	58 GPN 59 PBO	Not reported	GPN not better than PBO	Some subjects had undetectable serum GPN levels
	Frye et al. (2000)	6-week double-blind comparison of GPN, LTG, or PBO in refractory mood disorders	38 (crossover design)	Mean GPN dose = 3,987 mg/day	CGI-BP: 26% GPN; 52% LTG; 23% PBO	LTG > PBO; GPN = PBO
Topiramate	McIntyre et al. (2002)	8-week randomized comparison of TPM or mood stabilizers + BUP for bipolar depression	18 TPM 18 BUP	176 mg/day 250 mg/day	TPM = BUP	

Note. CGI-BP, Clinical Global Impressions Scale for Bipolar Disorder; MADRS, Montgomery–Asberg Depression Rating Scale; BUP, bupropion; CPZ, chlorpromazine; DVP, divalproex; GPN, gabapentin; HAL, haloperidol; Li+, lithium; LTG, lamotrigine; OXCBZ, oxcarbazepine; PBO, placebo; TPM, topiramate; VAL, valpromide.

[a]Double-blind monotherapy controlled trials of CBZ in acute mania are presented; numerous comparisons of CBZ to other agents, alone or in combinations, acutely and long-term, are summarized elsewhere (see Martin et al., 1994).

effects of these compounds. It is important to recognize that very few anticonvulsants have demonstrated antimanic efficacy in placebo-controlled studies (only divalproex and carbamazepine), and only one has demonstrated antidepressant efficacy (lamotrigine). Still less is known from rigorous studies about the effects of anticonvulsants in complex clinical states such as psychiatric or medical comorbid conditions. Psychotropic effects of newer anticonvulsants, therefore, should not be presumed in the absence of data from controlled trials.

Atypical Antipsychotics

Olanzapine

Olanzapine presently represents the only atypical antipsychotic drug approved by the FDA for the treatment of acute mania. Its efficacy was demonstrated in two placebo-controlled trials (Tohen et al., 1999; Tohen et al., 2000), with robust effects on mixed states (Tohen et al., 2000), rapid cycling (Gonzalez-Pinto et al., 2002), and prior nonresponse to lithium or divalproex (Baker, Goldberg, et al., 2002). One-year antimanic relapse prevention appears comparable to that of divalproex (Tohen et al., 2003) and superior to lithium (Tohen, Marneros, et al., 2002).

Ziprasidone

A 3-week placebo-controlled trial found that ziprasidone, rapidly dosed at 160 mg/day within 2 days, produced a superior acute antimanic response compared to placebo. Little empirical evidence exists to clarify whether ziprasidone could exacerbate an existing mania or induce manias or hypomanias over time.

Risperidone

Risperidone has demonstrated acute antimanic efficacy as monotherapy (Hirschfeld et al., 2002; Vieta, Khanna, et al., 2002) and as add-on therapy to lithium or valproate (Sachs, Grossman, et al., 2002). Open-label case reports of agitation or activation have not been validated by placebo-controlled trials, although dose-dependent akathisia (i.e., motor restlessness) may warrant dosage reductions in some instances. Clinicians may find it difficult sometimes to differentiate akathisia from the agitation associated with mania or hypomania.

Quetiapine

Acute antimanic efficacy with quetiapine as add-on therapy to lithium or divalproex has recently been demonstrated (Sachs, Mullen, et al., 2002). In addition, quetiapine (mean dose of 450 mg/day) added to lithium or valproate has been associated with a more robust 3-week antimanic response in hospitalized adolescents with bipolar disorder (DelBello et al., 2002).

Clozapine

Although not formally studied as monotherapy for bipolar disorder, open trials suggest value for clozapine, particularly in bipolar patients unresponsive to first-line medications. The sole randomized study in treatment-resistant bipolar patients (Suppes et al., 1999) found that clozapine (mean dose 355 mg/day) was significantly better than treatment as usual for reducing manic and psychotic symptoms, as well as overall psychopathology. Furthermore, recent data that support a distinct reduction in suicide risk among patients with schizophrenia taking clozapine (Meltzer et al., 2003) should prompt greater consideration of clozapine for suicide reduction in bipolar illness.

Aripiprazole

Aripiprazole is a new atypical antipsychotic with a novel mechanism of action. As a partial agonist of the dopamine D2 receptor, it is believed to modulate dopamine transmission by exerting antagonist action in hyperdopaminergic regions (e.g., mesolimbic tracts during psychosis) and agonist action in hypodopaminergic areas (e.g., mesocortical tracts associated with schizophrenic negative symptoms, or possible depressive features). As such, aripiprazole may serve to reduce psychosis while enhancing cognition and sparing motor (i.e., nigrostriatal) or tuberoinfundibular pathways. Antimanic efficacy was demonstrated in a 3-week placebo-controlled trial (Keck et al., in press), with reduction evident in both manic and depressive symptoms during mania. Response (> 50% reductions from baseline severity of mania) occurred in 41% of acute manic patients taking aripiprazole (15–30 mg/day) versus 19% taking placebo. Table 6.3 summarizes research on the use of atypical antipsychotics in bipolar depression.

TREATMENT OF BIPOLAR DEPRESSION: THE ANTIDEPRESSANT CONTROVERSY

There has been growing debate about whether treatment outcomes differ between bipolar and unipolar depression. Some authors have suggested that standard antidepressants may work less effectively in bipolar than unipolar depression (Malinger et al., 1999). Unfortunately, many studies prior to the 1980s failed to differentiate unipolar from bipolar depressed patients. At present, no medication has been approved by the FDA specifically

TABLE 6.3. Randomized Controlled Trials of Atypical Antipsychotics in Bipolar Disorder

Compound	Authors	Design	n	Dosing	Outcome
Olanzapine	Tohen, Sanger, et al. (1999)	3-week double-blind comparison of OLZ or PBO in acute mania	70 OLZ 66 PBO	OLZ begun at 10 mg/day	OLZ > PBO
	Tohen, Jacobs, et al. (2000)	4-week double-blind comparison of OLZ or PBO in acute mania	54 OLZ 56 PBO	OLZ begun at 15 mg/day; mean dose 16.4 mg/day	OLZ > PBO
	Tohen, Baker et al. (2002)	3-week double-blind comparison of OLZ or DVP in acute mania	125 OLZ 123 DVP	OLZ begun at 15 mg/day; DVP begun at 750 mg/day	OLZ > DVP
	Zajecka et al. (2002)	12-week double-blind comparison of OLZ or DVP in acute mania	57 OLZ 63 DVP	OLZ begun at 10 mg/day; DVP begun at 20 mg/kg/day	OLZ = DVP
	Tohen, Goldberg, et al. (in press)	12-week double-blind comparison of OLZ or HAL in acute mania	234 OLZ 214 HAL	OLZ mean dose = 15.3 mg/day; HAL mean dose = 8.2 mg/day	OLZ = HAL
	Tohen, Chengappa, et al. (2002)	6-week comparison of OLZ or PBO added to Li^+ or DVP in mania	229 OLZ 115 PBO	OLZ mean dose = 11.9 mg/day	OLZ > PBO
	Tohen et al. (2003)	47-week comparison of OLZ or DVP for bipolar relapse prevention	125 OLZ 125 DVP	OLZ mean dose = 16.2 mg/day; DVP mean dose = 1,584.7 mg/day	OLZ = DVP
	Tohen, Marneros, et al. (2002)	1-year comparison of OLZ or Li^+ for bipolar relapse prevention	217 OLZ 214 Li^+	OLZ mean dose = 11.9 mg/day; Li^+ mean dose = 1,103 mg/day	OLZ > Li^+ mania relapse; OLZ = $Li+$ for depression relapse
	Tohen, Suppes, et al. (2002)	18-month comparison of OLZ or PBO added to Li^+ or DVP for relapse prevention	51 OLZ+Li^+ or DVP; 48 PBO + Li^+ or DVP	OLZ mean dose = 8.6 mg/day	OLZ > PBO

	Study	Description	N	Dose	Result
	Baker, Vieta, al. (2002)	8-week double-blind comparison of OLZ, PBO, or OFC for acute bipolar depression	370 OLZ 377 PBO 86 OFC	OLZ mean dose = 8.7 mg/day; OLZ mean dose = 7.4 mg/day; FLX mean dose = 38.3 mg/day	OFC > OLZ > PBO
Ziprasidone	Keck, Versiani, et al. (2003)	3-week double-blind comparison of ZIP or PBO in acute mania	131 ZIP 64 PBO	ZIP mean dose = 135 mg/day	ZIP > PBO
Risperidone	Sachs, Grossman, et al. (2002)	3-week double-blind comparison of RIS, HAL, or PBO added to Li+ or DVP in acute mania	52 RIS 53 HAL 51 PBO	RIS mean dose = 3.8 mg/day; HAL mean dose = 6.2 mg/day	RIS = HAL > PBO
	Vieta, Khanna, et al. (2002)	3-week double-blind comparison of RIS or PBO monotherapy in mania	146 RIS 144 PBO	RIS mean modal dose = 5.6 mg/day	RIS > PBO
	Hirschfeld et al. (2002)	3-week double-blind comparison of RIS or PBO monotherapy in mania	134 RIS 125 PBO	RIS mean dose = 4.1 mg/day	RIS > PBO
Quetiapine	DelBello et al. (2002)	3-week double-blind comparison of QUET or PBO added to DVP in acute adolescent mania	15 QUET 15 PBO	QUET mean dose = 432 mg/day	QUET > PBO
	Sachs, Mullen, et al. (2002)	3-week double-blind comparison of QUET or PBO in acute mania	91 QUET 100 PBO	QUET: 200–800 mg/day	QUET > PBO
Clozapine	Suppes et al. (1999)	12-month randomized comparison of CLOZ + TAU or TAU alone	19 CLOZ 19 TAU	CLOZ mean dose = 355 mg/day	CLOZ > TAU
Aripiprazole	Keck et al. (in press)	3-week randomized comparison of ARI or PBO in acute mania	123 ARI 122 PBO	ARI mean dose = 28 mg/day	ARI > PBO

Note. ARI, aripiprazole; CLOZ, clozapine; DVP, divalproex; FLX, fluoxetine; HAL, haloperidol; Li+, lithium; OFC, olanzapine plus fluoxetine; OLZ, olanzapine; PBO, placebo; QUET, quetiapine; RIS, risperidone; TAU, treatment as usual; ZIP, ziprasidone.

for the depressed phase of bipolar illness, although as noted previously, relapse prevention data with lamotrigine appear more robust for depression than mania. Depression is the predominant mood state seen in individuals with bipolar disorder (Calabrese et al., 2001; Judd et al., 2002), yet remarkably, few standard antidepressants have been studied in randomized controlled trials for bipolar depression.

A central concern regarding antidepressant use in bipolar disorder involves their potential to induce mania or accelerate cycle frequency in about 20–40% of these patients (Altshuler et al., 1995; Goldberg & Whiteside, 2002). For this reason, controversy persists about their safety. Ghaemi, Lenox, and Baldessarini (2001) identified seven controlled trials of standard antidepressants used in bipolar patients and concluded that little justification exists for their use, above and beyond the antidepressant effects of mood stabilizers for depression. With regard to relapse prevention, there are no controlled data to support the view that long-term antidepressants help to avoid depression relapse any better than mood stabilizers alone, although recent noncontrolled data have challenged this assertion (Altshuler et al., 2001, 2003). Some authors suggest that newer antidepressants, such as the selective serotonin reuptake inhibitors (SSRIs), have a lower likelihood of inducing mania or hypomania than older tricyclic antidepressants (Peet, 1994), but other studies question this assumption (Post et al., 2001; Goldberg & Whiteside, 2002). Many clinicians believe that mood stabilizers in conjunction with antidepressants can reduce the risk of mania. This combination effect has been demonstrated more compellingly for lithium than divalproex (Henry et al., 2001), but several reports question whether mood stabilizers robustly protect against antidepressant-induced switches (Bottlender et al., 2001; Goldberg & Whiteside, 2002).

Still other authors raise the possibility that antidepressant-induced switches may be predicted more by patient characteristics than specific antidepressants. Antidepressant-induced manias tend to recur in a distinct subgroup of bipolar patients, regardless of antidepressant used (Goldberg & Whiteside, 2002). Preliminary genetic evidence suggests a possible biological susceptibility to antidepressant-induced mania based on a genetic variant or polymorphism of the protein responsible for transporting serotonin across the synapse (Mundo et al., 2001). Alcohol or other substance abuse also has been identified as a mood-destabilizing factor that may increase the risk for antidepressant-induced mania as much as sevenfold (Goldberg & Whiteside, 2002).

Based on these collective observations, current APA Practice Guidelines (American Psychiatric Association, 2002) advise against using antidepressants alone in patients with bipolar I disorder. The safety of antidepressants alone in patients with bipolar II disorder remains the subject of unresolved debate, since a limited database shows possible lesser risk of mood destabilization than in bipolar I depression (Amsterdam, 1998; Amsterdam et al., 1998). Lithium and lamotrigine are considered the first-line guideline-based treatments for bipolar depression (American Psychiatric Association, 2002). Table 6.4 summarizes research on the use of antidepressants in bipolar disorder.

Standard Antidepressants

As summarized in Table 6.4, few controlled studies have examined the use of standard antidepressants for bipolar depression. Bupropion often is regarded as among the safest and most effective of antidepressants for bipolar depression, but this conclusion derives mainly from a single randomized comparison of bupropion in nine patients versus desipramine in 10. Paroxetine is also often regarded as among the best-studied of SSRIs for bipolar depression, although Nemeroff and colleagues (2001) found that when serum lithium levels were dosed therapeutically (> 0.8 mEq/liter), the addition of paroxetine provided no antidepressant advantage over placebo.

Mood Stabilizers as Antidepressants

Even lithium has been shown to possess greater antimanic than antidepressant properties, and several long-term studies have found no advantage of lithium over placebo for preventing depressive relapses in patients with bipolar disorder (Prien, Caffey, & Klett, 1973; Dunner, Stallone, & Fieve, 1976; Bowden et al., 2003). Some of these studies may have reflected a high proportion of patients who rapidly cycle, for whom lithium may be less effective (Dunner et al., 1976). Preliminary data suggest that among depressed patients with bipolar I disorder, taking lithium or divalproex, a depressive episode is equally responsive to treatment with SSRI augmentation as it is with the addition of the second above mood stabilizer to the first (Young et al., 2000). The presence of a manic episode within a few months before the depression may predict a poorer response to antidepressant augmentation (MacQueen et al., 2001), affirming the importance of mood charting to document cyclic patterns.

For patients with bipolar disorder, lamotrigine is the only anticonvulsant that has been shown to possess antidepressant properties that are both acutely (Calabrese et al., 1999) and prophylactically (Bowden et al., 2003) superior to placebo. In a rigorous trial for acute bipolar depression, separation from placebo was evident after only 3 weeks (Calabrese et al., 1999), similar to the time course for response to standard antidepressants. In fact, because lamotrigine is the only anticonvulsant that has shown antidepressant efficacy relative to placebo (Ernst & Goldberg, 2003), it is considered a first-line agent for the treatment of bipolar depression (American Psychiatric Association, 2002). More limited data support a role for topiramate (shown as comparable to bupropion in one small study; McIntyre et al., 2002) and for divalproex (Sachs et al., 2001). No placebo-controlled data presently support the antidepressant properties of any other anticonvulsant drugs (Ernst & Goldberg, 2003). As an inhibitor of serotonin reuptake, it is possible that

TABLE 6.4. Randomized Controlled Trials of Standard Antidepressants for Bipolar Disorder

Medication	Authors	Design	n	Dosing	Outcome
Bupropion	Sachs et al. (1994)	8-week randomized controlled addition to standard mood stabilizers	9 BUP 10 DMI	BUP mean dose = 358 mg/day; DMI mean dose = 140 mg/day	BUP = DMI
Paroxetine	Nemeroff et al. (2001)	10-week addition of PAR vs. IMI vs. PBO added to Li$^+$	35 PAR 39 IMI 43 PBO	PAR mean dose = 32.6 mg/day; IMI mean dose = 166.7 mg/day	No significant differences; PAR or IMI > PBO if serum Li$^+$ < 0.8
	Young et al. (2000)	8-week comparison of Li$^+$ or DVP + PAR vs. 2nd mood stabilizer	11 PAR 16 Li$^+$ or DVP	PAR mean dose = 36 mg/day; Li$^+$ mean dose = 1,600 mg/day; DVP mean dose = 1,200 mg/day	PAR = Li$^+$ or DVP
Venlafaxine	Vieta, Martinez-Aran, et al. (2002)	6 week addition of PAR or VEN to standard mood stabilizers	30 PAR 30 VEN	PAR 32 mg/day; VEN 179 mg/day	PAR = VEN
Fluoxetine	Cohn et al. (1989)	3–6 week trial of FLX vs. IMI vs. PBO	30 FLX 30 IMI 29 PBO	FLX 62 mg/day; IMI not reported	
Tranylcypromine	Himmelhoch et al. (1991)	6-week randomized comparison with IMI	16 TRN 16 IMI	TRN mean dose = 37 mg/day; IMI mean dose = 246 mg/day	TRN = IMI but lower switch rate into mania

Note. BUP, bupropion; DMI, desipramine; DVP, divalproex; FLX, fluoxetine; IMI, imipramine; Li$^+$, lithium; PAR, paroxetine; PBO, placebo; TRN, tranylcypromine; VEN, venlafaxine.

ziprasidone may possess antidepressant properties, but this hypothesis remains underexplored (Keck, Versiani, et al., 2003).

Recent data suggest that some atypical antipsychotics may possess antidepressant properties in bipolar illness. Tohen, Vieta, et al. (in press) observed a 48% reduction from baseline Hamilton Depression Scale (HAM-D) ratings with olanzapine monotherapy for bipolar depression, and a 65% improvement when olanzapine was combined with fluoxetine; both strategies were superior to placebo. Among patients with refractory bipolar disorder, Suppes et al. (1999) found a near-significant reduction in HAM-D scores independent of reductions in psychosis or mania. On the other hand, risperidone—either alone or combined with paroxetine—did not significantly reduce depressive symptoms when added to standard mood stabilizers for bipolar depression (Stahl & Shelton, 2001).

NOVEL COMPOUNDS

A number of novel agents has begun to receive attention , although none has become established as a first-line alternative to standard psychotropics for acute or long-term treatment of bipolar illness. Calcium channel blockers such as verapamil, despite initial enthusiasm, have shown only modest efficacy in bipolar illness (Levy & Janicak, 2000). Exceptions may include a better response to verapamil in women than men (Wisner et al., 2002), and a role for the anticonvulsant calcium channel blocker nimodipine in patients with ultrarapid-cycling bipolar disorder (Goodnick, 2000). The omega-3 fatty acid ethyl-eicosapentanoate (EPA) was initially described in a preliminary 4-month study by Stoll and colleagues (1999) as being superior to placebo for relapse prevention among outpatients with bipolar disorder. However, more recently, EPA was found to be no better than placebo over an 8-week period among bipolar outpatients with depression or rapid cycling (Keck, McElroy, et al., 2003). Donepezil, a cholinergic drug used to treat Alzheimer's disease, was described in a preliminary open-case series as having potential value for both manic and depressive phases of bipolar illness (Burt et al., 1999). Thyroid hormone has been shown to provide some degree of antidepressant efficacy and may be of value in patients with rapidly cycling bipolar disorder (Bauer & Whybrow, 1990). Finally, the sugar inositol represents a biological target of lithium and may itself have therapeutic value for some patients with bipolar disorder (Chengappa et al., 2000).

SPECIAL POPULATIONS

Controlled pharmacotherapy trials are scarce in all phases of child and adolescent bipolar disorder. At present, only two randomized trials have been reported. Geller and colleagues (1998) studied 25 adolescent outpatients with bipolar disorder and comorbid substance abuse and found greater improvement in mood symptoms as well as substance use patterns on lithium compared to placebo for 6 weeks. DelBello et al. (2002) studied the atypical antipsychotic quetiapine versus placebo as add-on therapy to divalproex in 30 hospitalized adolescent inpatients with mania and found the combination to produce greater reductions in symptoms of mania but not depression.

Open trials preliminarily support the use of divalproex in children and adolescents (Paptheodorou et al., 1995), although controlled studies are lacking. Lamotrigine presents special concern in children and adolescents because of an increased risk in this age group for severe skin rashes, such as Stevens–Johnson syndrome.

Rapid cycling during the preceding 12-month period was added as a course specifier to bipolar illness in DSM-IV (American Psychiatric Association, 1994), denoting a subgroup of about one-fifth of patients with bipolar disorder, many of whom are women (Bauer et al., 1994). The concept of rapid cycling originated during studies designed to identify predictors of lithium prophylaxis failure; four or more distinct annual episodes emerged as the most robust predictor of subsequent relapse during lithium maintenance (Dunner & Fieve, 1974).

Antidepressant use is considered to be particularly high risk with patients who rapidly cycle, as noted above; when used, most experts advocate relatively short-term exposures (e.g., little more than several weeks after improvement in depression). In fact, the only existing placebo-controlled acute pharmacotherapy study in rapid cycling found that elimination of tricyclic antidepressants was superior to their continued use with respect to reducing cycle frequency (Wehr et al., 1988). Recent 6-month data also support the use of lamotrigine monotherapy to prevent recurrences among patients with rapid-cycling bipolar disorder, particularly in those with bipolar II disorder (Calabrese et al., 2000). A large open trial also found a high response rate with divalproex across varied illness phases among patients with rapid-cycling bipolar disorder (Calabrese et al., 1993). Additionally, a body of literature exists involving case reports and uncontrolled open trials with various other agents, including several anticonvulsants and atypical antipsychotics.

Finally, no controlled studies exist for the treatment of bipolar disorder during pregnancy or lactation, in the elderly, the medically ill, or in those with comorbid substance abuse or other Axis I disorders. These are crucial next steps for empirical study.

SUMMARY

Pharmacotherapy options for bipolar disorder have increased extensively amid the growing availability of newer anticonvulsants, atypical anti-

TABLE 6.5. Spectrum of Efficacy of Current Pharmacotherapies for Bipolar Disorder

Medication	Pure mania	Pure depression	Mixed state	Rapid cycling	Substance abuse	Anxiety	Bipolar II	Psychosis	Maintenance
Lithium	++	+	–	–	+[a]	+	+	+	M > D
Anticonvulsants									
Divalproex	++	+	++	+	+	+	+	+	D > M
Carbamazepine	++	+?	+	+	+	+	+?	–?	+?
Oxcarbazepine	+	?	?	?	?	?	+? (RC)	?	D > M
Lamotrigine	–	++	?	++	+/–[b]	+?	+	–	? ?
Gabapentin	–	+	?	?	+[c]	+	+?	–?	?
Topiramate	–	+	?	?	+[c]	?	?	?	?
Atypical antipsychotics									
Olanzapine	++	++	++	++	?	?	?	++	++
Risperidone	++	+	+	?	?	?	?	++	?
Quetiapine	++	+?	+	+	?	?	?	++	?
Clozapine	+	?	+	+	?	?	?	++	+
Aripiprazole	++	?	++	?	?	?	?	++	?
Ziprasidone	++	?	?	?	?	?	?	++	?

Note. ++, positive evidence in double-blind, placebo-controlled trials; +, positive evidence from open or randomized but not placebo-controlled trials, or else modest or mixed results from controlled trials; –, negative data from placebo-controlled trials; ?, no data available from open or controlled studies; M, mania; D, depression; RC, rapid cycling.

[a]Based on positive controlled data in adolescent bipolar disorder with substance abuse, though negative open trial data in adults with dual diagnosis comorbidity.

[b]Based on positive data in alcohol use disorders, although few data exist for bipolar disorder with comorbid substance abuse.

[c]Positive placebo-controlled data in primary alcohol dependence, though no data available in bipolar disorder with controlled substance abuse.

psychotics, and antidepressants. Recent controlled trials have provided an evidence base for differentiating efficacious agents for distinct illness subtypes, challenging older definitions of mood-stabilizing drugs.

As summarized in Table 6.5 (on p. 131), current medication options may best be viewed with regard to their "depth of spectrum" rather than their categorical ability to stabilize mood in all instances. Lithium remains an excellent treatment for classical and uncomplicated mania. Divalproex and carbamazepine are superior to placebo in acute mania, although controlled studies with other anticonvulsants have yet to demonstrate antimanic efficacy. Lamotrigine is the sole anticonvulsant that has been found to be superior for bipolar depression, without inducing manic symptoms. Controlled data support the monotherapeutic use of olanzapine, risperidone, ziprasidone, or aripiprazole in acute mania, and combination therapies with olanzapine, risperidone, quetiapine, and clozapine. An emerging role has become evident for a number of these compounds irrespective of their antipsychotic properties; some of these agents may exert antidepressant efficacy, and some may delay relapse as well as (if not better than) more standard agents such as lithium or divalproex. Antidepressant monotherapies are generally contraindicated for bipolar illness but may prove useful for a select patient subgroup when lithium, lamotrigine, and possibly other mood-stabilizing compounds prove suboptimal for bipolar depression. Future studies may help to (1) establish a stronger evidence base for choosing combination therapies and sequential medications, (2) target atypical symptoms in special populations, (3) combine medications with diagnosis-specific psychotherapies, and (4) bridge the gap between optimized efficacy and "real world" effectiveness for patients treated under ordinary circumstances.

REFERENCES

Altshuler, L., Kiriakos, L., Calcagno, J., Goodman, R., Gitlin, M., Frye, M., & Mintz, J. (2001). The impact of antidepressant discontinuation versus antidepressant continuation on 1-year risk for relapse of bipolar depression: A retrospective chart review. *Journal of Clinical Psychiatry, 62,* 612–616.

Altshuler, L. L., Post, R. M., Leverich, G. S., Mikalauskas, K., Rosoff, A., & Ackerman, L. (1995). Antidepressant-induced mania and cycle acceleration: A controversy revisited. *American Journal of Psychiatry, 152,* 1130–1138.

Altshuler, L., Suppes, T., Black, D., Nolen, W. A., Keck, P. E. Jr., Frye, M. A., McElroy, S., Kupka, R., Grunze, H., Walden, J., Leverich, G., Denicoff, K., Luckenbaugh, D., & Post, R. M. (2003). Impact of antidepressant discontinuation after acute bipolar depression remission on rates of depressive relapse at 1-year follow-up. *American Journal of Psychiatry, 160,* 1252–1262.

American Psychiatric Association. (1994). *Diagnostic and statistical manual of mental disorders* (4th ed.). Washington, DC: Author.

American Psychiatric Association. (2002). Practice guidelines for the treatment of patients with bipolar disorder (rev.). *American Journal of Psychiatry, 159,* 1–50.

Amsterdam, J. (1998). Efficacy and safety of venlafaxine in the treatment of bipolar II major depressive episode. *Journal of Clinical Psychopharmacology, 18,* 414–417.

Amsterdam, J., Garcia-Espana, F., Fawcett, J., Quitkin, F. M., Reimherr, F. W., Rosenbaum, J. F., Schweizer, E., & Beasley, C. (1998). Efficacy and safety of fluoxetine in treating bipolar II major depressive episode. *Journal of Clinical Psychopharmacology, 18,* 435–440.

Baker, R. W., Goldberg, J. F., Tohen, M., Milton, D. R., Stauffer, V. L., & Schuh, L. M. (2002). The impact of response to previous mood stabilizer therapy on response to olanzapine versus placebo for acute mania. *Bipolar Disorders, 4,* 43–49.

Bauer, M. S., Calabrese, J., Dunner, D. L., Post, R., Whybrow, P. C., Gyalai, L., Tay, L. K., Younkin, S. R., Bynaum, D., Lavori, P., et al. (1994). Multisite data reanalysis of the validity of rapid cycling as a course modifier for bipolar disorder in DSM-IV. *American Journal of Psychiatry, 151,* 506–515.

Bauer, M. S., & Whybrow, P. C. (1990). Rapid cycling bipolar affective disorder: II. Treatment of refractory rapid cycling with high-dose levothyroxine: A preliminary study. *Archives of General Psychiatry, 47,* 435–440.

Bottlender, R., Rudolf, D., Strauss, A., & Moller, H. J. (2001). Mood stabilisers reduce the risk of developing antidepressant-induced maniform states in acute treatment of bipolar I depressed patients. *Journal of Affective Disorders, 63,* 79–83.

Bowden, C. L. (2001). Strategies to reduce misdiagnosis of bipolar depression. *Psychiatric Services, 52,* 51–55.

Bowden, C. L., Brugger, A. M., Swann, A. C., Calabrese, J. R., Janicak, P. G., Petty, F., Dilsaver, S. C., Davis, J. M., Rush, A. J., Small, J. G., et al. (1994). Efficacy of divalproex vs. lithium and placebo in the treatment of mania: The Depakote Mania Study Group. *Journal of the American Medical Association, 271,* 918–924.

Bowden, C. L., Calabrese, J. R., McElroy, S. L., Gyulai, L., Wassef, A., Petty, F., Pope, H. G., Jr., Chou, J. C., Keck, P. E., Jr., Rhodes, L. J., Swann, A. C., Hirschfeld, R. M., & Wozniak, P. J. (2000). A randomized, placebo-controlled 12-month trial of divalproex and lithium in treatment of outpatients with bipolar I disorder: Divalproex Maintenance Study Group. *Archives of General Psychiatry, 57,* 481–489.

Bowden, C. L., Calabrese, J. R., Sachs, G. S., Yatham, L. N., Asghar, S. A., Hompland, M., Montgomery, P., Earl, N., Smoot, T. M., DeVeaugh-Geiss, J., & Lamictal 606 Study Group. (2003). A placebo-controlled 18-month trial of lamotrigine and lithium maintenance treatment in recently manic or hypomanic patients with bipolar I disorder. *Archives of General Psychiatry, 60,* 392–400.

Bowden, C. L., Janicak, P. G., Orsulak, P., Swann, A. C., Davis, J. M., Calabrese, J. R., Goodnick, P., Small, J. G., Rush, A. J., Kimmel, S. E., Risch, S. C., & Morris, D. D. (1996). Relation of serum valproate concentration to response in mania. *American Journal of Psychiatry, 153,* 765–770.

Burt, T., Sachs, G. S., & Demopulos, C. (1999). Donepezil in treatment-resistant bipolar disorder. *Biological Psychiatry, 45,* 959–964.

Calabrese, J. R., Bowden, C. L., Sachs, G. S., Ascher, J. A., Monaghan, E., & Rudd, G. D. (1999). A double-blind placebo-controlled study of lamotrigine monotherapy in outpatients with bipolar I depression: Lamictal 602 Study Group. *Journal of Clinical Psychiatry, 60,* 79–88.

Calabrese, J. R., Bowden, C. L., Sachs, G., Yatham, L., Behnke, K., Mehtonen, O. P., Montgomery, P., Ascher, J., Paska, W., Earl, N. L., DeVeaugh-Geiss, J., for the Lamictal 605 Study Group (in press). A placebo-controlled 18-month trial of lamotrigine and lithium maintenance treatment in recently depressed patients with bipolar I disorder. *Journal of Clinical Psychiatry.*

Calabrese, J. R., Shelton, M. D., Bowden, C. L., Rapport, D. J., Suppes, T., Shirley, E. R., Kimmel, S. E., & Caban, S. J. (2001). Bipolar rapid cycling: Focus on depression as its hallmark. *Journal of Clinical Psychiatry, 62*(Suppl. 14), 34–41.

Calabrese, J. R., Suppes, T., Bowden, C. L., Sachs, G. S., Swann, A. C., McElroy, S. L., Kusumaker, V., Ascher, J. A., Earl, N. L., Greene, P. L., & Monaghan, E. T. (2000). A double-blind, placebo-controlled, prophylaxis study of lamotrigine in rapid-cycling bipolar disorder: Lamictal 614 Study Group. *Journal of Clinical Psychiatry, 61,* 841–850.

Calabrese, J. R., Woyshville, M. J., Kimmel, S. E., & Rapport, D. J. (1993). Predictors of valproate response in bipolar rapid cycling. *Journal of Clinical Psychopharmacology, 13,* 280–283.

Chengappa, K. N., Levine, J., Gershon, S., Mallinger, A. G., Hardan, A., Vagnucci, A., Pollock, B., Luther, J., Buttenfield, J., Verfaille, S., & Kupfer, D. J. (2000). Inositol as an add-on treatment for bipolar depression. *Bipolar Disorders, 2,* 47–55.

Cohn, J. B., Collins, G., Ashbrook E., & Wernicke, J. F. (1989). A comparison of fluoxetine, imipramine and placebo in patients with bipolar depressive disorder. *International Clinical Psychopharmacology 4,* 313–322.

DelBello, M. P., Schwiers, M. L., Rosenberg, H. L., & Strakowski, S. M. (2002). A double-blind, randomized, placebo-controlled study of quetiapine as adjunctive treatment for adolescent mania. *Journal of the American Academy of Child and Adolescent Psychiatry, 41,* 1216–1223.

Denicoff, K. D., Smith-Jackson, E. E., Disney, E. R., Ali, O., Leverich, G. S., & Post, R. M. (1997). Comparative prophylactic efficacy of lithium, carbamazepine, and their combination in bipolar disorder. *Journal of Clinical Psychiatry, 58,* 470–478.

Dunner, D. L., & Fieve, R. R. (1974). Clinical factors in lithium carbonate prophylaxis failure. *Archives of General Psychiatry, 30,* 229–233.

Dunner, D. L., Stallone F., & Fieve, R. R. (1976). Lithium carbonate and affective disorders: VA double-blind study of prophylaxis of depression in bipolar illness. *Archives of General Psychiatry, 33,* 117–120.

Emrich, H. (1990). Studies with oxcarbazepine (Trileptal) in acute mania. *International Clinical Psychopharmacology, 5*(Suppl. 1), 83–88.

Ernst, C. L., & Goldberg, J. F. (2003). Antidepressant properties of anticonvulsant drugs for bipolar disorder. *Journal of Clinical Psychopharmacology, 23,* 182–192.

Freeman, T. W., Clothier, J. L., Pazzaglia, P., Lessem, M. D., & Swann, A. C. (1992). A double-blind comparison of valproate and lithium in the treatment of acute mania. *American Journal of Psychiatry, 149,* 108–111.

Frye, M. A., Ketter, T. A., Kimbrell, T. A., Dunn, R. T., Speer, A. M., Osuch, E. A., Luckenbaugh, D. A., Cora-Ocatelli, G., Leverich, G. S., & Post, R. M. (2000). A placebo-controlled study of lamotrigine and gabapentin monotherapy in refractory mood disorders. *Journal of Clinical Psychopharmacology, 20,* 607–614.

Geller, B., Cooper, T. B., Sun, K., Zimmerman, B., Frazier, J., Williams, M., & Heath, J. (1998). Double-blind and placebo-controlled study of lithium for adolescent bipolar disorders with secondary substance dependency. *Journal of the American Academy of Child and Adolescent Psychiatry, 37,* 171–178.

Ghaemi, S. N., Lenox, M. S., & Baldessarini, R. J. (2001). Effectiveness and safety of long-term antidepressant treatment in bipolar disorder. *Journal of Clinical Psychiatry, 62,* 565–569.

Goldberg, J. F., Garno, J., Leon, A. C., Kocsis, J. H., & Portera, L. (1999). A history of substance abuse complicates remission from acute mania in bipolar disorder. *Journal of Clinical Psychiatry, 60,* 733–740.

Goldberg, J. F., Harrow, M., & Sands, J. R. (1996). Lithium therapy in the longitudinal course of bipolar disorder. *Psychiatric Annals, 26,* 651–658.

Goldberg, J. F., & Whiteside, J. E. (2002). The association between substance abuse and antidepressant-induced mania in bipolar disorder: A preliminary study. *Journal of Clinical Psychiatry, 63,* 791–795.

Gonzalez-Pinto, A., Tohen, M., Lalaguna, B., Perez-Heredia, J. L., Fernandez-Corres, B., Gutirrez, M., & Mico, J. A. (2002). Treatment of bipolar I rapid cycling patients during dysphoric mania with olanzapine. *Journal of Clinical Psychopharmacology, 22,* 450–454.

Goodnick, P. J. (2000). The use of nimodipine in the treatment of mood disorders. *Bipolar Disorders, 2,* 165–173.

Henry, C., Sorbara, F., Lacoste, J., Gindrec, C., & Leboyer, M. (2001). Antidepressant-induced mania in bipolar patients: Identification of risk factors. *Journal of Clinical Psychiatry, 62,* 249–255.

Himmelhoch, J. M., Thase, M. E., Mallinger, A. G., & Houck, P. (1991). Tranylcypromine versus imipramine in anergic bipolar depression. *American Journal of Psychiatry, 148,* 910–916.

Hirschfeld, R. M. A., Allen, M. H., McEvoy, J. P., Keck, P. E. Jr., & Russell, J. M. (1999). Safety and tolerability of oral loading divalproex sodium in acutely manic bipolar patients. *Journal of Clinical Psychiatry, 60,* 815–818.

Hirschfeld, R. M., Keck, P. E. , Jr., Karcher, K., Kramer, M., Grossman, F., & Gershon, S. (2002, December). *Rapid antimanic effect of risperidone monotherapy: A 3-week multicenter randomized double-blind placebo-controlled trial.* Paper presented at the 41st Annual Meeting of the American College of Neuropsychopharmacology, San Juan, Puerto Rico.

Hollander, E., Allen, A., Lopez, R. P., Bienstock, C. A., Grossman, R., Siever, L. J., Merkatz, L., & Stein, D. J. (2001). A preliminary double-blind, placebo-controlled trial of divalproex sodium in borderline personality disorder. *Journal of Clinical Psychiatry, 62,* 199–203.

Ichim, L., Berk, M., & Brook, S. (2000). Lamotrigine compared with lithium in mania: A double-blind randomized controlled trial. *Annals of Clinical Psychiatry, 12,* 5–10.

Johnson, B., Ait-Daoud, N., Bowden, C. L., DiClemente, C. C., Roache, J. D., Lawson, K., Javors, M. A., & Ma, J. Z. (2003). Oral topiramate for treatment of alcohol dependence: A randomized controlled trial. *Lancet, 361,* 1677–1685.

Judd, L. L., Akiskal, H. S., Schettler, P. J., Endicott, J., Maser, J., Solomon, D. A., Leon, A. C., Rice, J. A., & Keller, M. B. (2002). The long-term natural history of the weekly symptomatic status of bipolar I disorder. *Archives of General Psychiatry, 59,* 530–537.

Keck, P. E., Jr., Marcus, R., Tourkodimitris, S., Ali, M., Liebeskind, A., Saha, A., Ingenito, G., & the Aripiprazole Study Group. (in press). A placebo-controlled, double-blind study of the efficacy and safety of aripiprazole in patients with acute bipolar mania. *American Journal of Psychiatry.*

Keck, P. E., Jr., McElroy, S. L., Freeman, M. P., Altshuler, L. L., Frye, M. A., Suppes, T., Mintz, J., Hwang, S., Kupka, R., Nolen, W., Grunze, H., Walden, J., Denicoff, K. D., Leverich, G. S., & Post, R. M. (2003, June). *Randomized, placebo-controlled trial of eicosopentanoic acid (EPA) in bipolar depression.* Poster presented at the 5th International Conference on Bipolar Disorder, Pittsburgh, PA.

Keck, P. E., Jr., McElroy, S. L., Richtand, N., & Tohen, M. (2002). What makes a drug a primary mood stabilizer? *Molecular Psychiatry, 7*(Suppl. 1), S8–S14.

Keck, P. E., Jr., Versiani, H., Potkin, S., West, S. A., Giller, E., Ice, K., & the Ziprasidone in Mania Study Group. (2003). Ziprasidone in the treatment of acute bipolar mania: A three-week, placebo-controlled, double-blind, randomized trial. *American Journal of Psychiatry, 160,* 741–748.

Ketter, T. A., & Calabrese, J. R. (2002). Stabilization of mood from below versus above baseline in bipolar disorder. *Journal of Clinical Psychiatry, 63,* 146–151.

Lambert, P. A., & Venaud, G. (1992). Comparative study of valpromide versus lithium in the treatment of bipolar disorder. *Nervure, 5,* 57–65.

Lerer, B., Moore, N., Meyendorff, E., Cho, S. R., & Gershon, S. (1987). Carbamazepine versus lithium in mania: A double-blind study. *Journal of Clinical Psychiatry, 48,* 89–93.

Levy, N. A., & Janicak, P. G. (2000). Calcium channel antagonists for the treatment of bipolar disorder. *Bipolar Disorders, 2,* 108–119.

MacQueen, G. M., Young, T. L., Marriott, M. J., & Joffe, R. T. (2001). Dr. MacQueen and colleagues reply. *American Journal of Psychiatry, 158,* 326.

Malinger, A. G., Frank, E., Barwell, M. M., Thase, M. E., & Kupfer, D. J. (1999). Effectiveness of traditional antidepressants is suboptimal in the depressed phase of bipolar disorder. *Bipolar Disorders, 1,* 41.

Manji, H. K., & Potter, W. Z. (1995). Signal transduction pathways: Molecular targets for lithium's actions. *Archives of General Psychiatry, 52,* 531–543.

Martin, L. S., Joffe, R. T, & Bebchuk, J. M. (1994). Clinical efficacy of carbamazepine. In R. T. Joffe & J. R. Calabrese (Eds.), *Anticonvulsants in mood disorders* (pp. 111–130). New York: Dekker.

McIntyre, R. S., Mancini, D. A., McCann, S., Srinivasan, J., Sagman, D., & Kennedy, S. H. (2002). Topiramate versus bupropion SR when added to mood stabilizer therapy for the depressive phase of bipolar disorder: A preliminary single-blind study. *Bipolar Disorders, 4,* 207–213.

Meltzer, H. Y., Alphs, L, Green, A. I., Altamura, A. C., Anand, R., Bertoldi, A., Bourgeois, M., Chouinard, G., Islam, M. Z., Kane, J., Krishnan, R., Lindenmayer, J. P., Potkin, S., & International Suicide Prevention Trial Study Group. (2003). Clozapine treatment for suicidality in schizophrenia: International Suicide Prevention Trial (InterSePT). *Archives of General Psychiatry, 60,* 82–91.

Mundo, E., Walker, M., Cate, T., Macciardi, F., & Kennedy, J. L. (2001). The role of serotonin transporter protein gene in antidepressant-induced mania in bipolar disorder: Preliminary findings. *Archives of General Psychiatry, 58,* 539–544.

Nemeroff, C. B., Evans, D. L., Gyulai, L., Sachs, G. S., Bowden, C. L., Gergel, I. P., Oakes, R., & Pitts, C. D. (2001). Double-blind, placebo-controlled comparison of imipramine and paroxetine in the treatment of bipolar depression. *American Journal of Psychiatry, 158,* 906–912.

Okuma, T., Inanaga, K., Otsuki, S., Sarai, K., Takahashi, R., Hazama, H., Mori, A., & Watanabe, M. (1979). Comparison of antimanic efficacy of carbamazepine and chlorpromazine: A double-blind controlled study. *Psychopharmacology, 66,* 211–217.

Pande, A. C., Crockatt, J. G., Janney, C. A., Werth, J. L., & Tsaroucha, G. (2000). Gabapentin in bipolar disorder—a placebo-controlled trial of adjunctive therapy: Gabapentin Bipolar Disorder Study Group. *Journal of Clinical Psychopharmacology, 2,* 249–225.

Pande, A. C., Davidson, J. R., Jefferson, J. W., Janney, C. A., Katzelnick, D. J., Weisler, R. H., Greist, J. H., & Sutherland, S. M. (1999). Treatment of social phobia with gabapentin: A placebo-controlled study. *Journal of Clinical Psychopharmacology, 19,* 341–348.

Pande, A. C., Pollack, M. H., Crockatt, J., Greiner, M., Chouinard, G., Lydiard, R. B., Taylor, C. B., Dager, S. R., & Shiovitz, T. (2000). Placebo-controlled study of gabapentin treatment of panic disorder. *Journal of Clinical Psychopharmacology, 20,* 467–471.

Paptheodorou, G., Kutcher, S. P., Katic, M., & Szalai, J. P. (1995). The efficacy and safety of divalproex sodium in the treatment of acute mania in adolescents and young adults: An open clinical trial. *Journal of Clinical Psychopharmacology, 15,* 110–116.

Peet, M. (1994). Induction of mania with selective serotonin reuptake inhibitors and tricyclic antidepressants. *British Journal of Psychiatry, 164,* 549–550.

Pope, H. G., Jr., McElroy, S. L., Keck, P. E., Jr., & Hudson, J. I. (1991). Valproate in the treatment of acute mania: A placebo-controlled study. *Archives of General Psychiatry, 48,* 62–68.

Post, R. M., Altshuler, L. L., Frye M. A., Suppes, T., Rush, A. J., Keck, P. E. Jr., McElroy, S. L., Denicoff, K. D., Leverich, G. S., Kupka, R., & Nolen, W. A. (2001). Rate of switch in bipolar patients prospectively treated with second-generation antidepressants as augmentation to mood stabilizers. *Bipolar Disorders, 3,* 259–265.

Post, R. M., Rubinow, D. R., & Ballenger, J. C. (1986). Conditioning and sensitization in the longitudinal course of affective illness. *British Journal of Psychiatry, 149,* 191–201.

Post, R. M., & Weiss, S. R. (1989). Sensitization, kindling, and anticonvulsants in mania. *Journal of Clinical Psychiatry, 50*(Suppl.), 23–30.

Prien, R. F., Caffey, E. M., Jr., & Klett, C. J. (1973). Prophylactic efficacy of lithium carbonate in manic–depressive illness: Report of the Veterans Administration and National Institute of Mental Health collaborative study group. *Archives of General Psychiatry, 28*, 337–341.

Sachs, G., Altshuler, L. L., Ketter, T., Suppes, T., Rasgon, N., Frye, M., & Collins, M. (2001, December). *Divalproex versus placebo for the treatment of bipolar depression*. Presented at the 40th Annual Meeting of the American College of Neuropsychopharmacology, Waikoloa, HI.

Sachs, G. S., Grossman, F., Ghaemi, S. N., Okamoto A., & Bowden, C. L. (2002). Combination of a mood stabilizer with risperidone or haloperidol for treatment of acute mania: A double-blind, placebo-controlled comparison of efficacy and safety. *American Journal of Psychiatry, 159*, 1146–1154.

Sachs, G. S., Lafer, B., Stoll, A. L., Banov, M., Thibault, A. B., Tohen, M., & Rosenbaum, J. F. (1994). A double-blind trial of bupropion versus desipramine for bipolar depression. *Journal of Clinical Psychiatry, 55*, 391–393.

Sachs, G. S., Mullen, J. A., Devine, N. A., et al. (2002, December). *Quetiapine versus placebo as adjunct to mood stabilizer for the treatment of acute bipolar mania*. Presented at the 41st Annual Meeting of the American College of Neuropsychopharmacology, San Juan, Puerto Rico.

Stahl, S. M., & Shelton, R. C. (2001, December). *Risperidone with and without paroxetine compared to paroxetine alone for bipolar depression*. Presented at the 40th Annual Meeting of the American College of Neuropsychopharmacology, Waikoloa, HI.

Stoll, A. L., Severus, W. E., Freeman, M. P., Rueter, S., Zboyan, H. A., Diamond, E., Cress, K. K., & Marangell, L. B. (1999). Omega-3 fatty acids in bipolar disorder: A preliminary double-blind, placebo-controlled trial. *Archives of General Psychiatry, 56*, 407–412.

Suppes, T., Swann, A. C., Dennehy, E. B., Habermacher, E. D., Mason, M., Crismon, M. L., Toprac, M. G., Rush, A. J., Shon, S. P., & Altshuler, K. Z. (2001). Texas Medication Algorithm Project: Development and feasibility testing of a treatment algorithm for patients with bipolar disorder. *Journal of Clinical Psychiatry, 62*, 439–447.

Suppes, T., Webb, A., Paul, B., Carmody, T., Kraemer, H., & Rush A. J. (1999). Clinical outcome in a randomized 1-year trial of clozapine versus treatment as usual for patients with treatment-resistant illness and a history of mania. *American Journal of Psychiatry, 156*, 1164–1169.

Swann, A. C. (1999). Treatment of aggression in patients with bipolar disorder. *Journal of Clinical Psychiatry, 60*(Suppl. 15), 25–28.

Swann, A. C, Bowden, C. L., Morris, D., Calabrese, J. R., Petty, F., Small, J., Dilsaver, S. C., & Davis, J. M. (1997). Depression during mania: Treatment response to lithium or divalproex. *Archives of General Psychiatry, 54*, 37–42.

Tohen, M., Baker, R. W., Altshuler, L. L., Zarate, C. A., Suppes, T., Ketter, T. A., Milton, D. R., Risser, R., Gilmore, J. A., Breier, A., & Tollefson, G. A. (2002). Olanzapine versus divalproex in the treatment of acute mania. *American Journal of Psychiatry, 159*, 1011–1017.

Tohen, M., Chengappa, K. N., Suppes, T., Zarate, C. A. Jr, Calabrese, J. R., Bowden, C. L., Sachs, G. S., Kupfer, D. J., Baker, R. W., Risser, R. C., Keeter, E. L., Feldman, P. D., Tollefson, G. D., & Breier, A. (2002). Efficacy of olanzapine in combination with valproate or lithium in the treatment of mania in patients partially nonresponsive to lithium or valproate monotherapy. *Archives of General Psychiatry, 59*, 62–69.

Tohen, M., Goldberg, J. F., Arillaga, A. M. G.-P., et al. (in press). A twelve-week double-blind comparison of olanzapine versus haloperidol in the treatment of acute mania. *Archives of General Psychiatry.*

Tohen, M., Jacobs, T. G., Grundy, S. L., McElroy, S. L., Banov, M. C., Janicak, P. G., Sanger, T., Risser, R., Zhang, F., Toma, V., Francis, J., Tollefson, G. D., & Breier A. (2000). Efficacy of olanzapine in acute bipolar mania—a double-blind, placebo-controlled study: The Olanzapine HGGW Study Group. *Archives of General Psychiatry, 57,* 841–849.

Tohen, M., Ketter, T. A., Zarate, C. A., Suppes, T., Frye, M., Altshuler, L., Zajecka, J., Schuh, L. M., Risser, R. C., Brown, E., & Baker, R. W. (2003). Olanzapine versus divalproex sodium for the treatment of acute mania and maintenance of remission: A 47-week study. *American Journal of Psychiatry, 160,* 1263–1271.

Tohen, M., Marneros, A., Bowden, C., Greil, W., Koukopoulos, A., Belmaker, H., Calabrese, J. R., Yatham, L. N., Jacobs, T., Baker, R. W., Williamson, D., Evans, A. R., Dossenbach, M., & Cassano, G. (2002, December). *Olanzapine versus lithium in relapse prevention in bipolar disorder: A randomized double-blind controlled 12-month clinical trial.* Presented at the 41st Annual Meeting of the American College of Neuropsychopharmacology, San Juan, Puerto Rico.

Tohen, M., Sanger, T. M., McElroy, S. L., Tollefson, G. D., Chengappa, K. N., Daniel, D. G., Petty, F., Centorrino, F., Wang, R., Grundy, S. L., Greaney, M. G., Jacobs, T. G., David S. R., & Toma, V. (1999). Olanzapine versus placebo in the treatment of acute mania: Olanzapine HGEH Study Group. *American Journal of Psychiatry, 156,* 702–709.

Tohen, M., Suppes, T., Baker, R. W., Risser, R. C., Evans, A. R., & Calabrese, J. R. (2002). Olanzapine combined with mood stabilizers in prevention of recurrence in bipolar disorder: An 18-month study. *Journal of European College of Neuropsychopharmacology, 12*(Suppl. 3), S307.

Tohen, M., Vieta, E., Calabrese, J., Ketter, T. A., Sachs, G., Bowden, C., Mitchell, P. B., Centorrino, F., Risser, R., Baker, R. W., Evans, A. R., Beymer, K., Dubé, S., Tollefson, G., & Breier, A. (in press). Efficacy of olanzapine and olanzapine/fluoxetine combination in the treatment of bipolar I depression. *Archives of General Psychiatry.*

Tondo, L., & Baldessarini, R. J. (2000). Reduced suicide risk during lithium maintenance treatment. *Journal of Clinical Psychiatry, 61*(Suppl. 9), 97–104.

Van Putten, T., & May, R. P. (1978). "Akinetic depression" in schizophrenia. *Archives of General Psychiatry, 35,* 1101–1107.

Vieta, E., Khanna, S., van Kammen, D., Lyons, B., Grossman, F., & Kramer, M. (2002, December). *Risperidone monotherapy in acute bipolar mania.* Presented at the 41st Annual Meeting of the American College of Neuropsychopharmacology, San Juan, Puerto Rico.

Vieta, E., Martinez-Aran, A., Goikolea, J. M., Torrent, C., Colom, F., Benabarre, A., & Reinares, M. (2002). A randomized trial comparing paroxetine and venlafaxine in the treatment of bipolar depressed patients taking mood stabilizers. *Journal of Clinical Psychiatry, 63,* 508–512.

Wehr, T. A., & Goodwin, F. K. (1987). Can antidepressants cause mania and worsen the course of affective illness? *American Journal of Psychiatry, 144,* 1403–1411.

Wehr, T. A., Sack, D. A., Rosenthal, N. E., & Cowdry, R. W.(1988). Rapid cycling affective disorder: Contributing factors and treatment responses in 51 patients. *American Journal of Psychiatry, 145,* 179–184.

Wisner, K. L., Peindl, K. S., Perel, J. M., Hanusa, B. H., Piontek, C. M., & Baab, S. (2002). Verapamil treatment for women with bipolar disorder. *Biological Psychiatry, 51,* 745–752.

Young, L. T., Joffe, R. T., Robb, J. C., MacQueen, G. M., Marriott, M., & Patelis-Siotis, I.(2000). Double-blind comparison of addition of a second mood stabilizer versus an antidepressant to an initial mood stabilizer for treatment of patients with bipolar depression. *American Journal of Psychiatry, 157,* 124–126.

Zajecka, J. M., Weisler, R., Sachs, G., Swann, A. C., Wozniak, P., & Sommerville, K. W.(2002). A comparison of the efficacy, safety, and tolerability of divalproex sodium and olanzapine in the treatment of bipolar disorder. *Journal of Clinical Psychiatry, 63,* 1148–1155.

CHAPTER SEVEN

COGNITIVE THERAPY

ROBERT L. LEAHY

The cognitive model of bipolar disorder focuses on the individual's phenomenological experience during the depressed and manic phases (Basco & Rush, 1996; Lam et al., 2000; Leahy, 1999, 2003; Leahy & Beck, 1988; Newman, Leahy, Beck, Reilly-Harrington, & Gyulai, 2002), with considerable empirical support for the model of depression (Clark, Beck, & Alford, 1999). According to this model, the physiological predisposition for bipolar disorder interacts with life events and coping abilities that are moderated by cognitive "styles" that confer vulnerability. Thus, the genetic predisposition for bipolar illness may be catalyzed by negative or positive events that are filtered through the individual's cognitive schemas (see Chapters 2 and 5, this volume). These cognitive schemas are reflected in the content and structure of the automatic thoughts and maladaptive assumptions that characterize either the depressed or manic phase (Lam et al., 2000; Leahy & Beck, 1988).

In this chapter I outline the characteristic cognitive content of depressed and manic thinking, review general treatment strategies for addressing both the depressed and manic phases, and provide a case example of the treatment of a bipolar individual. The treatment of bipolar individuals requires flexibility, strategic planning, awareness of comorbidity, the ability to handle crises as they occur, appropriate skills in the treatment of depression—with suicidal risk—and mania—with its risk-taking behavior and severe anger—in addition to skills in the treatment of substance abuse, family conflict, and nonadherence with medication regimens (Chapter 1, this volume; Freeman, Freeman, & McElroy, 2002; Goldberg, 2001; Suppes & Dennehy, 2002; Vieta et al., 2001).

AUTOMATIC THOUGHTS

The content of the cognitive schemas differs with mood: anxiety (threat and danger), anger (humiliation and domination), depression (loss and deprivation), and mania (extraordinary competence and opportunity). At the most immediate level are the automatic thoughts: These are thoughts that come spontaneously, appear plausible, and have a high probability of being associated with dysfunction. Depressed and manic individuals share similar cognitive distortions, except in the former the distortions are biased toward the negative, whereas in the latter they are biased toward the positive. For example, the depressed individual goes to a party and is flooded with negative thoughts: "I'll get rejected" (fortune telling), "I'm ugly" (labeling), "They think I'm a loser" (mind reading), "I never get along with people" (all-or-nothing thinking), and "I'm a loser at everything I do" (overgeneralizing). In contrast, the manic individual goes to the same party and is flooded with excessively positive thoughts: "I'll impress everyone" (fortune telling), "I'm beautiful and sexy" (labeling), "They think I'm a movie star" (mind reading), "I always get my way with people" (all-or-nothing thinking), and "Since someone said hello to me, I must be on a roll and everyone will love me" (overgeneralizing). Examples of typical automatic thought distortions in depression and mania are listed in Table 7.1.

Maladaptive Assumptions

Automatic thoughts are filtered through the individual's maladaptive assumptions, which are imperatives or rules that are rigid, unrealistic, and applied regardless of apparent consequences. For example, the depressive assumption "I should be successful at everything" is applied regardless of how difficult the task may be. Similarly, the imperative manic assumption "I should pursue every opportunity" is inflexibly applied, regardless of

TABLE 7.1. Automatic Thoughts in Depression and Mania

Cognitive distortion	Depression	Mania
Fortune telling	"I'll get rejected."	"Everyone will adore me."
Mind reading	"He thinks I'm a loser."	"He thinks I'm a genius."
Labeling	"I'm a loser."	"I'm a genius."
Discounting (positives/negatives)	"Anyone would have done well on that exam."	"Failing the exam means nothing."
Exaggerating outcomes	"It's awful not to do well."	"It's incredibly great that I did that."
Emotional reasoning	"I feel bad; therefore, everything is awful."	"I feel great; therefore, everything is great."

the possible risks entailed. Returning to the party example, the depressed person believes, "If one person doesn't like me, then I must be a loser" and "If people aren't enthusiastic about me, then that means they don't like me." This erroneous thinking may be followed by other assumptions, such as "I should avoid any possibilities of rejection" and "I should immediately escape from situations where people don't like me." In contrast to the depressive assumptions that reflect themes of inevitable rejection and loss, the manic assumptions emphasize unlimited opportunity, excitement, and boundless competence. These assumptions might include "If I feel it can work out, it will work out," "I should and I will be able to make anything a success," "Rejection and failure have no consequence for me, since I can absorb anything," and "If I feel I'm irresistible, then I must be irresistible."

Personal Schemas

These automatic thoughts and assumptions further support the underlying personal schema of the depressed or manic individual, reaffirming (in the person's mind) that he or she is indeed worthless and unlovable. The depressed individual who engages in mind reading—for example, "He thinks I'm a loser"—and who holds the assumption "If someone doesn't like me, then I must be a loser," will believe that his or her pessimism is repeatedly reinforced: "I went to a party; I know Bill thought I was a loser; therefore, my belief that I am a loser is confirmed." In contrast, the manic individual may find his or her overly positive thoughts and assumptions reaffirming his or her overly positive view of self: "I went to the party; Bill looked in my direction; he must think I'm a genius; his response proves what I've always thought—I'm a genius."

In the depressive phase, the personal schema is activated, along with the maladaptive assumptions and automatic thoughts, and the negative polarity and content of the ensuing cognitions are pervasive. In contrast, during the manic phase, the individual's schemas are polarized to the opposite extreme. Thus, the individual may view him- or herself as competent, strong, free of responsibility, and superior. It has been proposed that the schemas of these individuals alternate in polarity, such that the individual who believes he or she has no creative ideas when depressed will believe that he or she is the most creative genius in the world when manic (Leahy, 1999, 2000; Leahy & Beck, 1988; Newman et al., 2002).

The depressed individual, weighed down by his or her negative automatic thoughts, will engage in behavioral and interpersonal strategies to "cope" with all the negative beliefs. For example, he or she will leave parties or avoid them entirely in order to reduce the possibility of rejection. When interacting with others, he or she may attempt to compensate for his or her perceived unworthiness by remaining silent, casting his or her eyes downwards, or not asserting him- or herself. The result of these behavioral and interpersonal strategies is that others will find the person boring or rude and will avoid him or her, thereby reinforcing the belief that he or she is unlovable and worthless.

In contrast to the depressed individual, the manic individual, whose automatic thoughts are unduly positive, may misread the politeness of others as a "sure sign" that they are enthralled with everything he or she says. This misinterpretation results in behavioral and interpersonal strategies that may alienate others. For example, he or she might pace the room, gesticulating wildly, probably drinking heavily, in order to heighten his or her euphoric mood. He or she might speak too loudly—in order to impress people with the brilliance of his or her ideas. His or her interpersonal behavior might be provocative or aggressive, as he or she believes that he or she is sexually irresistible, always right in his or her opinion, and should always have things his or her way.

Whereas the depressed individual attempts to *compensate* for his or her perceived inadequacy and avoid being challenged, the manic individual attempts to *augment* his or her perceived superiority and seek out opportunities for self-aggrandizement. The depressed individual may act as if he or she is socially phobic—that is, he or she might avoid interactions with people. This person might attempt to compensate for the perceived inferiority by deferring to others, or, if he or she does interact with someone, it is likely to be the least attractive and appealing person, reflecting the belief that no one would want him or her. In contrast, the manic individual augments his or her behavior and seeks out greater opportunities with greater risk. Far from approaching others with downcast eyes, he or she elevates his or her voice, sings, laughs hysterically at his or her own jokes, and appears sexually provocative. Far from employing an avoidance strategy, the manic individual seeks out greater opportunities, approaching strangers with inappropriate propositions or challenging anyone who disagrees with him or her. Whereas the depressed individual takes on the role of submission, the manic individual attempts to dominate. This polarity reflects the contrast between depressive avoidance of further loss and manic pursuit of unlimited opportunity.

Comparisons of automatic thoughts, assumptions, schemas, and compensatory and augmentation strategies are shown in Tables 7.1, 7.2, 7.3, and 7.4. Although manic and depressive thinking appear to be diametrically opposed, there are structural similarities (Leahy, 1999; Leahy & Beck, 1988; Newman et al., 2002):

- Selective filtering and evaluation of information
- Exaggerated sense of personal causation
- Lack of differentiation
- Dependence on thoughts that are a reaction to emotion

TABLE 7.2. Maladaptive Assumptions in Depression and Mania

Depression	Mania
"If someone doesn't like you, it means you're worthless."	"If someone likes you, it means the whole world loves you."
"If you fail at something, you're a total failure."	"If you succeed at anything, you're the world's greatest success."
"It's terrible to make a mistake."	"It's terrible to miss an opportunity."

- Inferential leaps beyond the information available in the particular context
- Tendency to mislabel and overgeneralize
- Overuse of faulty inductive reasoning

In addition, bipolar individuals have overgeneral biographical recall and poorer problem-solving skills (Scott, Stanton, Garland, & Ferrier, 2000).

COGNITIVE THERAPY OF BIPOLAR DISORDER

Although I present a general plan of treatment, the specific sequencing and priorities depend on the "phase" presented in the initial contact with the patient. Given the considerable range of moods and problems that the patient may present, the initial treatment focus may need to address especially pressing concerns, such as reducing suicidal risk, obtaining patient's participation in substance abuse treatment, control of aggressive behavior, or medication nonadherence. Nonetheless, the outline presented in Table 7.5 may help clinicians organize their treatment framework when working with the bipolar patient.

TABLE 7.3. Compensatory and Augmentation Rules in Depression and Mania

Depression	Mania
Avoid conflict.	Tell everyone what to do.
Avoid rejection.	Approach everyone.
Avoid failure.	Pursue all opportunities.
Conserve energy.	Increase energy.
Quit before it's too late.	Persist, no matter what.
Keep yourself in line.	Do whatever you want.

TABLE 7.4. Personal Schemas in Depression and Mania

Depression	Mania
Ugly	Beautiful
Failure	Incredibly successful
No ability	Omnipotent
Don't know anything	Know everything

Preliminary Considerations

The treatment of depression for bipolar disorder follows many of the guidelines for cognitive therapy of unipolar depression (Beck, Rush, Shaw, & Emery, 1979; Leahy & Holland, 2000). Because of space limitations, the focus in this chapter is primarily on the treatment of the manic phase. Table 7.5 provides general guidelines for the treatment of the depressive phase. Table 7.6 provides examples of cognitive disputations that are useful for self-critical and hopeless thoughts typically exhibited by bipolar individuals.

The emphasis here is on treating patients with mania when they are euthymic—that is, between episodes and not mood-symptomatic. However, in the real world of clinical practice, the therapist often first meets the patient when he or she is dramatically symptomatic. Once the manic phase is activated, it may be difficult to implement these interventions, unless the patient and therapist have arrived at a case conceptualization and plan of treatment prior to the episode. A hallmark of mania is the associated lack of insight and the perception that one does not need help. Consequently, in the euthymic phase, it is useful to review previous manic phases ("What can be learned?") and plan how to minimize the risk for future manic phases.

Case Conceptualization

A central component of the treatment of mania is adherence to a medication regimen. The overall treatment approach might be explained, as follows: "This is an illness—a chronic illness—for which you need continued treatment. Our treatment efforts will focus on the management of the illness through medication and therapy. Medication will help reduce mood fluctuations, and therapy will help you manage the moods if they occur." Patients are asked if, during the manic phase, they recall believing that they had unlimited resources and would be able to achieve unlimited benefits in the future. Their beliefs that they can predict with certainty, control all outcomes, and act without costs are also examined. Their love of risk, during the manic phase, and the specific risks pursued are also evaluated. Their overemphasis on their high energy and enthusiasm as "proof" that their

TABLE 7.5. General Plan of Treatment

Conduct initial evaluation.
Consult with family and significant individuals in patient's life.
Socialize the patient to the treatment process.
Interventions: Depression
  Reducing suicidal risk
  Overcoming hopelessness
  Monitoring mood
  Cost–benefit analysis of mood/behavior
  Implementing behavioral activation
  Eliciting and modifying cognitive distortions
  Inoculating against future depressive thinking
Interventions: Mania
  Evaluating current risk behaviors
  Evaluating previous manic episodes: What can be learned?
    Individual symptom patterns
    Event triggers
    Lack of insight during episode
  Conducting cost–benefit of mania
    Short-term versus long-term consequences
    How others view consequences
    Review prior regrets
  Precommitment strategies
  Activity scheduling
  Self-calming and relaxation technique
  Reduced opportunity
  Delaying and distracting
    Reminders—cue cards
    Distraction strategies
    48-hour rule
    Three-person rule
  Inoculating against future manic thinking

boundless motivation will lead to positive outcomes is identified. Their sense of urgency and rejection of disappointment or regret, during the manic phases, are also evaluated in terms of the costs and benefits. Underlying schemas of control, entitlement, competence, and/or sexual gratification are examined, as these relate to risks encountered during the manic phase.

Precommitment Strategies

All of us recognize that there are certain temptations we cannot resist. If we try to resist once the tempting stimulus is in front of us, then we are lost—and we know it. For example, some people have part of their salary automatically transferred to a savings account because they know that they will spend it if they have it. Others demonstrate a precommitment to avoid

TABLE 7.6. Challenging Depressive Cognitive Distortions Related to
Bipolar Disorder

Automatic thought	Distortion	Rational response
"My moods will never be stable."	Dichotomous thinking Overgeneralizing Fortune telling	"Once I am on a mood stabilizer, I will have relatively more stable moods. No one has the same neutral mood all the time."
"I will never be able to control my moods."	Fortune telling Dichotomous thinking	" 'Control' is an all-or-nothing term. I might be able to have a lot more control over my moods, but no human being has total control. I can keep a record and see if my moods vary less now that I am getting the proper treatment."
"I am just a bipolar 'nut.' "	Dichotomous thinking Mislabeling Discounting positives	"I can think of my problem as a specific vulnerability. I have many qualities in addition to my mood fluctuations. Half of the population has a history of a mental illness. Everyone has some specific problems. There are many talented and interesting people who have bipolar disorder. I <u>have</u> bipolar disorder—"<u>I am not 'bipolar disorder.'</u> "
"People will look at me and think, 'He's bipolar. Stay away.' "	Mind reading Fortune telling	"I don't know what people are thinking. Most people will never know. Many people will see this disorder as only one part of me. In a sense, for those people who know me, this is really nothing new—they already know me."
"I will never be able to have a life."	Fortune telling Dichotomous thinking	"Having problems is one part of everyone's life. I have had a life so far—in fact, my life could be better now that I know what the problem is and can get the proper treatment. Millions of people have bipolar disorder and tens of millions of people have other problems. They all have lives."

temptation by avoiding the problematic environment or substance—the liquor, drugs, or high-calorie pastry. Precommitment simply reflects our recognition of our all-too-human weakness to act myopically in response to our emotions and appetites. It is helpful to point out to bipolar patients that, during a manic phase, several internal and behavioral shifts occur— there is an increased sense of empowerment, increased risk-taking behavior, decreased insight and awareness of the disorder, and increased sense of urgency— which can be modified and even contained by thoughtful precommitment strategies.

For excessive spending, the patient's precommitment statement might read: "I will do a mood check daily for any manic symptoms. If I detect more than three manic symptoms, then I will leave the credit cards with my husband, I won't go to the mall, won't spend more than $100 without first reviewing it with my husband, and I'll wait 24 hours after 2 nights of good sleep before shopping" (see Newman et al., 2002, for detailed descriptions of these self-control strategies). For patients with other manic outlets, precommitment strategies might include promising not to drive, not to call prostitutes, or to review unconventional decisions with the therapist and two friends before taking any action. The therapist and patient can refer back to the precommitment agreement when the patient enters a manic phase. Having said that, it must be added that although this strategy may be a desirable approach, it does not always work!

INOCULATION AGAINST DISTORTED MANIC THINKING

During the calmer euthymic phase, the therapist can examine the patient's idiosyncratic symptoms of mania, as noted in the case conceptualization shown in Table 7.5. The therapist and patient can weigh the costs and benefits of acting out manic impulses and the consequences of prior manic episodes. The patient's specific cognitive distortions used to justify the acting-out behavior, illusions of unlimited resources and power, emotional rationalizations, time urgency, and selective focus on, and exaggeration of, the positive can be identified. These rationalizing perspectives can be recorded on flash cards in the office and reviewed daily by the patient.

As indicated, manic cognition is polarized toward the positive extreme, which usually (always?) means ignoring real risks. The goal in the inoculation stage is finding the normative middle, located somewhere between the poles of unlimited power and unrelenting failure. I refer to this position as the "normative middle" in order to shift the patient's attention away from extreme, rigid, and emotionally laden cognition. Finding the normative middle recognizes (1) differentiation (e.g., "I'm not entirely power*ful* or power*less*"), (2) independence of events (e.g., "My success (or failure) on this one task will not necessarily generalize to all other tasks"), and (3) distribution of causal forces ("It's not entirely my fault or entirely my credit"). The goal of the inoculation phase is to encourage patients to avoid the belief that they are either superior or inferior to the norm.

Inoculation entails active role-plays in which the therapist alternates between enacting the tempting and energizing distortions of mania and the tempering rational response. The patient plays the alternative. Thus, the therapist can "bait" the patient with luring assertions of unlimited abilities, assets, and the risks/thrills awaiting him or her, while the patient disputes these distortions:

THERAPIST: Let's imagine that you're feeling manic. You've slept 2 hours a night for the past 2 nights, you feel wired and irritable, and you want to go to the mall. I'll present the manic position: "You have a tremendous amount of money. Just go to the mall and buy whatever you want."

PATIENT: I don't have a lot of money. I'll regret it.

THERAPIST: You're manic, you don't regret anything.

PATIENT: I'll come out of the manic mood, then I'll get depressed about what I've spent.

THERAPIST: But you feel invincible. Just go with your feelings.

PATIENT: When I'm manic, my feelings are a poor guide.

THERAPIST: You've got to have those things now!

PATIENT: No, I can wait. The mood will pass. Then I won't want them.

DEVELOPING REALISTIC DECISION PROCESSES

The overly positive valence of the manic pole results in an exaggeration of resources, predictability, and control, and an indifference to regret and decreased need for information. Specific interventions for varieties of high-risk thinking are shown in Table 7.7. Given the overly optimistic, opportunity-driven thinking of the individual in a manic phase, we can see that the clinical task is to focus the patient on the following realizations:

- Your current resources are limited—what are they?
- Your future resources—especially in the near future—are also limited. What are they?
- You think that you can predict the future. How wrong have you been in the past about your predictions?

- You think that you can control events. How wrong have you been in the past about your ability to control outcomes?
- When you are manic, you think that risk is low. But what has really happened when you did risky things in the past? Are there even worse things that could have happened, but you were lucky to avoid them?
- You have thought that things that you achieved, bought, or consumed were going to be terrific. How valuable were they—in reality? Now that you are not in a manic phase, do you think those things were worth the risk or price you paid?
- You thought you could just keep going, that nothing could stop you. In reality, have you learned that you do not have unlimited energy or time to make things work out?
- You often think, when you are in a manic phase, that you have an unlimited range of different resources and rewards in your life. In reality, have the losses you experienced when you were in a manic phase had a negative impact on you?

CASE STUDY

Initial Interview

Susan called the office and indicated to the intake coordinator that she needed help because she was a "compulsive shopper." She had spent thousands of dollars during shopping sprees, and now she and her husband had to file for bankruptcy. The therapist noted from her remarks that Susan often had periods when she needed almost no sleep and that she had racing thoughts. Like many patients with bipolar disorder, Susan's initial presentation revealed that she had no idea what could be wrong with her. She indicated that she was a 30-year-old woman married, with a 5-month-old daughter, and that she wanted help with her impulsivity and regret. Her score on the Beck Depression Inventory was 29 and on the Beck Anxiety Inventory, 26. She showed indications of some dependent, avoidant, obsessive–compulsive, and histrionic traits on the SCID-II.

Susan reported that during her shopping sprees, she often felt empowered, terrific, attractive, and smarter than other people. She reported decreased need for sleep, boundless energy, a pressure to talk, and increased sociability. There were no identifiable triggers, and she was not using drugs or alcohol. She had a long history of frequent manic episodes, beginning in college, that focused on drinking, partying, impulsive travel, and overspending. These sprees were followed by periods of depression and then by 2 weeks to a month of euthymia. The depressed and manic phases each lasted about 2 to 3 weeks. Since the birth of her baby, she had not gone on any shopping sprees.

TABLE 7.7. Specific Problem Areas in Mania

Manic cognition	Questions to reduce manic cognitions
"She likes me. She went nuts over me."	"Is it possible that she was just being friendly? What are the consequences to you if you overestimate how much she likes you? Why not wait a while to see what she really feels?"
"I'll succeed—everything I touch turns to gold."	"Is it possible that you might not do as well as you think? What could the consequences be if you did fail? Would you be able to absorb the loss?"
"It's terrific. It's the most terrific opportunity of a lifetime."	"Does everyone else seem to think it's terrific? Why not ask five people if they think it's as great as you think it is? Have you had these thoughts about how terrific things are and found our later, when you are not manic, that things were not terrific?"
"I'm a genius."	"You may be very smart, but what does it imply to think that you are a 'genius' ? Are there some areas in which you are not a genius? Do you think you have special powers of thought? Do you think that others share this view of you? Why don't they?"
"My losses don't matter— I can handle them."	"Have you had these thoughts before and found that the costs were more than you could bear?"
"Look at all the people who love me the moment they meet me."	"Could you be misreading things? When you say that they 'love you,' could it really be that they are simply polite or that they like you? If you think they love you, are you more likely to say or do something provocative?"
"This always happens to me—I succeed at everything."	"When you have come out of your manic phases, have you found that some things did not go as well?"
"Everyone loves me."	"What are the consequences of being wrong about how people respond to you? Do you always feel this way— even when you're not manic? Could you be misinterpreting how people really think and feel? What actions would you take, based on this thinking? Would you be willing to refrain from taking any action for a while?"
"I feel great. I have a hunch I'll really excel."	"*Feeling great* and *doing well* are not always the same thing. Could you be using emotional reasoning and overly positive prediction? Does everyone else agree with you, or do some people think that you are exaggerating?"

(continued)

"I should never pass up an opportunity."	"Why not? What would happen if you did? If you pursue everything, do you run the risk of doing nothing well? Of overextending yourself?"
"The relationship ended. It was entirely his/her fault."	"What is the consequence of believing this one-sided view? Is this an overgeneralized thought? Could it be that both of you share some of the blame?"
"I'm more successful than they are."	"Perhaps on some things, but on everything? Is it possible that you are overestimating your success and that you might overextend yourself as a result?"
"There's no sense in regretting anything. It doesn't matter."	"What will happen when you come out of your manic state? Will you run the risk of regretting some of these things? Will this lack of regret have a negative effect on other people?"
"What if I'm an incredible success?"	"It could happen, but has it happened before? Have you had this thought when you were manic before, but things turned out not to be as successful or as great as you thought?"
"I did great. I'm terrific. Nobody comes even close!"	"You may be a good person, and you may have had some success, but is it possible that it is just 'OK' and not 'terrific'? Do other people think that what you did is the greatest thing in the world? Why do their opinions differ from yours?"

Diagnosis

Susan was told that she had bipolar disorder. The therapist photocopied the DSM-IV criteria for manic episode and bipolar disorder. She and the therapist reviewed each of the symptoms of mania and the criteria for bipolar disorder. She was told that she had a rapid-cycling variation, with several episodes each year. Given the possibility that the personality dimensions on the SCID-II might be affected by the Axis I diagnosis of bipolar disorder, the Axis II diagnosis was deferred. As the bipolar disorder was stabilized, the Axis II diagnosis was discounted. Her apparent histrionic and obsessive–compulsive traits seemed more attributable to mood instability than to a true personality disorder. (This example underscores the importance of deferring diagnosis for personality disorder until the bipolar disorder can be treated.)

Socialization to Treatment

Concurrent with providing her with the diagnosis, Susan was told that bipolar disorder is a biological illness that is largely inherited, but which can be treated with a combination of medication and cognitive therapy. The therapist indicated that it was a chronic, lifelong illness, similar to diabetes or essential hypertension. And as is the case with other systemic disorders, if left untreated, serious negative effects could ensue. However, if treated, many of these negative effects could be lessened and some normalcy might be restored to her life.

As a result of the chronicity of this disorder, she would need to take medication for the rest of her life. The medication had a good chance of reducing the frequency, intensity, and duration of manic as well as depressive episodes, but she should not expect a "100%" cure. Discontinuing the medication might result in a "breakthrough" episode. She was told that earlier episodes in her life might have been triggered by stressful events, but that the later episodes might have simply "started on their own." Consequently, it was important for her to be an active participant in her treatment. This active participation would require her learning how to monitor her manic and depressed moods and identifying what precommitment strategies would be appropriate.

Periods of mood swings and regret over prior acting out were related to the episodic nature of bipolar disorder. Her alcohol abuse when younger was explained as her attempt to self-medicate her manic moods with the depressant effects of alcohol. When Susan understood the nature of bipolar disorder, she began to believe that her mother, who was divorced from her father, also had bipolar disorder. She recalled that her mother indulged in extravagant shopping sprees and had severe mood swings, coupled with agitation, euphoria, and depression.

At first, Susan was skeptical of the diagnosis. She was encouraged to "surf" Internet websites on bipolar illness to see if she had anything in common with the people who described the illness and their experiences with it. When she read the material on these Websites and observed the "chat rooms," she was struck by the similarities between herself and many of the people. She was also somewhat relieved to find out that she was not as badly off as some of these people. Susan also was asked to read the *Feeling Good Handbook* (Burns, 1989) and Jamison's *Unquiet Mind* (1997), and she was encouraged to continue doing searches on the Internet regarding bipolar illness. Susan's husband and her father arranged separate consultations with the psychopharmacologist, who gave them a detailed description of bipolar illness.

Medication

As noted, Susan was referred to a psychopharmacologist, who concurred with the diagnosis of bipolar disorder and reinforced the need for combined treatment. Because she was entering treatment in a depressed phase, she was started on lithium and Paxil. Three weeks later, the Paxil was discontinued because of emerging hypomanic symptoms. The necessity to comply with all medication requirements was carefully stressed. Both the therapist and the psychopharmacologist explained the chronic, systemic nature of the bipolar illness. The therapist indicated that, even though she might be feeling better, the medication was necessary for ongoing treatment of the illness. The medication would serve a prophylactic function, preventing many future episodes of manic–depression. The therapist also indicated that the medication was no guarantee against some mood variations and even a possibility of breakthrough episodes of mania and depression. Because of the likelihood of mood variation, it would be important for Susan to take an active role in her treatment, including monitoring both manic and depressed moods, developing self-help techniques for handling these moods, and informing her doctor of the need to readjust the medication. She was told that certain medications could be added for the treatment of manic moods and other medications could be added for the treatment of depressed moods.

Self-Monitoring

Two weeks after the intake, Susan noted that she had experienced some hypomanic symptoms over the prior week. These included feeling hot, agitated, and overly energetic. In session, she developed her own mood checklist for mania and hypomania, which she was to keep on her refrigerator door, and about which she was to tell her husband. She listed the following: "Sweating, feeling overheated, increased, rapid movement, more talkative, shifting topics, talking rapidly, nervous, upset stomach, loss of appetite, thirsty, less need for sleep (3–4 hours), energized, grandiose, feeling like I have unlimited assets, desire to shop, and overly generous."

In addition to monitoring her mood for manic symptoms, Susan developed a checklist for signs of depression. She listed the following: "Unhappy, feeling something is hanging over my head, hopelessness, thoughts of suicide, negative thoughts, loss of energy, self-critical, avoidance, sleeping too much (10 hours or more), indecisive, no interest in things or people, lower pleasure, lowered sex drive, eating less, wearing dark colors, guilt and regret."

Evaluating and Modifying Guilt

Susan indicated that she felt extremely guilty about her past behavior. She had lied to her husband, father, and friends. She had written checks and used credit cards, with no money or credit to cover these debts. Along with filing for bankruptcy, she had been charged with a felony related to her check-cashing practices. Even though no one (except her) had lost any money, she was sure that she had ruined her life and her marriage. She recalled that during one manic phase she had purchased $50,000 worth of gems on her AMEX card, believing that she really had the money. The total amount of bounced checks and bad credit exceeded $200,000. She had forged a check once, believing that she actually had the money to cover the debt. As a result of these behaviors, she was being prosecuted for a felony.

Susan was encouraged to translate regret and self-criticism into "self-correction" and "what I have learned." For example, rather than criticize herself for her manic behavior, she was encouraged to examine what she had been learning in treatment (i.e., the biological basis of bipolar illness, the availability of medication and therapy). She considered how the bankruptcy and marital conflict that resulted from her overspending could be helpful in motivating her to continue with her self-help therapy and with compliance with medication.

Susan developed a self-defense statement to handle her self-criticism:

- "Manic–depression is a biological disorder that you inherit and that you did not ask for."
- "Manic–depression can be successfully treated, and you are doing so."
- "Manic–depression is part of who you are and is nothing to be ashamed of."
- "Manic–depression affects millions of people, including some of the most successful artists and business people in history."
- "You were ill when you did things that hurt other people. Now you are getting better."

Hopelessness

Like many bipolar patients, Susan had feelings of hopelessness and suicidal ideation. Her thoughts of hopelessness included the beliefs that "I won't feel better," "I'm a terrible person," "Because I feel badly now, my life must be terrible," and "I've ruined my marriage, and my husband will never forgive me." We developed a checklist of rational responses that included the following:

- "I have lots of things to look forward to . . . my baby, traveling to Europe, scuba diving, surfing. I've seen myself come out of depressive moods before. Medication might help me. Being bipolar means that you change."
- "I'm not a terrible person. I inherited bipolar illness. I didn't mean to hurt anyone. I'm taking my medication in order to get

better. I'm actually a thoughtful and considerate person. I wouldn't blame someone else for her illness."

- "Just because I feel badly doesn't mean anything about the way things have to be. My life isn't so bad right now. My daughter is healthy. I'm getting the help I need from my doctors and from medication. My husband and some of my friends understand what happened to me."

Suicidal Risk

Even though she was not actively suicidal when she entered therapy, and even though there was no history of suicidal behavior in the past, it was essential to address any risk of suicide in the event of a depressive shift. We examined the costs and benefits of living—especially after she was stabilized on medication. The advantage in addressing this issue was that the treatment itself provided hope of a better life—since she had received no treatment prior to this time. We also examined the costs and benefits for her husband and daughter of her living. Susan realized that her daughter would need her—and, despite the strain on her marriage, that her husband did love her and did need her. The therapist role-played the suicidal thoughts, and Susan was able to defend her reasons for living. In addition, Susan agreed to call both her therapist and her psychopharmacologist in the event of any strong suicidal ideation.

Self-Control for Mania

In order to develop a self-control method of dealing with the mania, Susan was encouraged to create flash cards containing instructions that she would keep near her mood checklist for mania. She was urged to discuss the instructions with her husband. These included the following:

- Self-monitor any signs of mania. If more than three symptoms appear, use these techniques; even if there are not three symptoms, think about these techniques anyway.
- List the costs and benefits of spending money NOW.
- List the costs and benefits of spending money 2 days from now.
- Discuss any spending more than $100 with husband or therapist.
- Use distraction: relaxation, warm baths, reading, playing with daughter, exercising, housecleaning, and watching TV.

We focused on her temptation to shop by examining the costs and benefits of going to the mall and spending a lot of money. The benefits were that "it's exciting, fast-paced, stimulating, and I can feel powerful and rich." The costs were that "it led to higher bills—which had led to bankruptcy, my husband was angry, I regretted it later, and this would aggravate the mania." The therapist role-played the manic thoughts, while Susan played the role of rational responding. She was encouraged to review these therapy notes when she felt the urge to go on a spending spree. In addition, the therapist role-played "self-help resistance"—for example: "Don't bother to look at those boring flash cards. You deserve a spending spree. Your therapist is uptight and rigid. You don't have to do anything he tells you to do. Just go ahead and spend as much as you want." Susan then engaged the rational response role and verbalized the reasons these thoughts were fallacious and self-destructive.

After 3 months, Susan's moods began to stabilize, although she occasionally experienced some hypomania and some days on which she felt down. Up to this point she and her husband had agreed that she was not to go to the shopping mall with her credit card, lest she begin another shopping spree. We examined the pros and cons of experimenting with "controlled spending"—that is, going to the mall with a set limit on shopping. Susan concluded that this would be helpful in making her feel that she was more normal and that both she and her husband could "trust" her behavior again. She agreed to a plan that required her to do a mood check for mania (if she had more than two symptoms, she agreed to avoid the mall). We developed a flash card that identified her manic spending thoughts: "Just go out and spend as much as you want to. It'll feel good." Susan then referred to her flash card that identified the costs of manic spending: "Hurts marriage. Hurts parenting. Causes financial distress. Causes legal problems. Causes other people to suffer." We also examined how she would feel after going to the mall and spending very little or nothing. She indicated that she would feel proud of herself and that she was in control. The exposure to controlled spending worked: She went to the mall, shopped around at different stores, and decided to buy a pair of shoes for $78.

Behavioral Interventions for Depression

Given her initial depressive episodes, we focused on activity scheduling and graded task assignments. She indicated it was hard to get out bed and difficult to get motivated to do anything during the day. Her inactivity thoughts were "It's hard to push myself" and "I can't do it, I don't have the energy." We examined the costs and benefits of staying in bed. The benefits included "conserving energy, don't have to push myself, it's too hard," whereas the costs included "prolong feeling depressed, don't get anything done, nothing changes."

Susan constructed a "reward menu" of past and possibly current rewards that she could pursue when she was feeling down. Her reward menu included thoughts and images of her husband, her daughter, scuba diving in Australia, ballooning in Italy, and friends whom she cherished.

Her "assigned activity" list included exercising, walking the dog, watching George Carlin and Robin Williams' movies, calling a friend, looking at her wedding photo album, and looking at pictures of her daughter on her first and second birthdays. She kept this list next to her refrigerator list of mood checks.

In addition to these positive behaviors, Susan was instructed in the value of "self-reward." This form of reinforcement included emphasizing positive statements about herself for getting the right help, keeping track of her moods, practicing positive behaviors, challenging her negative thoughts, and working collaboratively with her doctors. In addition, she was encouraged to remind herself of the fact that she was basically a very honest and decent person who was trying to help herself. Finally, to augment self-reward, she was asked to think of the supportive things she would say to a friend with the same problem.

Family Interventions

During the first few weeks of treatment, Susan felt the need to contact her mother, whom she had not seen in 12 years. Susan believed that her mother also suffered from untreated bipolar disorder. When Susan was 16 her parents had separated, after conflicts involving her mother's overspending, forgery, and driving around aimlessly for hours. Her mother alternated between "normality" and intense alcohol abuse. Unfortunately, her attempt to contact her mother resulted in frustration for Susan, because her mother had very little interest in speaking with her daughter. Susan's relationship with her father also was problematic. He was a successful businessperson, with a controlling, no-nonsense approach to relationships. Susan's psychopharmacologist spoke with him about the nature of her illness. His response was, "I'm glad it's not something I did in raising her." He also indicated that her mother's behavior now made more sense to him. He continued to invalidate Susan, however, often criticizing her or speaking to her sarcastically. He would say, "You're damaged goods. I got rooked when it came to children. You're stupid." We examined her automatic thoughts when her father acted this way: "He'll make me miserable. He doesn't value me. He doesn't care about me. I need my father's approval." We examined the advantages and disadvantages of "needing Father's approval," and she concluded that she would be better off accepting the possibility that she could not get his approval: "It's more important that I have approval from myself." She also recognized that she received approval from other people in her life and that the reason her father was so critical and invalidating had more to do with him than with her. Finally, Susan was encouraged to establish clear guidelines for conversations with Dad. She wrote—and told her father—the following: "If you are critical or verbally abusive with me, then our conversation will be ended. I'll hang up. If you are visiting me, and you are verbally abusive, then you will have to leave immediately." Her father listened to this assertion in silence, but his verbally hostile behavior declined.

Susan's relationship with Tom, her husband, was dramatically affected by her bipolar disorder. Both of them had been working hard to develop some financial security, which had been devastated by the bankruptcy. Understandably, even after Tom had spoken with her psychopharmacologist, both of them worried about her ability to control her spending in the future. Much to his credit, Tom was quite open to learning more about Susan's illness, but it activated thoughts about his own financial position: "Other people I know have more money than I do. They're further ahead." Furthermore, Tom began to worry about Susan's business pursuits, which she began about 1 year after starting treatment: "Is she becoming manic again?" This led Susan to feel that he was overcontrolling and distrustful.

Tom's worries about a reccurrence of mania and Susan's feelings of being controlled and not trusted were understandable reactions for both of them. Susan and the therapist discussed how she could be an active listener with Tom, both by empathizing with his feelings and validating some of his perceptions, but also by indicating how she had changed since treatment had begun.

After a year of treatment, Susan decided to take a full-time job, which meant that her daughter (Nancy) would be in day care for the entire day. Her daughter began to cry more at the day-care center and acted more aloof when Susan came to pick her up. The therapist explained to Susan that it was hard for Nancy, who was so young, to understand that " 'Mommy is returning'—she doesn't have the ability yet to keep that image intact in her mind." The therapist suggested a "cognitive transitional object" to help Nancy with the separation during the day. Susan chose a stuffed frog that Nancy was fond of and placed a picture of herself and her husband on the frog. She told Nancy, "Be sure and look at Froggy and think of me and Daddy." Susan was surprised at how effective this little stuffed animal was in reducing Nancy's separation anxiety while in day care.

Maintenance Treatment

After 1 year, therapy was phased back for Susan, although it was still required as part of a legal agreement with the district attorney. Many of the sessions after the first year were primarily focused on family adjustments to work arrangements, plans on moving out of state, how to deal with her father, her concerns about being away from her daughter, and her feelings that she "really did not need this much treatment."

She continued to use her mood checks, self-instructions, rational responding, and problem-solving skills. She found it helpful to take her medication at almost exactly the same time each day. Her relationship with her husband improved substantially, but her relationship with her father reached a "standoff," which she accepted. She disclosed to many of her closer friends that she was being treated for bipolar illness and that she was much improved. Most of her friends were quite supportive, but a few appeared to distance themselves from her. Initially angry with this distancing behavior, she was able to recognize that this behavior reflected the shortcomings—indeed, naiveté—of some friends, and it allowed her to determine who her real friends were. The therapist indicated to her that national surveys show that 50% of the general public has a history of a mental illness during their lifetime, suggesting that many of these friends who rejected her would, themselves, be likely to experience a mental illness. The difference, she realized, was that she was honest about it and was getting appropriate treatment.

Summary (in Susan's Words)

Perhaps the best way to summarize Susan's experience is to give her the opportunity to speak in her own words:

> "In the movie *Contact,* there is a scene where actress Jodie Foster plummets, with no peripheral vision, through galactic 'worm holes' of bright, racing colors. At the other end, she meets an alien disguised as her late father and proceeds to converse with him. When she 'returns' to Earth, her account of these events is not believed, and she's shown a video indicating that her body never left the planet. She's accused of defrauding the government for the cost of the space vehicle. If I were Jodie Foster, this would have been a manic episode.
>
> "I wouldn't remember much of the space ordeal except the bright, fast colors and maybe some snippets of conversation, but I do know that I would have said something, done something, or encouraged something completely out of character during the mania. In fact, there is a moment when you 'return to Earth,' so to speak, after a manic episode to find that, generally, everyone is pissed off at you.
>
> "As an untreated, rapid-cycling manic–depressive, I was probably out of touch with reality two to three times per week. Pregnancy exacerbates the disorder, and there are approximately 7 months in 1996 that I barely remember, during which I bought $55,000 in diamonds. Not rings or bracelets or necklaces, just plain, loose diamonds for which I had no use.
>
> "While manic episodes get the most attention and cause the most damage to others, depression is no picnic. I spent many afternoons sitting on our terrace, looking at Central Park and planning my suicide. If I had known that sleeping pills are barbiturates, I'd be long

gone. Furthermore, my drinking in college was so out of control that I don't remember my 18th, 19th, or 20th birthdays, and I was asked to live off campus after violating the school's alcohol policy more than three times.

"That said, being diagnosed as a person with bipolar disorder and given a bottle of pills was a huge relief. It took 13 weeks of careful monitoring and nasty side effects, but I now swallow five capsules a day and experience normalized behavior—no vicious mood swings, no holes in my memory, no outlandish spending sprees, no heavy drinking, no desire to die. In fact, I donated a blood sample for research, and it appears I inherited markers for the disorder. After graphing my family tree, this is not surprising: My mother exhibits extreme moodiness, alcoholism, and other reckless behavior; my great-uncle committed suicide; and my great-grandmother had numerous nervous breakdowns. I also found out I was 12.5% Navajo Indian, which is just really neat and has nothing to do with manic–depression.

"Which brings me to the present day and the healthy, happy life to which my diagnosis led. My home is lovely, my husband and I have fun planning romantic weekends, and we adore watching our little girl grow and change. Our life is filled with friends who were supportive during truly tough parts of my illness, and we ignore certain friends who were meanspirited about the diagnosis. I've learned to enjoy and utilize a hypomanic day: I save up all my laundry, cleaning, household projects, and other "to do" items and wait until I'm feeling a bit too excited. Then I pull out my list and go to it. Never fails. The projects get done, and the mania is put to good use. Meanwhile, I'm so stable, my girlfriends suffering from PMS wonder if lithium would work for them!

"I realize, however, that my experience is not the norm. First, I was lucky to be correctly diagnosed. In addition, there was no overlapping drug or alcohol dependence issue, I made a concerted effort to stay on medication and have continued it religiously, I have a tremendously supportive husband and two of the finest doctors treating me, plus medical insurance. Unlike most, I have no shame about the disorder either. Frankly, while untreated, manic–depression created havoc in my life. Nowadays, it just isn't a big deal."

REFERENCES

Basco, M. R., & Rush, A. J. (1996). *Cognitive-behavioral therapy for bipolar disorder.* New York: Guilford Press.

Beck, A. T., Rush, A. J., Shaw, B. F., & Emery, G. (1979). *Cognitive therapy of depression.* New York: Guilford Press.

Burns, D. D. (1989). *The feeling good handbook: Using the new mood therapy in everyday life*. New York: Morrow.

Clark, D. A., Beck, A. T., & Alford, B. A. (1999). *Scientific foundations of cognitive theory and therapy of depression*. New York: Wiley.

Freeman, M. P., Freeman, S. A., & McElroy, S. L. (2002). The comorbidity of bipolar and anxiety disorders: Prevalence, psychobiology, and treatment issues. *Journal of Affective Disorders, 68*(1), 1–23.

Goldberg, J. F. (2001). Bipolar disorder with comorbid substance abuse: Diagnosis, prognosis, and treatment. *Journal of Psychiatric Practice, 7*(2), 109–122.

Jamison, K. R. (1997). *An unquiet mind*. New York: Random House.

Lam, D. H., Bright, J., Jones, S., Hayward, P., Schuck, N., Chisholm, D., et al. (2000). Cognitive therapy for bipolar illness: A pilot study of relapse prevention. *Cognitive Therapy and Research, 24*, 503–520.

Leahy, R. L. (1999). Decision making and mania. *Journal of Cognitive Psychotherapy, 13*(2), 83–105.

Leahy, R. L. (2000). Mood and decisions: Implications for bipolar disorder. *Behavior Therapist, 23*(3), 62–63.

Leahy, R. L. (2003). *Cognitive therapy techniques: A practitioner's guide*. New York: Guilford Press.

Leahy, R. L., & Beck, A. T. (1988). Cognitive therapy of depression and mania. In R. Cancro & A. Georgotas (Eds.), *Depression and mania* (pp. 517–537). New York: Elsevier.

Leahy, R. L., & Holland, S. J. (2000). *Treatment plans and interventions for depression and anxiety disorders*. New York: Guilford Press.

Newman, C. F., Leahy, R. L., Beck, A. T., Reilly-Harrington, N. A., & Gyulai, L. (2002). *Bipolar disorder: A cognitive therapy approach*. Washington, DC: American Psychological Association.

Scott, J., Stanton, B., Garland, A., & Ferrier, I. (2000). Cognitive vulnerability in patients with bipolar disorder. *Psychological Medicine, 30*(2), 467–472.

Suppes, T., & Dennehy, E. B. (2002). Evidence-based long-term treatment of bipolar II disorder. *Journal of Clinical Psychiatry, 63*(Suppl. 10), 29–33.

Vieta, E., Colom, F., Corbella, B., Martinez-Aran, A., Reinares, M., Benabarre, A., et al. (2001). Clinical correlates of psychiatric comorbidity in bipolar I patients. *Bipolar Disorders, 3*(5), 253–258.

CHAPTER EIGHT

INTERPERSONAL AND SOCIAL RHYTHM THERAPY

ELLEN FRANK
HOLLY A. SWARTZ

When we set out to develop a psychotherapeutic intervention that could en-hance or complement drug therapy for manic–depressive illness, we began by asking ourselves, "What kinds of things do first-rate clinicians do with patients who have this disorder, in addition to prescribing appropriate med-ications?" We realized that most expert pharmacotherapists also recom-mended a series of lifestyle changes in addition to careful adherence to the medication regimen they prescribed. Furthermore, we realized that these lifestyle modifications were all consistent with a model of the illness that posits physiological instability as central to the pathology of bipolar I dis-order. Thus, our theoretical rationale for interpersonal and social rhythm therapy has its foundation in our understanding of the pathophysiology of all recurrent mood disorders and in our clinical research experience with recurrent unipolar and bipolar patients.

THEORETICAL BACKGROUND

In their classic textbook on manic–depressive illness, Goodwin and Jamison (1990) argued that an integrated theory for understanding bipolar disorder can be based on an "instability model." Indeed, they "postulate that [insta-bility] is the fundamental dysfunction in manic–depressive illness" (p. 594).

Although it may not be immediately apparent how psychosocial and biological components that appear to be responsible for the onset of illness episodes relate to one another, we believe that such an integration is essential to understanding and treating the disorder and that interpersonal and social rhythm therapy (IPSRT; Frank et al., 1994; Frank, Kupfer, Malkoff-Schwartz, 2000) provides a rationally integrated approach.

Another key component supporting instability models is derived from empirical data relating the sleep abnormalities observed in both depression and mania to the pathophysiology of the disorder. Moving to the next level of integration, we sought to place these sleep changes in the broader context of the pervasive circadian disturbances hypothesized as associated with bipolar disorder. Our work (Ehlers, Frank, & Kupfer, 1988; Ehlers, Kupfer, Frank, & Monk, 1993) has emphasized the relationship between psychosocial stressors (and, equally important, alterations in the patterning of daily life that are not psychologically stressful) and changes in biological rhythms.

Circadian rhythm researchers refer to those exogenous environmental factors that set the circadian clock as *zeitgebers* or "time givers" (Aschoff, 1981). The primary and most powerful zeitgeber is the rising and setting of the sun; however, especially in urban, industrialized society, social factors such as the timing of work, meals, and even television programs have an important influence on circadian rhythms. We have hypothesized that, in vulnerable individuals, disruptions in such social zeitgebers may lead to affective episodes, and that a treatment that encourages regularity in such daily routines could shore up the vulnerable circadian systems of individuals with recurrent mood disorders, thus protecting them from new illness episodes.

Prior to our description of our "social zeitgeber hypothesis," few attempts had been made to integrate the available body of knowledge on the importance of circadian rhythm disturbances with that on the role of stressful life events in provoking new episodes of affective illness (Brown, Harris, & Peto, 1973; Brown & Harris, 1986; Dohrenwend & Dohrenwend, 1981).

We argue that major (and minor) life events may act as specific precipitants by inducing the rhythm disruptions that form a direct link to the biomedical features of mood episodes. It may be that some of the specific psychosocial precipitants of depressive disorder, particularly those initially identified by Brown and colleagues (Brown et al., 1973; Brown & Harris, 1986), are particularly potent in their ability to trigger these biological desynchronizations through the capacity of interpersonal relationships and social demands to act as potent synchronizing factors for our biological rhythms. More recently, we have shown that life events that result in disruptions in social routines, whether psychologically stressful in the traditional sense or not, are significantly associated with the onset of manic episodes in individuals with bipolar disorder (Malkoff-Schwartz et al., 2000; Malkoff-Schwartz et al., 1988).

As can be seen in Figure 8.1, we propose that specific social prompts, or social *zeitgebers*, be treated as unobservable variables that are implied from the relationship between the occurrence of a life event and a change in the stability of social rhythms. Although the major hypotheses of our theoretical model are indicated by the cascading sequence shown in Figure 8.1, it is also important to examine factors such as coping skills, social support, gender, and temperament as intervening variables. In the primary path of the model, there is a chain of events in which instability of social rhythms can lead to instability in specific biological rhythms, particularly sleep. The extent of instability is likely to be a function of the power of a particular relationship, task, or demand to set biological rhythms, that is, to act as a zeitgeber. The extent of instability and the appearance of consequent somatic symptoms are modulated by protective and vulnerability factors from both the psychosocial and the psychobiological spheres. These factors include the individual's coping skills, available social supports, and temperament, as well as the flexibility of his or her particular biological clock, as exemplified by the individual's ability to adapt, for example, to a nighttime work shift, the time-zone changes associated with travel, or even the change from standard time to daylight saving time, and vice versa.

In vulnerable individuals—those with "delicate" clocks—the manic or depressive state then becomes the final psychobiological response to changes

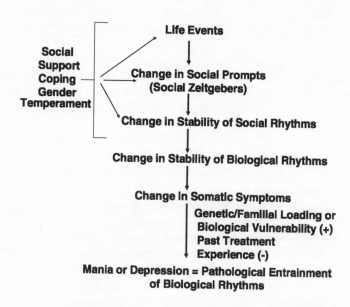

FIGURE 8.1. Schema for social zeitgeber theory.

in the regularity of daily routines or social rhythms. In nonvulnerable individuals, biological rhythm disruption is self-limiting and experienced only as mild somatic symptoms, such as those observed under conditions of jet lag, or, in some cases, as having no effect at all. In individuals vulnerable to mood disorder, however, the biological instability that leads to these somatic symptoms is not easily reversed. We believe that such individuals literally get stuck in a state of ongoing desynchronization or pathological entrainment of biological rhythms such as that observed in major depression and mania.

Interpersonal psychotherapy (IPT; Klerman, Weissman, Rounsaville, & Chevron, 1984), as developed for unipolar disorder, focuses on improving the quality and number of interpersonal relationships in the patient's life and the patient's degree of comfort with his or her primary social roles. It is noteworthy that in the process of doing so, interpersonal psychotherapy also often serves to regulate daily and weekly social interaction and activity. In this way, then, IPT may serve indirectly to reestablish social zeitgebers and probably to re-entrain circadian rhythms.

In interpersonal and social rhythm therapy, we have taken a more direct approach to applying social rhythm theories to therapy for affective disorder. We sought to develop a therapy that would help patients "regularize" their social rhythms through direct monitoring and modification of routines, while, at the same time, improving the quality of the patient's interpersonal relationships and his or her satisfaction with social roles. It is through this multipronged effort that we hoped to help to protect patients with bipolar I disorder against the development of new episodes.

A final assumption central to IPSRT is that bipolar disorder can almost never be treated effectively without pharmacotherapy. Unfortunately, the concept of a lifelong "dependence" on medication is abhorrent to many individuals with this condition, especially those newly diagnosed. Nevertheless, pharmacotherapy remains the cornerstone of treatment for bipolar disorder. Education about the disorder, in general, and about the individual patient's particular pattern of symptoms and episode onsets can greatly enhance acceptance of the need for medication and the ability to work collaboratively with the physician in the prevention of new onsets.

OVERVIEW OF IPSRT

Built on the foundation of three overlapping paradigms, IPSRT fuses a triad of distinct interventions into one: psychoeducation, social rhythm therapy, and interpersonal psychotherapy. IPSRT focuses on helping patients optimize the regularity of daily routines, resolve social and interpersonal problems, and understand their illness. By intervening with respect to each of these potential pathways to recurrence, IPSRT attempts to prevent new illness episodes and reduce interepisode symptom fluctuation. In the following material, each component of the treatment intervention (i.e., psychoeducation, social rhythm therapy, IPT) is described separately; however, in practice, the clinician is continually interweaving these components. During the course of a single session, the therapist moves seamlessly among the components, according to the particular needs of the patient at the time. Thus, IPSRT represents a true integration of what may seem like disparate approaches. Table 8.1 summarizes these three components and the treatment techniques associated with them.

IPSRT is administered in four phases: initial phase, intermediate phase, maintenance phase, and termination. The specific tasks of each phase are outlined below. Each phase requires the therapist to use all three of the strategies associated with IPSRT—psychoeducation, social rhythm therapy, and interpersonal psychotherapy. Thus, the therapist will utilize these intervention strategies throughout the phases of treatment, advancing central themes that are identified as important during the initial phase.

PHASES OF IPSRT

In the initial phase of IPSRT, the therapist focuses on (1) history taking, (2) educating the patient about bipolar disorder, (3) completing what is known as the "interpersonal inventory," and (4) identifying the interpersonal problem area or areas that will become the focus of the interpersonal interventions. These activities allow the therapist to arrive at an initial case formulation. The case formulation sets the stage for the treatment that follows by defining a treatment focus that incorporates both the medical model of bipolar disorder and a patient-specific interpersonal problem area.

Once the case formulation is complete and the therapist and patient have agreed on an initial interpersonal problem area on which to focus, the intermediate phase of the treatment begins. The goals of this phase are (1) regularization of the patient's social rhythms, and (2) resolution of the identified interpersonal problem. The expectation is that these interventions, along with appropriate pharmacotherapy, will be associated with remission of mood symptoms.

The third phase of treatment, which may last for years, focuses on (1) maintaining regularity in social rhythms, (2) anticipating and resolving interpersonal problems before they cause distress, and (3) maintaining euthymic mood.

When treatment termination is appropriate, the final phase of IPSRT focuses on the process of termination.

TABLE 8.1. Components of Interpersonal and Social Rhythm Therapy

Component	Techniques

Psychoeducation	Provide education regarding:
	    Medication and side effects
	    Course and symptoms of bipolar disorder
	Teach patients to recognize:
	    Prodromal symptoms
	    Early signs of impending episodes
	    Stressors likely to lead to episodes
	Encourage patients to:
	    Become experts on their own illness
	    Work collaboratively with clinician to manage illness

Social rhythm therapy	Balance stimulation and stability
	Complete Social Rhythm Metric
	    Monitor regularity of routines
	    Monitor frequency/intensity of social interactions
	    Monitor daily mood
	Search for specific triggers of rhythm disruption
	Gradually regularize social rhythms

Interpersonal psychotherapy	Take in-depth psychiatric and social history
	Link mood changes to interpersonal/social problems
	Establish interpersonal case formulation (focus on one
	    or two problem areas):
	    Grief
	    Role transition
	    Role dispute
	    Interpersonal deficits
	Grieve the lost "healthy self," if indicated

History Taking and Psychoeducation

The therapist's first tasks in the initial phase are history taking and psychoeducation. The history taking covers symptomatic and interpersonal aspects of earlier episodes, with particular emphasis on the most recent episodes. As indicated above, the philosophy of and rationale for IPSRT assume a close and interdependent relationship between interpersonal distress and disruption in the social rhythms of the patient's life. In taking the history, therefore, we look for evidence of alterations or disruptions in the patient's daily routine and interpersonal interactions that *preceded* the development of symptoms. Teasing apart the relationship between early symptoms and any lifestyle alterations that may have preceded those symptoms may be difficult; however, it is often possible to separate externally caused disruptions in routine from prodromal symptoms of mania or depression.

We typically construct an *illness history time-line* that includes episodes of illness, treatment, important life events, lifestyle alterations, and any other information that seems relevant to understanding the precipitants of episodes and what kinds of treatments have been helpful in the past. An example of such a time-line is provided in Figure 8.2.

During the history taking, the time-line construction, and, in fact, throughout the initial phase of treatment, the IPSRT therapist is engaged in educating the patient about the disorder and the ways in which interpersonal problems and lifestyle disruption may have been related to the onset and continuation of episodes. Even patients who have suffered from bipolar disorder for many years and who have read extensively about the disorder may not see the connections among interpersonal problems, rhythm disruption, and symptom exacerbation.

Case Example

Carla is a 41-year-old female, separated from her husband, who entered IPSRT treatment following her fourth manic episode. In session two, she and her therapist were reviewing the events that had led up to each of her manic episodes. Although she had never made the connection previously, it became apparent that the common thread preceding each of her episodes was sleep deprivation, often combined with missing a single dose of lithium. At her job as a critical care nurse, Carla was often required to work double shifts when her unit was full and the patients were particularly ill. On the night prior to three of her onsets of mania, her head nurse had insisted that she work the 11–7 shift following a full and exhausting day on the 3–11 shift. On each of these occasions, intensely focused on the critically ill patients for whom she was caring, she also forgot to take her evening dose of lithium. Her fourth episode followed a time when she had stayed up all night studying for an exam she needed to take to renew her license. Again, she completely forgot about taking her evening dose. Although the similarities among the events leading up to each of her episodes was obvious when she reviewed them with her therapist, she had previously failed to see the connections among her sleep deprivation, missing doses, and the onset of her manic episodes.

Taking the Interpersonal Inventory

The interpersonal inventory was created as part of interpersonal psychotherapy for unipolar depression (Klerman et al., 1984); it refers to a review of the important relationships in the patient's life. In the initial phase of IPSRT, the clinician takes the interpersonal inventory with an eye toward understanding the nature of these relationships, whether there are any consistent positive or negative patterns in them, and particularly whether prob-

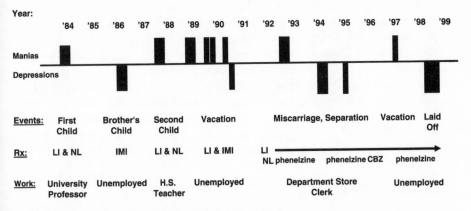

FIGURE 8.2. Example of a history of illness time-line.

lems in any of these relationships are linked to the onset or persistence of the most recent episode of illness. The completion of the interpersonal inventory is the last part of the extended history-taking process and leads directly to the individual case formulation.

There is no set formula for taking the interpersonal inventory. Frequently, patients who have had a good deal of experience in therapy more or less structure this part of the assessment for the therapist. When patients have had less treatment experience, however, the therapist makes certain that, by the time the interpersonal inventory is completed, he or she has a clear picture of the people who are currently important to the patient, the people who have been important to the patient in the past, and the nature of each of these relationships. In working with patients who have bipolar disorder, we also find it is important to inquire about people who once were very important to the patient but with whom the patient now has no relationship. The nature of bipolar symptomatology often leads to permanent breaks or "cutoffs" in important relationships. If the patient describes such cutoffs, we explore whether reconnecting with this person might be something that would be beneficial to him or her.

Identifying an Interpersonal Problem Area

After the interpersonal inventory is completed, the therapist determines which interpersonal issues are most central to the patient's current mood symptomatology. Under ideal circumstances, the therapist and patient collaboratively identify a primary (and sometimes a secondary) problem area from among the four interpersonal problem areas originally associated with interpersonal psychotherapy for unipolar disorder: unresolved grief, interpersonal disputes, role transition, or interpersonal deficits (cf. Klerman et al., 1984; for a full discussion of the conceptual basis for the interpersonal problem areas, see also Weissman, Markowitz, & Klerman, 2000). To the four problem areas of IPT, we have added a fifth subarea: grief for the lost healthy self. This area is often the initial focus of intervention with patients with bipolar disorder who are in psychotherapy for the first time and who see their lives (and themselves) as divided into "before my illness" and "since my illness." Each of these problem areas is described in some detail below.

Unresolved Grief

Unresolved grief becomes the focus of treatment when the current affective episode is connected to the death of an important person in the patient's life. Treatment strategies utilized during the intermediate phase of treatment include facilitating the mourning process by reviewing the full nature of the relationship with the deceased person, encouraging the expression of previously suppressed affect, helping the patient recognize distorted (either overly positive or overly negative) memories of his or her relationship with the deceased, and encouraging behavior change in terms of forming new relationships and interests.

Case Example

Jeanette is a 49-year-old widow, mother of two, who works full-time and lives alone. She has a history of bipolar illness dating from age 18. She has had three manic episodes and three episodes of depression. Raised in a strict religious household, early on, she turned to the church for the support she did not get from her distant parents. Jeannette married a young man she had met in church activities and had her first child at the age of 20. Over the course of the marriage, Jeannette became mother and father to her children, as her husband gradually became unhappy, withdrawn, and began to drink. Her religious beliefs reinforced her personal conviction that she had to please others to be worthy of their love.

Her last depressive episode occurred in the aftermath of her husband's sudden suicide. Prior to his death, he had become very critical of Jeannette and their sons for seemingly minor failures. Jeannette blamed herself not only for all of her supposed failings, but for those of her sons as well. Following her husband's suicide, Jeannette quickly readjusted and did not show the normal signs of grieving. She resisted the efforts of friends to comfort her, and she became severely depressed 6 months later. Jeannette described her depression as a collapse into guilt over not having been a good enough wife and mother.

In IPSRT, Jeannette came to understand that she had been taking responsibility for the feelings of others since she was a small child. Her religious beliefs had meshed with her interpersonal style in such a way as to produce enormous guilt for not having been a better wife. In questioning this belief in the context of her IPSRT treatment, the guilt that had stood in the way of normal mourning began to resolve. Early in the treatment, Jeannette was able to become angry with her husband for his "abandonment" of the family, first through alcohol and then through suicide. She was also able to experience sadness over her loss. Throughout the remainder of therapy she continued to grieve in a more normal way and worked hard on developing new interests and relationships. She became closer to her grown sons and came to recognize that she had done an excellent job of raising them and to feel very competent in her mother-of-adult-children role. Finally, she was able to turn once again to her church as a source of satisfying social activity and support.

In standard IPT, the problem area of grief is selected only when an important person in the patient's life has died. Individuals with bipolar disorder, however, often experience the symbolic loss of *the person they would have become* had they not been afflicted with bipolar disorder. As noted, we refer to this as grieving the lost healthy self. We have included this work under the broader category of grief because many of the therapeutic strategies and tactics are similar, although it could just as well be thought of as a form of role transition. The work involves helping patients explore limits placed on their life by the illness, lost hopes, and missed opportunities. After mourning these losses, the patient is helped to recognize his or her strengths (rather than focusing on the losses) and gently encouraged to set new, realistic goals.

Case Example

John was a brilliant 20-year-old music student with a clear future as a concert violinist when he had his first manic episode. Completely confused about what was happening to him, but wildly psychotic, he was brought to the psychiatric emergency room by the campus police. Following a brief hospitalization, he returned to school and entered IPSRT treatment. Although his manic symptoms had been brought under quick control, with ongoing treatment he began to experience severe tremor related to his lithium treatment. Every other drug regimen was tried, but after many, many months of experimentation, he and his treatment team were forced to conclude that only lithium kept his illness under control. His choices were to stay on lithium and give up the violin or take something less effective and hope that he could continue his studies while his moods fluctuated wildly.

With the help of his IPSRT therapist, he was able to grieve the loss of his dream of a concert career (acknowledging that while fame and fortune might have been nice, the life of a concert musician was a difficult one indeed ... especially for someone who needed regular routines) and make plans for a career that would enable him to make use of his musical talent and love of music, while still being able to take care of his health. Today, John is a happy, euthymic music teacher in a fine arts high school who enthusiastically gives his gifts of skill and knowledge to young people very much like he once was, while leading a very orderly life.

Role Transition

A role transition is defined as a major change in a life role. Examples of role transitions include starting a first job, getting married, becoming a parent, getting divorced, etc. Although such transitions are a normal part of life experience, in individuals who are vulnerable to mood disorders, such changes are often associated with episode onset. Patients with bipolar disorder are especially vulnerable to change, even in the face of relatively minor perturbations in their environment. IPT strategies for addressing a role transition during the intermediate phase include helping the patient to develop more realistic views of both the old and new roles, in light of the tendency to idealize the old role and devalue the new one, and to acquire the skills needed to master the new role.

Bipolar illness itself may bring about role transitions: job loss resulting from inappropriate manic behavior and marital breakup resulting from either depressive or manic symptoms that are intolerable to the spouse. Finally, and quite paradoxically, achieving mood stability may represent a challenging role transition for patients who have known no such stability since childhood. In particular, patients whose manias have not been particularly destructive frequently miss the pleasurable hypomanic episodes associated with more mood variability. In this case, the therapist is called upon to help the patient mourn the loss of these episodes, identify their negative consequences, and help the patient find pleasures associated with new-found mood stability.

Case Example

Lakshmi is a 28-year-old business student of Indian origin. When she entered IPSRT treatment, she was engaged to an Indian graduate student, who had been chosen by her parents, and was interviewing for jobs around the United State and Canada. Although in a depressed phase when she was diagnosed with bipolar disorder, it was clear from her history that she had experienced at least two relatively mild manias earlier, in her 20s, that had gone unrecognized.

Her IPSRT treatment initially focused on educating her about the disorder and preparing her for the multiple role transitions she was anticipating in the coming months: graduation from business school, entering the work world, and marriage—all important expectations of her parents. When her worried parents traveled from India to meet with the treatment team, it became apparent that the most important transition she needed to negotiate was the developmental shift from dependent child to mature adult occurring against the complex (and often conflicting) cultural expectations of her Indian parents and her American peers. Although she had been quite satisfied with her treatment, her parents strongly questioned both the diagnosis and our methods of intervention and urged her to discontinue her Western medicines in favor of traditional Eastern treatments. Whereas she was planning to take a lower-salaried job that would leave her some leisure time and some say in the amount of work that would be expected of her, her parents could not understand why she wasn't considering any of the high-power, high-salaried jobs she was being offered.

Perhaps most important, she was in no hurry to marry the young man her parents had chosen for her, while they were busy planning the wedding. The remainder of her IPSRT treatment focused on her grieving the lost role of favored and obedient child and making the transition to independent adulthood while still remaining as respectful as possible of her loving, if demanding, parents.

Role Dispute

An interpersonal role dispute occurs when nonreciprocal role expectations are present in intimate relationships, leading to overt or covert disputes with a significant other. The goals of this phase of treatment include identification of the dispute, alteration of role expectations and communication patterns, and development of a change plan. Therapeutic strategies used during the intermediate phase include role-play, investigation of realistic options, and communication analysis. As acknowledged, role disputes are a normal part of close relationships, but they also are a common sequela of bipolar disorder. The irritability and entitled attitude associated with bipolar symptomatology can wreak havoc in close relationships. Similarly, the loss of interest and social withdrawal associated with bipolar depressions can leave the other party feeling that he or she is bearing all the responsibility for the relationship.

Case Example

Will was a 42-year-old divorced male when he entered IPSRT, following his fifth episode of bipolar illness. He had been unemployed for 1 year. During that year he had had a prolonged manic episode, toward the end of which he was hospitalized for several weeks. His wife had insisted on a separation earlier in the year, when the mania became evident, and had subsequently divorced him. He had lost his job as a carpenter, working for a local construction company.

When he was discharged from the hospital, he'd had nowhere to go. He decided to relocate to the town where he'd grown up, moving in temporarily with his parents until he could find work and get his personal life in order. This was a difficult decision for a man who had been living independently for 26 years. From the time he returned home, his relationship with his parents was conflicted. Both parents had difficulty understanding his illness and what had happened to "the apple of their eye." They tried to tell him how to live his life and what activities he should do each day. Will deeply resented all this advice, but he felt trapped in his situation. He was actively job hunting, looking for a work as a carpenter, but construction work was at a virtual standstill in his parents' small town. They kept insisting that he consider other careers and broaden his job search. Because of his illness and his age, Will felt he needed to stick with what he knew he was capable of doing well and not worry so much about the length of time it was taking him to find work.

Will used the IPSRT therapy to discuss his frustration about living at home, his anger at his parents' intrusiveness, and their attempts at controlling his life. He was able to recognize that because he was living in his parents' home again and was being supported by them financially, there was a tendency for them to treat him like a teenager. Understanding that his parents were acting out of concern for him, his illness, and his need to gain employment helped to diffuse his anger. He and his IPSRT therapist discussed ways to cope with his parents' intrusiveness and to establish role expectations that were more appropriate to his age and life experience. He chose to not react to most of their nagging, but when it became too difficult, he tried to help them see he was now an adult—albeit an adult with *some* of the needs of a child— and he needed to direct his own life and career path. He also learned to pair such comments with his thanks for his parents support and concern, rather than with the angry outbursts that had characterized his behavior toward them prior to beginning IPSRT.

Interpersonal Deficits

Patients with interpersonal deficits are those who have long histories of unsuccessful relationships or are completely socially isolated. This problem area is generally used as a "default" category, applied only when the three other problem areas do not apply to the patient's circumstances. Patients with longstanding bipolar disorder who have destroyed virtually all of their close relationships may be best characterized as experiencing interpersonal deficits. The therapeutic work in the intermediate phase focuses on strategies for forming new relationships and keeping them from deteriorating once they are formed. This is the one problem area in which the therapeutic relationship itself may become a focus of discussion.

Case Example

Meredith is a 30-year-old single female who has worked, on and off, in travel agencies since graduating from high school. Meredith's interpersonal deficits dovetailed with the need for symptom management, particularly in the area of social stimulation. Meredith had worked in relatively isolated settings, where she might be one of only two agents, as well as in large offices, with dozens of coworkers. When working alone, she had a tendency to feel understimulated and to put off taking care of details that needed attention. She seemed to need others around and watching over her, to some extent, to stay on task.

On the other hand, when she worked in an office with many coworkers, her pattern was to immediately divide them into a "good" and "bad" group. Both groups, however, produced problems for her. She was attracted to the "good" coworkers as companions, enjoyed socializing with them, but often found that she became so overstimulated in their company that she was unable to concentrate on her work when she returned to the office from lunch or a coffee break. If she went out with them after work, sometimes she was unable to fall asleep when she got home after a night on the town. The "bad" coworkers irritated her with their inefficiency, lack of attention to detail, and "stupidity." She frequently got into petty arguments with them. Sometimes she became so preoccupied with their failings that she could not concentrate on her own work.

IPSRT focused first on helping her to see both groups of coworkers in a more balanced way, to recognize that some members of the "good" group also occasionally failed to pay attention to details or get things done, and to see that there were positive things about each of the members of the so-called "bad" group. She was eventually able to put some limits on her rumination about the "bad" colleagues, even to see some of their deficits as similar to her own. Most important, she was able to downscale the conflict she created with them and concentrate on her own work. She and her therapist then began working on setting some limits on her interaction with her more appealing coworkers, limiting the number of days each week that she went out to lunch or engaged in after work social activities with them. While she missed the fuller social life that she had enjoyed before, she acknowledged that her mood was more stable as a result.

REGULARIZING SOCIAL RHYTHMS

The social rhythm component of IPSRT focuses on developing strategies to promote regular, rhythm-entraining social zeitgebers and manage the negative effects of disrupting *zeistörers* (or entrainment-disturbing factors). Most of the social rhythm work occurs during the intermediate and maintenance phases of treatment—although an assessment of baseline social rhythms is routinely conducted in the initial phase.

Each week patients are asked to complete an instrument, the Social Rhythm Metric (SRM), which is designed to help them optimize the regularity of their daily rhythms. The original SRM was designed to track the occurrence of 15 prespecified activities and two individually selected activities (such as a particular leisure activity, prayer, or dog walking) that the person completing the instrument reports taking part in more days than not (Monk, Flaherty, Frank, Hoskinson, & Kupfer, 1990; Monk, Kupfer, Frank, & Ritenour, 1991). We have subsequently developed two new versions of the SRM, both for use in the treatment of individuals with bipolar disorder. The first of these adaptations, called the SRM-II, differs from the original in that it makes the *patterning* of daily activity apparent to the person completing the form, and it enquires about the extent to which the patient found his or her involvement with others stimulating (See Figure 8.3). We have demonstrated that the use of interpersonal and social rhythm therapy is associated with changes in the regularity of the activities recorded on the SRM-II (Frank et al., 1994). Because the 17-item version of the SRM-II can prove impractical in many treatment contexts, and because we found that the majority of the variance in the SRM score was accounted for by a small number of items (Monk, Frank, Potts, & Kupfer, 2002), we developed a five-item version of the SRM-II (Figure 8.4). This version is currently being used in the large, national, multicenter Systematic Treatment Enhancement Program for Bipolar Disorder (STEP-BD) study of treatments for bipolar disorder.

In the initial phase of treatment, the patient is asked to complete the SRM weekly. The first 3 to 4 weeks of SRM records are used to establish the patient's baseline social rhythms. The therapist and patient jointly review the SRMs, identifying both stable and unstable daily rhythms. For instance, the therapist will want to know whether the patient went to bed at a reasonable hour during the week but then stayed out late on the weekend, disrupting what was otherwise a fairly regular bedtime. Does the patient's mood change for the worse on days when he or she skips meals? By examining the SRMs, the therapist and patient can begin to identify behaviors that negatively influence the stability of the patient's rhythm or mood.

Once baseline SRMs are collected and patterns of irregularity identified, the therapist and patient begin working toward rhythm stabilization through graded, sequential lifestyle changes. This work typically occurs in the intermediate phase of IPSRT. The therapist and patient identify short-term, intermediate, and long-term goals to gradually make social rhythms less variable. For example, a short-term goal might be getting out of bed in the morning at a fixed time for a period of 1 week. In order to achieve that goal, the patient may need to make changes in other social behaviors (e.g., curtailing late-night social activities).

The Social Rhythm Metric (SRM)
MacArthur Foundation Mental Health Research Network I
Please Fill This Out At The End Of The Day

Respondent #	Day of Week:	Date:

PEOPLE
0 = Alone
1 = Others just present
2 = Others actively involved
3 = Others very stimulating

ACTIVITY	TIME	AM or PM	DAY OF WEEK						
OUT OF BED	Earlier								
	Exact Earlier Time								
Mid-point of your normal range →				0		0			
					0				
	Later								
	Exact Later Time								
	Check if did not do								
FIRST CONTACT (IN PERSON OR BY PHONE) WITH ANOTHER PERSON	Earlier								
	Exact Earlier Time								
Mid-point of your Normal range →									
					2				
	Later								
	Exact Later Time								
	Check if did not do								

FIGURE 8.3. Page 1 of the SRM-II (17-item version). From Frank et al. (1994). Copyright 1994 by the Association for Advancement of Behavior Therapy. Reprinted by permission.

177

DIRECTIONS

Please complete this form at the end of each day for the period of two consecutive weeks. *Write day of the week (Su, M, T, W, H, F, Sa) and write date (mm/dd/yy)* for which the form was completed. For each activity, *indicate the time you started it. Circle "AM" or "PM"* so we know whether the time you entered is in the morning or evening. If you did not do a particular activity, *place an "X" over the box for that activity.*

Day of Week	Date	Out of Bed	First Contact (in Person or by Phone) with Another Person	Start Work, School, Housework, Volunteer Activities, Child or Family Care	Have Dinner	Go to Bed
Su	05 / 23 / 02	6 : 30 (AM) PM	7 : 00 (AM) PM	9 : 00 (AM) PM	⊠ AM PM	11 : 00 AM (PM)
	__ / __ / __	__:__ AM PM	__:__ AM PM	__:__ AM PM	__:__ AM PM	__:__ AM PM
	__ / __ / __	__:__ AM PM	__:__ AM PM	__:__ AM PM	__:__ AM PM	__:__ AM PM
	__ / __ / __	__:__ AM PM	__:__ AM PM	__:__ AM PM	__:__ AM PM	__:__ AM PM
	__ / __ / __	__:__ AM PM	__:__ AM PM	__:__ AM PM	__:__ AM PM	__:__ AM PM
	__ / __ / __	__:__ AM PM	__:__ AM PM	__:__ AM PM	__:__ AM PM	__:__ AM PM
	__ / __ / __	__:__ AM PM	__:__ AM PM	__:__ AM PM	__:__ AM PM	__:__ AM PM
	__ / __ / __	__:__ AM PM	__:__ AM PM	__:__ AM PM	__:__ AM PM	__:__ AM PM

FIGURE 8.4. SRM-II (five-item version).

Intermediate goals might include sleeping at least 7 hours a night, with no naps during the day, or decreasing the amount of overstimulating activity the patient packs into the weekends. In order to accomplish these goals, the patient builds on the gains of the short-term goal attainments as well as instituting some new behaviors (e.g., agreeing to a regular afternoon tennis game to decrease napping).

Longer-term goals might include finding a new job that never requires shift work or extended overtime. The therapist also monitors the frequency and intensity of social interactions and identifies connections between mood and activity level. If the patient is depressed, the therapist encourages him or her to participate in more stimulating and satisfying activities; if hypomanic, the patient is encouraged to minimize any overstimulation that might lead to further mood elevation.

Throughout all phases of treatment, the therapist continues to review SRMs on a regular basis. The weekly SRM provides the therapist with the opportunity to review progress toward identified social rhythm goals and address impediments to change. In addition, the SRM is used to help the patient self-monitor for evidence of any change in mood symptoms. Thus, the SRM functions as both a measure of therapeutic change and a mechanism for monitoring changes in symptomatic status.

Case Example

Nancy was a 58-year-old widowed woman with a 34-year history of bipolar disorder when she began IPSRT treatment. Whereas most of her early episodes were manic, for the decade prior to entering therapy she had primarily experienced depressions associated with high levels of anxiety and occasional agoraphobia. Her social anxiety had prompted her to severely limit her interpersonal contacts.

When Nancy's therapist reviewed her first few weeks of SRMs, she noted that Nancy had very little social stimulation in her life. Initially the therapist focused on getting her to schedule one out-of-the-house activity each week. Toward the end of each session, they would plan the activity for the coming week. Her therapist then pointed out how much brighter her mood seemed to be on the day before the activity (in anticipation of it), on the day of the activity, and on the day after the activity. This correlation led to a discussion of the relationship between out-of-the-house activities and improved mood. Moving quite slowly, the IPSRT therapist then suggested a second activity every other week. When Nancy realized that she could tolerate this level of activity without additional anxiety, she and her therapist then agreed on two regular out-of-the-house activities each week. Over the course of several months, Nancy expanded her activity schedule to the point where she was frequently planning social activities on four or five days of each week. Her response to this intervention was a marked improvement in both her mood and her self-esteem.

INTEGRATING SOCIAL RHYTHM AND INTERPERSONAL INTERVENTIONS: A MODULAR APPROACH

As noted, the interpersonal and social rhythm components of the treatment, although discussed separately in this chapter, in actual practice are integrated throughout the intervention. Once the initial psychoeducation is complete, the therapist focuses on obtaining the necessary interpersonal information to identify an interpersonal problem area on which to focus. If the patient's social routines are very disturbed, they might focus exclusively on efforts to regularize those routines for the next several weeks. If not, the therapist may turn immediately to the interpersonal problem area, reviewing the SRMs each week to be certain that the patient is maintaining stable routines while making the desired interpersonal changes. Once a remission is achieved, treatment moves to the maintenance phase, and the focus of treatment shifts to prevention of relapse, with alternating emphasis on preventing new interpersonal difficulties or meeting the challenges of new roles the patient has taken on and keeping social rhythms stable. Should the patient experience a new episode of mania or depression, many of the strategies and tactics used early in the treatment may be employed again. Thus, the therapist will draw on different components in different sequences, depending upon what is happening in the patient's life at the time and what the patient's mood state is.

PROBLEMS IN THE IMPLEMENTATION OF IPSRT

Motivating the patient to participate in IPSRT and make the changes in routine prescribed in the treatment can represent a substantial challenge, especially with younger patients and those experiencing a first episode of illness. Younger patients naturally want to deny that they have a lifelong illness that will require lifelong treatment. Those in a first episode, whether they are young or old, may not yet have suffered sufficiently negative consequences of the illness to be motivated to participate in treatment. For most other patients, completing the illness history time-line and the interpersonal inventory, with the consequent recognition of the costs of *not* making changes, is usually sufficient motivation to keep them engaged in treatment. With younger and first-episode patients, often the best the clinician can do is leave the door open for a return to treatment at any future point in time.

Concerning nonadherence to treatment, many of the same issues apply; however, the clinician must always be careful to try to distinguish willful nonadherence from symptoms of an incipient episode of mania or depression. A developing depression may mean that the patient simply does not have the energy or organizational capacity to do everything that the therapist is asking. An incipient mania may be equally disorganizing, or may lead to loss of insight regarding the need for treatment adherence.

The sheer emotional intensity associated with bipolar disorder and, in particular, the irritability to which individuals with bipolar disorder are prone can make the clinician's job very difficult and frustrating. In such cases, we often give ourselves the same advice we offer to patients' families: Consider whether this provoking behavior is the patient or the illness talking. Nevertheless, a clinician working along with numerous patients suffering from high levels of bipolar symptomatology can come to feel overwhelmed. In such instances, it can be helpful for the IPSRT clinician to work in the context of a group or team practice so that he or she can turn to other clinicians for support, or, if such a context is unavailable, to participate in regular peer supervision groups, where cases are discussed and techniques for the management of difficult cases are shared.

As is the case with virtually every other psychiatric disorder, comorbidity can complicate treatment. Particularly common in patients with bipolar disorder are panic and substance use comorbidities on Axis I and Cluster B comorbidities on Axis II. Panic disorder or panic spectrum (see Frank et al., 2002) comorbidity can complicate treatment because of the patient's low tolerance for side effects of drugs and resultant medication nonadherence. Substance use obviously can serve to produce the very symptoms the treatment is trying to address. Cluster B personality disorders, especially borderline features, require that the clinician move much more slowly and carefully in the area of making changes in the patient's interpersonal life and be considerably less demanding in terms of the kinds of changes the patient is asked to make and the speed with which he or she can make them.

CONCLUSIONS

We see the zeitgeber/*zeitstörer* hypothesis as an explanation of some of the considerable variability in human response to a wide range of psychosocial events, in terms of biological rhythm change and alterations in psychological or psychiatric symptoms.

The clinical implications of an instability model for recurrent mood disorders are obvious. The model suggests that clinicians should be directed to intervene early and aggressively, emphasize long-term treatment approaches that include prophylactic components, and seek to enhance circadian integrity, especially the regular scheduling of daily activities and avoidance of any activities (even those that are not perceived as obvious stressors) or substances that disrupt rhythms.

According to our model, there are likely to be three paths to recurrence in patients with bipolar disorder maintained on lithium carbonate or other so-called mood stabilizers: (1) medication noncompliance, (2) stressful life events, and (3) disruptions in social rhythms. IPSRT specifically addresses each of these potential pathways to new episodes of illness. IPSRT reduces denial and increases acceptance of the lifelong nature of the illness and its never-to-be-underestimated propensity to recur by providing (1) standard medication compliance training, and (2), more important, a forum in which the patient can explore his or her individual feelings about the disorder, grieve for the lost healthy self, and come to terms with how the disorder has altered his or her life. By addressing interpersonal problem areas in the patient's life, IPSRT attempts to reduce the number and severity of interpersonally based stressors the patient experiences. By paying careful attention to the regularity of daily routines (both the timing of events and the amount of stimulation they produce) and the extent to which both positive and negative life events may influence these daily routines (i.e., social rhythms), IPSRT increases the regularity of patients' lives and their vigilance with respect to maintaining that stability.

We have found that IPSRT, a psychotherapeutic intervention that specifically targets these three prominent pathways to new episodes, is associated with (1) low rates of episode recurrence, (2) increased stability of mood between episodes, and (3) perhaps most important, significant reductions in suicidal behavior (Rucci et al., 2002) in patients with bipolar I disorder (and the consequent improvements in the quality of long-term remission they experience).

REFERENCES

Aschoff, J. (1981). *Handbook of behavioral neurobiology: Vol. 4. Biological rhythms.* New York: Plenum Press.

Brown, G. W., & Harris, T. (1986). Stressor, vulnerability and depression: A question of replication. *Psychological Medicine, 16,* 739–744.

Brown, G. W., Harris, T. O., & Peto, J. (1973). Life events and psychiatric disorders: II. Nature of causal link. *Psychological Medicine, 3,* 159–176.

Dohrenwend, B. S., & Dohrenwend, B. P. (Eds.). (1981). *Stressful life events and their contexts.* New York: Watson.

Ehlers, C. L., Frank, E., & Kupfer, D. J. (1988). Social zeitgebers and biological rythms. A unified approach to understanding the etiology of depression. *Archives of General Psychiatry, 45*(10), 948–952.

Ehlers, C. L., Kupfer, D. J., Frank, E., & Monk, T. H. (1993). Biological rhythms and depression: The role of zeitgebers and zeitstörers. *Depression, 1,* 285–293.

Frank, E., Cyranowski, J. M., Rucci, P., Shear, M. K., Fagiolini, A., Thase, M. E., Cassano, G. B., Grochocinski, V. J., Kostelnik, B., & Kupfer, D. J. (2002). Clinical significance of lifetime panic spectrum symptoms in the treatment of patients with bipolar I disorder. *Archives of General Psychiatry, 59,* 905–912.

Frank, E., Kupfer, D. J., Ehlers, C. L., Monk, T. H., Cornes, C., Carter, S., & Frankel, D. (1994). Interpersonal and Social Rhythm Therapy for bipolar disorder: Integrating interpersonal and behavioral approaches. *Behavior Therapist, 17,* 143–149.

Frank, E., Kupfer, D. J., & Malkoff-Schwartz, S. (2000). Life stress and bipolar disorder: Is the dimension of social rhythm disruption specific to onset of manic episodes? In T. Harris (Ed.), *Where inner and outer worlds meet* (pp. 263–274). London: Routledge.

Frank, E., Swartz, H. A., & Kupfer, D. J. (2000). Interpersonal and social rhythm therapy: Managing the chaos of bipolar disorder. *Biological Psychiatry, 48,* 593–604.

Goodwin, F. K., & Jamison, K. R. (1990). *Manic–depressive illness.* New York: Oxford University Press.

Klerman, G. L., Weissman, M. M., Rounsaville, B. J., & Chevron, E. S. (Eds.). (1984). *Interpersonal psychotherapy of depression.* New York: Basic Books.

Malkoff-Schwartz, S., Frank, E., Anderson, B. P., Hlastala, S. A., Luther, J. F., Sherrill, J. T., Houck, P. R., & Kupfer, D. J. (2000). Social rhythm disruption and stressful life events in the onset of bipolar and unipolar episodes. *Psychological Medicine, 30,* 1005–1016.

Malkoff-Schwartz, S., Frank, E., Anderson, B., Sherrill, J. T., Siegel, L., Patterson, D., & Kupfer, D. J. (1998). Stressful life events and social rhythm disruption in the onset of manic and depressive bipolar episodes: A preliminary investigation. *Archives of General Psychiatry, 55,* 702–707.

Monk, T. H., Flaherty, J. F., Frank, E., Hoskinson, K., & Kupfer, D. J. (1990). The social rhythm metric: An instrument to quantify the daily rhythms of life. *Journal of Nervous and Mental Disease, 178,* 120–126.

Monk, T. H., Frank, E., Potts, J. M., & Kupfer, D. J. (2002). A simple way to measure daily lifestyle regularity. *Journal of Sleep Research, 11*(3), 183–190.

Monk, T. H., Kupfer, D. J., Frank, E., & Ritenour, A. M. (1991). The social rhythm metric (SRM): Measuring daily social rhythms over 12 weeks. *Psychiatry Research, 36,* 195–207.

Rucci, P., Frank, E., Kostelnik, B., Fagiolini, A., Mallinger, A. G., Swartz, H. A., Thase, M. E., Siegel, L., & Wilson, D. (2002). Suicide attempts in patients with bipolar I disorder during an acute and maintenance clinical trial. *American Journal of Psychiatry, 159,* 1160–1164.

Weissman, M. M., Markowitz, J. C., & Klerman, G. L. (2000). *Comprehensive guide to interpersonal psychotherapy.* New York: Basic Books.

CHAPTER NINE

FAMILY THERAPY

DAVID J. MIKLOWITZ

Psychoeducational approaches to the treatment of recurrent psychiatric disorders have a long and distinguished history. Psychoeducation literally means "psychological education," which entails providing information to consumers about coping with psychiatric illness while simultaneously addressing their reactions to that information. Family psychoeducational approaches have their roots in schizophrenia research. Numerous controlled trials have indicated that combining family psychoeducation and skills training with neuroleptic regimens can delay relapses, reduce symptom severity, and improve functioning among patients with schizophrenia (for a review, see Goldstein & Miklowitz, 1995). Only recently, however, has psychoeducation been applied to families containing a member with bipolar disorder (Clarkin, Carpenter, Hull, Wilner, & Glick, 1998; Miklowitz et al., 2000; Miklowitz & Goldstein, 1997).

This chapter reviews one such approach, family-focused treatment (FFT). FFT is a 9-month, 21-session outpatient program consisting of five consecutive modules: assessment of the family, education about bipolar disorder, communication-enhancement training, problem-solving skills training, and termination. The theoretical and empirical background of the approach is reviewed briefly, followed by an exposition of the clinical techniques of the core modules. Recommendations on dealing with clinical complexities—notably, resistances to treatment—are presented. Appropriate modifications of the model to fit the developmental needs of patients with childhood-onset bipolar disorder are discussed. In the sections that follow, I am addressing the clinical practitioner—"you"—who wants to apply this approach to patients in "your" mental health setting.

THEORETICAL BACKGROUND

Early studies of families of patients with bipolar disorder presumed a primarily psychosocial origin of the illness (Cohen, Baker, Cohen, Fromm-Reichmann, & Weigert, 1954). These clinical observations of families were all but forgotten when research demonstrated the strong genetic, neurophysiological, and neuroanatomical bases of the disorder (Goodwin & Jamison, 1990). But as previous chapters in this volume have shown, the course of bipolar illness over time is strongly affected by provocative psychosocial agents that interact with genetic and neurophysiological vulnerabilities. Particularly relevant to the planning of family interventions is the observation that patients with bipolar disorder who are associated with family or marital environments characterized by high expressed emotion (EE; highly critical, hostile, or overprotective attitudes among caregivers) have more frequent relapses than patients associated with more benign low EE environments (Miklowitz, Goldstein, Nuechterlein, Snyder, & Mintz, 1988; Priebe, Wildgrube, & Muller-Oerlinghausen, 1989; O'Connell, Mayo, Flatow, Cuthbertson, & O'Brien, 1991; see Chapter 5, this volume).

High EE attitudes in caregivers are best conceptualized as "leading indicators" of strife within the family as a whole, particularly during the postepisode stabilization period. A laboratory study of family interaction indicated that, following a patient's acute episode, high EE relatives and patients are prone to negative, back-and-forth cycles of escalation on both verbal and nonverbal levels (Simoneau, Miklowitz, & Saleem, 1998). Furthermore, high EE caregivers are prone to attribute negative behaviors (e.g., irritability, poor employment records) of patients to personal and controllable factors (notably, personality or lack of effort) rather than uncontrollable factors (i.e., the bipolar illness; Hooley & Licht, 1997; Wendel, Miklowitz, Richards, & George, 2000). Accordingly, the FFT model assumes that increasing the efficiency and emotional tone of the family's communication and problem-solving styles and encouraging greater tolerance and acceptance of the illness among caregivers will enhance the patient's mood stability over time.

EMPIRICAL STUDIES OF FAMILY-FOCUSED TREATMENT

FFT has received support in one open trial and two randomized trials (for further details on these studies, see Chapter 11, this volume). In the first of these, nine patients who were discharged from the hospital after a manic episode were treated with FFT, consisting of 21 sessions of psychoeducation, communication training, and problem-solving training. A group of 23 patients from an earlier study served as a comparison group. All patients received aggressively delivered regimens of mood stabilizers and, when appropriate, adjunctive agents. Rates of relapse (new episodes that developed after states of remission or partial remission) were higher in the historical controls (14/23, 61%) than in the FFT patients (1/9, 11%; Miklowitz & Goldstein, 1990).

An investigation at the University of Colorado randomized 101 acutely ill patients to 9 months of FFT (n = 31) or a treatment-as-usual condition called crisis management (CM; n = 70), using a 1:2 allocation strategy (Miklowitz et al., 2000; Miklowitz, George, Richards, Simoneau, & Suddath, in press). Patients in CM received two sessions of family education and crisis intervention sessions, as needed, over 9 months. All patients received pharmacotherapy delivered by community physicians. Over 2 years, patients in FFT demonstrated a threefold higher rate of survival without relapse (52%) than patients in CM (17%). Patients in FFT also evinced lower levels of depressive and manic symptoms and better adherence to medication regimens than patients in CM. An analysis of laboratory-based interactional behavior revealed that families in FFT showed greater increases in positive verbal and nonverbal interactional behavior over 9 months of treatment than families in CM (Simoneau, Miklowitz, Richards, Saleem, & George, 1999).

Were the effects in the Colorado trial due to the greater intensity of therapist–patient contact in the FFT than the comparison intervention? This question was answered, in part, by a randomized trial conducted at UCLA (Rea et al., 2003). This study assigned 53 patients with bipolar, manic disorder to FFT and medication or to a comparably paced (21 sessions) supportive individual therapy. The individual therapy modality focused on illness management, medication adherence, and coping with life stressors, without direct family involvement. Patients in FFT had longer periods of sustained remission and fewer hospitalizations than patients in individual therapy, but only during a 1-year posttreatment interval. Patients in FFT and individual therapy were equally likely to relapse or be hospitalized during the 9-month period of active psychosocial treatment. It appears that the didactic information and skills training provided by FFT must be "absorbed" by families before patients realize benefits relative to equally intensive individual interventions.

The results of these studies indicate that adding FFT to a standard regimen of mood stabilizers increases long-term mood stability among patients. Its mechanisms of action may include encouraging drug compliance among patients and enhancing the use of positive communication skills among patients and their family members.

POPULATIONS TARGETED BY
FAMILY-FOCUSED TREATMENT

FFT targets patients with bipolar I or bipolar II disorder who are currently in, or have begun to stabilize from, an acute episode of mania, hypomania, mixed disorder, or depressive disorder (including rapid cycling). The episode need not have included a hospitalization, although most of the treatment research reviewed above focused on patients who began treatment in a hospital setting. If you are the treating clinician, it is helpful to verify the patient's diagnosis by administering the Structured Clinical Interview for DSM-IV (SCID-IV; First, Spitzer, Gibbon, & Williams, 1995). In addition to increasing diagnostic certainty, this interview increases your awareness of the clinical presentation of the patient's most recent episode and the early warning signs of future episodes.

Two additional inclusionary criteria are necessary for involvement in FFT. First, the patient must be taking medication. There is no evidence that bipolar disorder can be managed with psychosocial intervention alone. Second, FFT requires that family members be available and willing to participate in treatment, although the patient may be living in a different household. We have included parents, spouses, siblings, romantic partners, and roommates. Treatment is usually most applicable to relatives who have at least 4 hours of face-to-face contact with the patient each week and consider it a part of their role to help the patient manage the illness.

FFT includes patients with a variety of comorbid conditions, including anxiety, personality, eating, or psychotic disorders. Current substance abuse and dependence is usually an exclusion. In our experience, patients with active drug or alcohol problems need to achieve abstinence through chemical dependency programs before their bipolar disorder can be appropriately diagnosed and treated.

Special issues arise in child or adolescent patients with bipolar disorder. First, children with bipolar disorder often have comorbid attention-deficit/hyperactivity disorder, oppositional defiant disorder, conduct problems, or other disorders that may need medical or psychosocial intervention. Second, adult patients usually have episodic courses with relatively distinct onsets and offsets, whereas juvenile patients often have brief, frequent, and intense cycles of mood instability with no clear euthymic intervals. In extreme cases, juvenile patients show "ultrarapid cycling," involving switches of polarity that occur every 24 hours. Child patients also are more prone to mixed or dysphoric mania, psychosis, and aggressiveness (Geller & Luby, 1997; Geller et al., 2002; Lewinsohn, Seeley, Buckley, & Klein, 2002). These different patterns of cycling have implications for the conduct of FFT treatment. For example, the chronicity of childhood-onset bipolar illness may lead parents to doubt the validity of the diagnosis, especially when comparing their child's disorder to the adult forms of the disorder. In turn, relapse prevention planning in families with juvenile patients may require identifying and attempting to derail "bad moods," "hyper periods," or "meltdowns" rather than discrete episodes.

GOALS AND STRUCTURE OF TREATMENT

The overriding goals of FFT are to assist patients and their relatives to (1) make sense of the current episode of illness and its precipitants; (2) recognize and plan for the likelihood that the illness will recur; (3) accept the need for an ongoing program of medication to maintain stability; (4) distinguish the disorder from the patient's premorbid personality; (5) learn to cope with stressors that provoke episodes of illness; and (6) maximize the functionality of family or marital relationships in the aftermath of an illness episode.

Note that these objectives do not contain any presumption that the family or marriage was "dysfunctional" prior to the onset of the illness or that the family played a causal role in the disorder's onset. Rather, our evidence indicates that understanding the illness and its precipitants, learning skills to minimize family conflict, and following an illness management program (which, for the patient, includes taking medication) facilitates a better outcome of the disorder. Outcome is measured in several domains: (1) the duration of time the patient maintains partial or full remission, (2) the degree of severity of his or her intermorbid symptoms and level of adaptive functioning, (3) his or her consistency with medications, and (4) the quality and efficiency of family communication and problem solving.

The 21 sessions of FFT are administered in a tapered format, with the most intensive treatment occurring in the first 3 months (12 weekly sessions) followed by 6 biweekly sessions and 3 monthly sessions. For adolescent patients, we have begun experimenting with a format that includes trimonthly maintenance sessions following the 9-month active treatment period. This adjustment reflects our observation that communication and problem-solving skills tend to decay over time as new challenges present themselves. Booster sessions can remind families of the coping strategies they have learned.

Phase 1: Assessing the Family

The assessments conducted in FFT identify antecedent–behavior–consequence chains that cause problems in the family environment. How much do the participants know about bipolar illness already? How do caregiving relatives understand and react to the patient's symptom states? Have their reactions been helpful or hurtful? How has the patient responded to relatives? Does he or she provoke them? Does he or she understand the difficult bind in which relatives find themselves? How do his or her reactions to caregiving efforts affect the relatives?

Family assessments in the research laboratory include the Camberwell Family Interview for rating EE (Vaughn & Leff, 1976), a 1 to 1½-hour semistructured interview that examines the development of the patient's most recent episode and its effects on the family. For childhood patients, the EE interview may be modified so that an episode is redefined as a period in which the child was more irritable/hyper/aggressive than usual. The EE interview, if coded according to research criteria, yields ratings of criticism, hostility, emotional overinvolvement, warmth, and positive remarks. In nonresearch clinical settings, the interview can be administered less formally to clarify the history of the illness, the overall level of negative affectivity in the caregiver–patient relationship, and the relative's attributions regarding the causes of the patient's behaviors. For example, when describing manic behavior, a relative said, "If he could only slow down and focus on one thing at a time, he might actually get something done." This is an example of a "controllability attribution."

Planning FFT sessions is also aided by obtaining an interactional sample from the family or couple. In our research, we have asked the family to participate in two 10-minute problem-solving discussions that are videotaped and later transcribed. These interactions are coded on dimensions such as the amount of relative-to-patient or patient-to-relative criticism, guilt-induction, intrusiveness, self-disclosure, acceptance, acknowledgment, and problem solving (Simoneau et al., 1998; Miklowitz et al., 1989).

In one of our studies (Miklowitz, Goldstein, & Nuechterlein, 1995), the families of recently ill young adult patients with bipolar disorder were engaged in cycles of communication that involved criticism and intrusiveness from parents and counterattacks from patients. In contrast, the families of recently ill patients with schizophrenia were engaged in cycles involving criticism and intrusiveness from parents and self-critical or self-denigrating statements by patients (e.g., "I know how hard I've made things for you guys"). These styles can change as the patient becomes more fully remitted, but observing interactions during a pretreatment period gives the clinician a sense of the likely targets for communication training. Does the patient need to learn how *not* to provoke his or her relatives, and vice versa? Can family members be taught to listen actively and acknowledge each other's viewpoints? Do they know how to deliver constructive criticisms or are their criticisms more personal and global? In other words, which skills are already extant and which need to be developed?

Phase 2: Psychoeducation

Psychoeducation (approximately 7–10 weekly sessions) is placed first on the FFT agenda because patients and family members are most able to make use of illness information when the patient's symptoms are still evident. The major objectives of this module are to help the family make sense of the most recent episode, make plans to prevent or at least minimize the severity of the next episode, and teach the patient wellness-maintaining strategies.

Reviewing the Symptoms of the Disorder

In the first one to two sessions, review the symptoms of bipolar disorder with the family. Focus your review on the most recent episode (for adults) or the most recent period of moodiness and poor functioning (for children and adolescents). The best way to review the symptoms is to pass out a handout showing the typical symptoms of manic and depressive episodes (see Miklowitz & Goldstein, 1997, for handouts). Then say to the patient: "You are the one who has gone through all of this, so maybe that makes you more of an expert on the disorder than the rest of us. Maybe you can help educate me and the rest of your family on what it is like when you experience high or low periods." Ask him or her to describe the feelings of elated mood, intense irritability, grandiosity, racing thoughts, sadness, or hopelessness. Encourage each relative to chime in with his or her own observations. The patient—especially if he or she is a child—may not be fully aware of how his or her behavior changes when he or she is ill.

Pay particular attention to the way the prodromal symptoms of the most recent illness are described. For example, the parents of juvenile patients often recall irritability, aggression, frenetic behavior, impulsiveness, and decreased sleep. The child may describe feeling great, wound up, or just plain mad at everything. Adults describe a similar constellation of symptoms but also may be more attuned to internal processes (e.g., racing thoughts, confidence and extra intelligence, feeling "tired but wired"). Do the same for the depressive pole of the illness (if the patient experiences it) and see if you can identify a prodrome.

For pediatric patients, we include a videotape called "Teens with Bipolar Disorder: In Their Own Words" (Josselyn Foundation, 2000). This tape can be shown in segments during the educational sessions, or you can send it home with them to watch and discuss on their own. The film features very articulate, insightful teenagers who have gone through manic and depressive episodes. The child or teen who sees the film often realizes that he or she is not alone, that bipolar disorder is not the province of "nerdy" kids, and that many function well despite the disorder and its treatments. One 14-year-old girl, after watching the film, had the following interchange with her therapist:

THERAPIST: What did you think, Stacy? Can you relate to any of this?

STACY: Yeah, I think so. I agree with the fact that it's a family issue and not an individual issue. I appreciated the film because I have trouble being understood sometimes when I try to explain this stuff . . . like when I get really hyper and threaten to hit someone, and an hour later I'll say to my dad and my stepmom, "I'm so sorry, I can't even explain what was going on, I was in a different state of mind," but that's really hard to explain. That's one of my goals for treatment, for everyone to understand that most of the time *I* can't control it, but maybe we could think of some ideas of how *we* could control it, because my dad feels helpless when he tries to hold me back, because there's nothing he can say or do to soothe me. . . . I don't even know how to deal with it.

THERAPIST: So a goal for you is to recognize that some of this behavior is uncontrollable on your part and try to figure out some ways for the family to help you control it.

STACY: Right! Because if it is uncontrollable, we should find out ways to, like, totally break it down and make it a controllable situation.

Etiology, Risk, and Protection

As the psychoeducation module progresses, focus the family's attention on genetic and biological predispositional factors (e.g., ask, "Who else in your family had bipolar disorder? Can you describe his/her episodes?"). Communicate the notion that there are chemical imbalances in the brain that lead to symptoms, and that these imbalances are largely uncontrollable by the ill person. Simultaneously, help the family to understand that social–environmental stressors are important in provoking symptom states. Take them through the most recent illness period and determine if life changes (e.g., new romantic relationships or breakups, extensive travel across time zones, school or social pressures, job losses or promotions) precipitated the flare-up of symptoms. Note to yourself that certain stressful events (e.g., losing one's job) may have been brought about by the patient's symptomatic behavior rather than the reverse. Once you have identified these stressors, the family can begin to see pathways from specific life stressors to prodromal symptoms to the onset of manic or depressive episodes.

With the aid of a handout (see copies in Miklowitz & Goldstein, 1997), explain to the family that risk and protective factors modulate the interaction between biological vulnerability and stress. Risk factors include alcohol and drug usage, sleep deprivation, family distress and other interpersonal conflicts, and inconsistency with medications. Protective factors include self-monitoring of moods and triggers for fluctuations, maintaining consistent daily and nightly routines, relying on social and family supports, and engaging in regular drug and psychosocial treatment.

The Mood Chart

At this point, you can introduce the patient to the idea of keeping a mood chart. Mood charts vary in their complexity and coverage. We usually encourage people to download the mood chart used in the Systematic Treatment Enhancement Program for Bipolar Disorder (STEP-BD; Sachs, 1998; Sachs et al., 2003) from *www.manicdepressive.org* (see Appendix 2). This chart asks patients to track their moods on a −3 (severely depressed) to 0 (euthymic) to +3 (severely manic) state. For each day, the patient makes at least one overall rating, or, better yet, a best and a worst rating. There are separate spaces to record psychosocial stressors, medications taken, psychotherapy received, hours of sleep, and other associated symptoms (e.g., irritability, anxiety, psychosis). After keeping the charts for a month or more, patients and relatives begin to see the interrelationships between stress and social stimulation, sleep changes, medication compliance, and mood stability (Frank, Swartz, & Kupfer, 2000).

Mood charts for children are available (*www.bpkids.org/learning/ mood.htm*), or you can ask the child or parents to develop one of their own. Ask both the child and the parent to fill one out each week. If the child seems unable or unwilling to do it, sit next to the child in the next session and fill one out with him or her.

How the Family Can Help

Family caregivers often benefit from a handout that summarizes the steps to take to get help for their ill relative (see Table 9.1). Pass this out to the family and patient and ask them to discuss the items one by one. How can the parents of a 15-year-old adolescent with bipolar disorder help him or her get regular sleep/wake hours? To what extent should a spouse be involved in helping her husband get to psychiatry appointments or necessary lab tests? What level of reduced expectations should a parent or spouse have during the patient's recovery? This handout also previews two important components of FFT: the relapse drill and communication skill modules.

The Relapse Drill

The purpose of the relapse drill is to develop a plan, as a family, for handling the escalation of symptoms (or, in the case of children, bad moods or meltdowns). For adults, review the prodromal symptoms of the most recent episode and the circumstances in which these occurred. For example: "You started to escalate in your mood after you stayed up late two nights in a row studying for finals. Your first signs were irritability, your thoughts going faster, and feeling like you had more energy." Or: "You became depressed after you broke up with Katrina. Your first sign was that you became tired and lethargic, and then you started feeling slowed down in your thinking." Then ask the patient and relatives to list various alternative responses they could engage if these prodromal symptoms were to reap-

TABLE 9.1. How Can the Family Help?

- Help your relative to obtain treatment and keep all appointments.
- Help him or her to be consistent about taking medications.
- Help him or her to maintain regular daily routines and sleep cycles.
- Get help for yourself or other members of the family who are having a difficult time.
- Learn as much as you can about bipolar illness so that you can recognize early warning signs of relapse.
- Develop a plan as a family for controlling the escalation of mood swings.
- Maintain a tolerant and low-key home atmosphere.
- Reduce expectations of what he or she should be able to accomplish during recovery; recognize that, for most medical illnesses, recovery is a gradual process.
- Try to continue on with normal family life as much as possible; attend to the needs of other kids in the family.
- Use good communication skills:
  - Praise good behaviors or positive changes.
  - Listen actively.
  - Express anger as constructively as possible.
  - Use collaborative problem solving.
  - Exit interactions that are becoming unproductive.

pear. Typical plans the patient can implement to prevent full-blown mania include calling the physician to arrange a modification of the medication regimen (e.g., adding an atypical antipsychotic drug to derail manic escalation or psychotic thinking), or permitting his or her spouse to do so; arranging to get his or her medication blood levels tested; temporarily giving up credit cards and car keys; and taking friends along on night outings to avoid getting into risky sexual situations.

Relatives also can support the patient by (1) serving as a sounding board when he or she wishes to talk about internal conflicts (especially when depression is beginning to worsen), (2) helping the patient avoid taking on too much social stimulation or making foolish financial or business decisions, (3) encouraging him or her to avoid alcohol or street drugs, and (4) helping him or her to stay intellectually and physically active when becoming depressed. Some caregivers, particularly spouses, can help the person with bipolar disorder restabilize the sleep–wake cycle by helping him or her get to bed and wake up on time. Once the family has generated several preventive options, write them down on a piece of paper and ask everyone to sign the plan. Note that this is often the family's first exposure to active problem solving.

For adolescent or child patients, the relapse drill is done differently. Stand next to a flip chart or dry erase board and ask each participant (including the parents and any siblings who might be present) to describe "having a bad day." Asking each person to admit to his or her negative moods takes pressure off of the child, who may feel unfairly stigmatized as the only one in the family with problems. Ask each person to list his or her triggers (for example, Roy, a 13-year-old boy with bipolar disorder, listed "when my brother gets in my way," and "when my parents ground me") and what bad moods look like for him or her (he listed "grouchy," "hyper," and "bummed" and his parents chimed in with "testy," "angry," and "obnoxious"). Then ask each person to list "what would help" when those moods are present. Options for Roy included being left alone (his preference) or being allowed to "chill out and listen to music." His mother felt that sitting with him and talking him through his anger was more effective. Between sessions, type up the responses and present it to the family as a relapse prevention plan.

Remind the parents and child that the physician may suggest altering the medication regimen when moods escalate to a certain level of dysfunction. Medication adjustments are usually an alternative when the child is a danger to self or others, has shown an increase in irritability at home, or is deteriorating in school.

Dealing with Resistances to Psychoeducation: The "Psychotherapeutic Attitude"

It is important to conduct FFT as a psychotherapist rather than a teacher. In so doing, you may be able to derail the resistances to treatment that often arise, particularly in the young. Think of your task as following two separate but interactive tracks: providing information and skill training while simultaneously dealing with the affective reactions of the participants to this information. In this section, techniques for addressing resistances are described.

Dealing with Resistances to the Diagnosis

Adult patients who have only had a few episodes and most juvenile patients have significant doubts about the validity of the diagnosis and see no need to talk about it with their family members. Talking about the illness makes them feel immature and under their parents' thumb. They complain of feeling overexamined, intruded upon, or "picked apart." When they feel this way, they sometimes behave in childlike and uncooperative ways in family sessions.

It is usually helpful to comment on patients' negative emotional reactions to the diagnostic label, their anger in response to criticisms from other family members, or their discomfort about being "an object of discussion." Anticipate the negative reactions of patients by making good use of normalizing and reframing techniques. For example, you might say: "I suspect that when we talk about the illness, there are times when you feel under the microscope, or that you're the only one in the family who has any problems. You may start to wonder whether the diagnosis is really accurate or whether what we cover here really applies to you. It's natural and understandable, and even healthy to have these reactions. Are you having any of these reactions now? If so, would you care to talk about them?" If the patient says "no," then you can add: "If you do feel like talking about this in our future sessions, I hope you'll let me know so that we can figure out a way for you to be more comfortable here." Simple statements such as these go far in bolstering a treatment alliance with the patient and cutting through resistances.

Another way to address the patient's discomfort is to "spread the affliction." Ask other members of the family whether they have had experiences with depression or anxiety. Explore prior episodes of depression in a mother, father, or spouse. Ask questions such as: "Which of the mood symptoms did you have? How did you handle them? What did others do that helped or didn't?" You can conclude the discussion by saying: "So, maybe dealing with depression is an issue for several of you. Let's figure out some strategies for dealing with mood problems as a family."

Medical analogies are often helpful to destigmatize the diagnostic label and the requirement of long-term medication. For example, draw similarities between bipolar disorder and other long-term, recurrent medical illnesses like diabetes or hypertension. Point out that other medical illnesses require medication and lifestyle management (for example, eating low-salt foods) and that medical patients also are ambivalent about making these sacrifices. Patients and family members are often relieved to think of bipolar disorder on a continuum with other physically based illnesses.

Addressing Caregivers Who Feel Blamed

Be aware that parents of adults and children with bipolar disorder often feel unfairly blamed for their offspring's disorder. Spouses feel blamed or guilty as well, especially if they have been accused by the patient of not having provided adequate support. Spouses may believe that they should have seen their partner's episodes coming long before they did. Even if caregivers do not raise these issues, you can show your awareness of them. For example, you might say: "I know that many relatives who take part in family counseling feel that they're being told they've done things wrong. I want to be clear that I'm in no way blaming you as parents [or as a spouse] or implying that I would have done things differently. Bipolar disorder can be quite taxing to a family that is trying to do its best. My goal here is to help you develop strategies that will make you even more efficient in communication and problem solving than the average family, given the challenges you face. How does this sound to you?"

Communicating Flexibility, Optimism, and Hope

Be flexible in your approach: Have an agenda but be willing to depart from it, as the situation requires. Be willing to accept a degree of ambiguity—feelings on the part of family members that do not quite make sense, relationships that have love–hate components, seemingly contradictory approaches to the illness (e.g., "There's nothing wrong with me, but I know I have to take medication"), or problems that do not get neatly solved. Ambiguity and unpredictability are core features of bipolar disorder, and families usually function better when they do not become overly tied to one vision of the patient's illness and future.

Lastly, express optimism and hope. Families and couples understandably want to hear that they can look forward to the future. Take the stance that, although the illness is likely to recur at some point, the patient is armed against this likelihood through taking medications, using lifestyle management techniques, and making good use of family or marital support.

Phase 3: Communication Enhancement Training

The second and third modules of FFT address the family's communication and problem-solving skills and deficits. By this point, you have probably developed a rapport with the family, and the participants are more open to direct behavioral intervention. You also have a better idea of the family's or couple's strengths and weaknesses in communication. The communication enhancement training (CET) module (approximately seven sessions, the first of which are weekly, up to session 12, and then biweekly) begins with an explanation of how healthy communication will help the family to cope with bipolar illness:

"Remember a few sessions ago we talked about protective factors? Well, good communication and problem solving can help protect you as a family [or couple] against stress and improve your relationships, and may even help with [the patient's name's] illness. I want to help you communicate in the clearest and least stressful manner possible, so that everyone's voice is heard and problems get solved. I'll be asking you to 'role play' with each other some new ways of talking and listening. You'll begin to see how these ways of talking make you feel like you are all on the same team."

Four skills are taught: expressing positive feelings, active listening, making positive requests for change, and expressing negative feelings. The basic technique for learning all of these skills is role-playing. Ask two members of the family to volunteer to be speaker and listener, and to turn their chairs toward each other. Then coach them to use a specific skill according to the steps listed on a series of associated handouts (see Miklowitz &

Goldstein, 1997). For example, if you want to teach active listening, ask the speaker to relate a relatively nonthreatening event from his or her day (e.g., a father of a 17-year-old girl with bipolar disorder talked of his frustration on his construction job). Then instruct the listener to nod his or her head and ask clarifying questions (e.g., "So when did all of this happen?") and to paraphrase or listen reflectively (e.g., "So it was frustrating because your boss was telling everyone to do things differently and then blaming you when the job didn't get done right"). When teaching the skill of making positive requests, ask one participant to make a specific request of another, along with a feeling statement (e.g., "I'd really appreciate it if, when you want something from me, you'd ask in a nice tone of voice so that I can feel better about giving it").

You can expect a certain degree of resistance to the role-play process. Typically, people do not feel natural about role-playing, and adolescents feel particularly uncomfortable with it. Nevertheless, it is really the only way to learn communication skills in a way that facilitates their generalization to other settings. Among the various strategies for dealing with resistance, three are central:

1. Serve as the speaker or listener yourself and model the skill before asking the participants to do it.
2. Ask the more active members of the family to role-play before asking the more reticent members.
3. Inject humor into the process (e.g., "I'm trying to get you all to talk just like therapists. Isn't that what you've always wanted?").

All CET sessions should conclude with a homework assignment. Ask all family members to keep track of instances in which they praised or made requests of other members of the family, delivered constructive criticisms, or listened actively. Ask them to choose a time during the week to meet as a family and practice the skills, and then bring in completed worksheets. Once again, you can expect resistance to this process, and many families go several weeks before actually practicing the skills between sessions. Remind them of the purposes of learning the skills and acknowledge that "it can be difficult to get everyone together in the same room, especially to practice talking in a way that may feel foreign." Problem solve with them about how they could choose a convenient time to practice, and give them a lot of praise when they succeed in even minor ways (e.g., "We didn't practice, but we talked together more").

Most of all, keep giving them encouragement to try out the new skills. Our experience has been that families who actively practice and make use of communication skills in the home setting benefit most from FFT in terms of reductions in family tension. In fact, one of our studies showed that increases in the use of positive verbal and nonverbal communication styles, particularly by the patient, predicted the patients' improvement over 1 year of treatment (Simoneau et al., 1999).

Phase 4: Problem-Solving Skills Training

The final module of FFT focuses on problem solving (four or five biweekly and then monthly sessions). This is the process by which family members are taught the following skills:

1. Identify and define problems that have arisen in the aftermath of a period of illness.
2. Generate a list of solutions to these problems ("brainstorming") without evaluating their viability yet.
3. Submit each proposed solution to an analysis of advantages and disadvantages.
4. Choose a best solution or combination of solutions.
5. Develop an implementation plan (Falloon, Boyd, & McGill, 1984; Liberman, Wallace, Falloon, & Vaughn, 1981).

One assumption of problem solving is that high levels of EE prior to, during, or following an acute illness are, at least in part, the result of problems that could be broken down into smaller components and successfully negotiated. The patient, however, may need to achieve a degree of clinical stability before addressing problems associated with the illness—which is why the problem-solving module is positioned last.

In our experience, families of patients with bipolar disorder usually have problems in one or more of the following domains: (1) disagreements over illness management (e.g., the patient's inconsistency in medication usage, erratic sleep–wake routines, work, school, and play hours, drug/alcohol abuse); (2) problems related to the resumption of work, school, or social responsibilities; (3) disagreements over household management, rules, or finances; and (4) relational problems, including disagreements about intimacy (for couples) or boundaries (for parent–offspring pairs). Problem solving also can be applied to relapse prevention, as illustrated above.

For juvenile patients, problem solving can be used to develop behavior management plans. For example, one adolescent girl repeatedly swore at her mother in public. Through problem solving, she and her mother defined the circumstances in which it was likely to occur (typically, when her mother denied her something she wanted), discussed preventative plans (e.g., determining when her anger was starting to spiral and redirecting her), and developed a list of possible consequences for the behavior (e.g., being grounded, lack of access to money or her car, writing her mother a letter of apology).

Here is an example of how problem solving was used in one family to address school truancy.

The patient, Carmela, was a 17-year-old Hispanic female who lived with her father, his girlfriend, and her two younger brothers. She had been cutting her final class period nearly every day. Her clinical condition was reasonably stable on her regimen of oxcarbazepine (Trileptal) and olanzapine (Zyprexa). She was somewhat ashamed of her behavior, explaining that many of her friends did not have a final class period, so it had become easy to skip class to "hang with them." Her father added that Carmela had found the school day to be very long and stressful, and that she needed a break by day's end. Skipping class had provided her both a social outlet and a relief from stress, but she had been placed on academic probation. She had had other problems in public school since transitioning from a special education environment, such as inappropriate outbursts of anger toward teachers.

Carmela and her father proposed a number of possible solutions: (1) introducing rewards for completing school days (e.g., her father taking her out once a week to her favorite fast-food restaurant) or consequences for failing to complete the day (e.g., not being able to go out with her boyfriend that night); (2) going to see a school psychologist to learn stress management techniques to employ during the school day; (3) arranging to get together with friends to do something fun after her final class period, giving her an incentive to follow through with the day; (4) taking brief relaxation breaks or naps at the nurse's office (in addition to stress, she suffered fatigue from her antipsychotic medication); (5) her father checking in with the school dean every week to see how many classes she had missed; and (6) her father's girlfriend dropping by school at the beginning of Carmela's last period to make sure she had made it to class.

Upon evaluating the pros and cons of each solution, Carmela and her father quickly eliminated the second option (too time intensive) and the fifth and sixth options (required too much intrusion by her parents). Item 3 was attractive to Carmela but difficult to arrange with friends on a regular basis. The solutions chosen were a combination of the first and fourth options—obtaining rewards and accepting consequences from her father that were contingent on her classroom attendance, and arranging brief breaks at the nurse's office to rest and relieve stress. The latter solution required preplanning with the school nurse, which became part of their implementation plan. These solutions did not fully eliminate the problem but made it occur less frequently, such that she was able to get off of academic probation.

Learning the steps of problem solving gives the family a sense of competence in mastering its own difficulties. When the family communication is progressing well, the therapist can take a less active role as members structure their own discussions. Because the frequency of sessions has been tapered to once a month by the end of the problem-solving module, between-session homework assignments become critical to the generalization of the skills.

Phase 5: Termination

In the last sessions of FFT, review the progress the family has made in treatment, with a focus on the six overall goals listed earlier. Review the relapse prevention contract and modify it with the family, as needed. Discuss the patient's plans for continued pharmacological treatment and alert the physician that more regular monitoring of symptoms and compliance may now be necessary. The last point is critical, because patients have been known to discontinue medications when their psychotherapy ends.

Termination sessions also allow you to discuss follow-up treatment options with the patient and relatives. These may include individual therapy (preferably with a clinician who is knowledgeable about bipolar disorder), support groups (e.g., the National Alliance for the Mentally Ill; see *www.nami.org*), or additional family or marital therapy. You also may wish to offer the family booster sessions every few months to help solidify their gains in treatment. You can expect that many families will keep in touch with you for years after termination to seek support for new challenges brought about by the illness.

FUTURE DIRECTIONS

Although FFT has demonstrated efficacy in two randomized trials, much is still to be learned about its application to patients with bipolar disorder and their families. The subgroups of patients who benefit most, FFT's mechanisms of action, and its effects on functional outcomes are currently being examined. The multisite STEP-BD study may be able to answer questions about the effectiveness of FFT relative to comparison individual therapy approaches, such as interpersonal or cognitive-behavioral therapy. STEP-BD also may clarify the difficulties encountered when transporting family interventions to community settings that differ in the orientation and background of therapists, the socioeconomic status of the communities served, the availability of family members, and the clinical complexity of the patient populations.

Another ongoing study (Oquendo, Barrera, & Mann, 2001) is examining FFT as adjunctive to different pharmacotherapy strategies in an ethnically diverse sample of patients with bipolar disorder who have mixed or depressed episodes and suicidality. Finally, the efficacy of FFT for adolescent patients with bipolar disorder is undergoing examination in a two-site randomized trial (Miklowitz, 2001). Results from these studies should generate revised clinician's manuals to help adapt the intervention to a diversity of clinical settings and populations.

ACKNOWLEDGMENTS

Preparation of this chapter was supported in part by a grant from the National Institute of Mental Health (MH62555) and a Distinguished Investigator Award from the National Alliance for Research on Schizophrenia and Depression.

REFERENCES

Clarkin, J. F., Carpenter, D., Hull, J., Wilner, P., & Glick, I. (1998). Effects of psychoeducational intervention for married patients with bipolar disorder and their spouses. *Psychiatric Services, 49,* 531–533.

Cohen, M., Baker, G., Cohen, R. A., Fromm-Reichmann, F., & Weigert, V. (1954). An intensive study of 12 cases of manic–depressive psychosis. *Psychiatry, 17,* 103–137.

Falloon, I. R. H., Boyd, J. L., & McGill, C. W. (1984). *Family care of schizophrenia: A problem-solving approach to the treatment of mental illness.* New York: Guilford Press.

First, M. B., Spitzer, R. L., Gibbon, M., & Williams, J. B. W. (1995). *Structured clinical interview for DSM-IV axis I disorders.* New York: New York State Psychiatric Institute.

Frank, E., Swartz, H. A., & Kupfer, D. J. (2000). Interpersonal and Social Rhythm Therapy: Managing the chaos of bipolar disorder. *Biological Psychiatry, 48,* 593–604.

Geller, B., Craney, J. L., Bolhofner, K., Nickelsburg, M. J., Williams, M., & Zimerman, B. (2002). Two-year prospective follow-up of children with a prepubertal and early adolescent bipolar disorder phenotype. *American Journal of Psychiatry, 159,* 927–933.

Geller, B., & Luby, J. (1997). Child and adolescent bipolar disorder: A review of the past 10 years. *Journal of the American Academy of Child and Adolescent Psychiatry, 36,* 1168–1176.

Goldstein, M. J., & Miklowitz, D. J. (1995). The effectiveness of psychoeducational family therapy in the treatment of schizophrenic disorders. *Journal of Marital and Family Therapy, 21,* 361–376.

Goodwin, F. K., & Jamison, K. R. (1990). *Manic–depressive illness.* New York: Oxford University Press.

Hooley, J. M., & Licht, D. M. (1997). Expressed emotion and causal attributions in the spouses of depressed patients. *Journal of Abnormal Psychology, 106,* 298–306.

Josselyn Foundation (2000). *In their own words: Teens with bipolar disorder* [videotape]. Chicago, IL: Josselyn Foundation.

Lewinsohn, P. M., Seeley, J. R., Buckley, M. E., & Klein, D. N. (2002). Bipolar disorder in adolescence and young adulthood. *Child and Adolescent Psychiatric Clinics of North America, 11,* 461–475.

Liberman, R. P., Wallace, C. J., Falloon, I. R. H., & Vaughn, C. E. (1981). Interpersonal problem-solving therapy for schizophrenics and their families. *Comprehensive Psychiatry, 22,* 627–629.

Miklowitz, D. J. (2001). *Family-focused psychoeducation for bipolar adolescents.* (NIMH grant R21–MH62555). Rockville, MD: National Institute of Mental Health.

Miklowitz, D. J., George, E. L., Richards, J. A., Simoneau, T. L., & Suddath, R. L. (in press). A randomized study of family-focused psychoeducation and pharmacotherapy in the outpatient management of bipolar disorder. *Archives of General Psychiatry.*

Miklowitz, D. J., & Goldstein, M. J. (1990). Behavioral family treatment for patients with bipolar affective disorder. *Behavior Modification, 14,* 457–489.

Miklowitz, D. J., & Goldstein, M. J. (1997). *Bipolar disorder: A family-focused treatment approach.* New York: Guilford Press.

Miklowitz, D. J., Goldstein, M. J., Doane, J. A., Nuechterlein, K. H., Strachan, A. M., Snyder, K. S., & Magana, A. (1989). Is expressed emotion an index of a transactional process? I. Parents' affective style. *Family Process, 28,* 153–167.

Miklowitz, D. J., Goldstein, M. J., & Nuechterlein, K. H. (1995). Verbal interactions in the families of schizophrenic and bipolar affective patients. *Journal of Abnormal Psychology, 104,* 268–276.

Miklowitz, D. J., Goldstein, M. J., Nuechterlein, K. H., Snyder, K. S., & Mintz, J. (1988). Family factors and the course of bipolar affective disorder. *Archives of General Psychiatry, 45,* 225–231.

Miklowitz, D. J., Simoneau, T. L., George, E. L., Richards, J. A., Kalbag, A., Sachs-Ericsson, N., & Suddath, R. (2000). Family-focused treatment of bipolar disorder: 1-year effects of a psychoeducational program in conjunction with pharmacotherapy. *Biological Psychiatry, 48,* 582–592.

O'Connell, R. A., Mayo, J. A., Flatow, L., Cuthbertson, B., & O'Brien, B. E. (1991). Outcome of bipolar disorder on long-term treatment with lithium. *British Journal of Psychiatry, 159,* 123–129.

Oquendo, M. A., Barrera, A., & Mann, J. J. (2001). Psychopharmacologic strategies for the prevention of suicidal behavior in bipolar patients. *Clinical Neuroscience Research, 1,* 387–393.

Priebe, S., Wildgrube, C., & Muller-Oerlinghausen, B. (1989). Lithium prophylaxis and expressed emotion. *British Journal of Psychiatry, 154,* 396–399.

Rea, M. M., Tompson, M., Miklowitz, D. J., Goldstein, M. J., Hwang, S., & Mintz, J. (2003). Family-focused treatment vs. individual treatment for bipolar disorder: Results of a randomized clinical trial. *Journal of Consulting and Clinical Psychology, 71,* 482–492.

Sachs, G. (1998). *Treatments for bipolar disorder.* (NIMH contract no. N01MH80001). Rockville, MD: National Institute of Mental Health.

Sachs, G. S., Thase, M. E., Otto, M. W., Bauer, M., Miklowitz, D., Wisniewski, S. R., Lavori, P., Lebowitz, B., Rudorfer, M., Frank, E., Nierenberg, A. A., Fava, M., Bowden, C., Ketter, T., Marangell, L., Calabrese, J., Kupfer, D., & Rosenbaum, J. F. (2003). Rationale, design, and methods of the Systematic Treatment Enhancement Program for Bipolar Disorder. *Biological Psychiatry, 53,* 1028–1042.

Simoneau, T. L., Miklowitz, D. J., Richards, J. A., Saleem, R., & George, E. L. (1999). Bipolar disorder and family communication: Effects of a psychoeducational treatment program. *Journal of Abnormal Psychology, 108,* 588–597.

Simoneau, T. L., Miklowitz, D. J., & Saleem, R. (1998). Expressed emotion and interactional patterns in the families of bipolar patients. *Journal of Abnormal Psychology, 107,* 497–507.

Vaughn, C. E., & Leff, J. P. (1976). The influence of family and social factors on the course of psychiatric illness: A comparison of schizophrenic and depressed neurotic patients. *British Journal of Psychiatry, 129,* 125–137.

Wendel, J. S., Miklowitz, D. J., Richards, J. A., & George, E. L. (2000). Expressed emotion and attributions in the relatives of bipolar patients: An analysis of problem-solving interactions. *Journal of Abnormal Psychology, 109,* 792–796.

CHAPTER TEN

SUPPORTING COLLABORATIVE PRACTICE MANAGEMENT
The Life Goals Program

MARK S. BAUER

As summarized elsewhere in this book and in our other contributions (e.g., Bauer & McBride, 2003; Bauer et al., 2001; Wells et al., 2002), manic–depressive (bipolar) disorder* is a severe, chronic, and costly illness. Moreover, it is a treatable disorder, but the impact of treatments fall far short of established efficacy in general clinical practice (Bauer et al., 2001). This chapter introduces the reader to the Life Goals Program, a group-based psychoeducational program designed to assist individuals with manic–depressive disorder to become better collaborators in their own illness management. The development and orientation of this intervention derives from a somewhat different source than many of the psychotherapies for major mental illnesses, since its roots lie primarily in the optimization of medical-model treatment of chronic medical diseases, rather than in specific psychological theories of mood disorders. Because of this somewhat different orientation, I first discuss the concepts of chronic disease management, then focus on the patient-centered component of this complex task. In this context, the Life Goals Program is presented in detail, with case material interspersed to illustrate the concepts and interventions of the program.

*Note that throughout this chapter, I have used the term "manic–depressive disorder" rather than "bipolar disorder." For this discussion, manic–depressive disorder is the more accurate term in terms of describing the symptoms the patients actually experience (Bauer, 2003b).

Although the concepts of chronic disease management may appear to pertain mainly to working within complex systems, evidence indicates that simple collaborative patient-level interventions alone can have substantial impact on outcome. In a recent generalist's psychiatric assessment treatment manual, we make the point that a collaborative approach focused on patient education can be implemented by individual practitioners treating patients with various mental disorders (Bauer, 2003a). Thus, understanding these "big picture" system-based concepts and data is in the service of supporting the practice of individuals in office-based practice. Appendix 5 contains a basic outline of how the collaborative approach can be applied to all dyadic provider–patient interactions in treating mental illness.

OUR INITIAL FORAYS INTO COLLABORATIVE DISEASE MANAGEMENT OF MANIC–DEPRESSIVE DISORDER

Recognizing the existence of an "efficacy-effectiveness gap" (Institute of Medicine, 1985) in the treatment of manic–depressive disorder, in the early 1990s we developed a tripartite disease management program that emphasized collaboration with patients to improve outcome (described in Bauer et al., 1997, 2001; Bauer, 2001b). The three facets of the program address patient, provider, and system contributions to the efficacy-effectiveness gap: (1) patient illness self-management skills using the Life Goals structured group program (Bauer & McBride 1996, 2003); (2) provider support through national practice guidelines (Bauer et al., 1999) in simplified form (Bauer, 2001b); and (3) improved access to, and continuity of care through, primary nurse providers working in conjunction with psychiatrists (Shea, McBride, Gavin, & Bauer, 1997). As noted, in its explicit focus on patient, provider, and system factors, the program more closely resembles disease management programs that were concurrently developed for treatment of chronic medical illnesses (Wagner, Austin, & Von Korff, 1996; Wagner et al., 2001; Von Korff, Gruman, Schaefer, Curry, & Wagner, 1997). What were some of the precedents that helped us to develop the Life Goals component of this disease management program?

RELATION TO COLLABORATIVE MANAGEMENT PROGRAMS FOR OTHER CHRONIC DISEASES

As we designed this program in the early 1990s, disease management programs for a broad spectrum of chronic medical illnesses also were being developed. A large number of randomized controlled trials (RCTs) demonstrated that multifaceted disease management programs can improve outcome and quality of care for patients with diabetes, hypertension, lung disease, arthritis, and oncologic conditions (reviewed in Center for the Advancement of Health, 1996; Renders et al., 2003; Von Korff et al., 1997; Wagner et al., 1996; Wagner et al., 2001). Clinical practice guidelines for mental health underscore the impression that multifaceted interventions can improve process quality and outcome for mental illnesses (Bauer, 2002). The core components of virtually all these disease management programs include a focus on patient self-management skills, accompanied by varying degrees of emphasis on provider and system factors. Self-management components typically emphasize development of skills and collaboration between patient and provider in goal setting and treatment planning.

Consideration of these various sources, in particular their emphasis on the patient taking an active role in his or her treatment, led us to focus on the theme of *collaboration* in designing the intervention. We subsequently articulated a definition for *collaborative disease management* as an organization of care that (1) emphasizes the development in the patient of disease self-management skills and (2) supports provider capability and availability to (3) engage patients in timely, joint decision making regarding their illness (Bauer, 2001b). What are the precedents for a collaborative approach, particularly the patient-centered component, in managing chronic illnesses?

An extensive literature on patient education also indicates that interventions focusing exclusively on the *patient behavior* component of care also can be effective in improving the process and outcome of care. First, it is important to note that deficiencies in patient–provider communication and collaboration are the rule rather than the exception in medical care (e.g., Beisecker, 1990; Braddock, Edwards, Hasenberg, & Laidley, 1999; Ciechanowski, Katon, Russo, & Walker, 2001; Cooper-Patrick et al., 1999; Kaplan, Gandek, Greenfield, Rogers, & Ware, 1995; Kaplan, Greenfield, Gandek, Rogers, & Ware, 1996; Little et al., 2001; Roter, 1989; Starfield et al., 1981; Stewart, McWhinney, & Buck, 1979) as well as psychiatric care (e.g., Estroff, 1981; Karp, 1996; Katz, 1984; Lazare, Eisenthal, & Wasserman, 1975; Levinson, Merrifield, & Berg, 1967; Lidz, Meisel, & Zerubavel, 1984; Lish, Dime-Meenan, Whybrow, Price, & Hirschfeld, 1994; NDMDA, 2001). Moreover, there is substantial evidence that patient–provider communication problems are associated with worse outcome (reviewed in Simpson et al., 1991).

Further, the broad patient education literature indicates that patient-centered interventions in chronic medical illnesses can indeed lead to improved process quality and outcome (reviewed in Bayer Institute, 1996–2000; Center for the Advancement of Health, 1996; Ong & deHaes, 1995; Stewart, 1995; The Worthlin Group, 1995), including outcome for several chronic diseases (e.g., Greenfield, Kaplan, & Ware, 1985; Greenfield et al., 1988; Inui et al., 1979; Lorig, Mazonson, & Holman, 1993; Montgomery, Lieberman, Singh, & Fries, 1994). Interestingly, several studies indicate that consumer-led interventions also may improve outcome in patients with chronic medical or psychiatric illnesses (e.g., Dixon et al., 2002; Lorig et al., 1999; Reissman & Banks, 2001). It is important to note that such patient-centered interventions achieve significant effects without intervening directly with providers or systems. Accordingly, Wagner and colleagues point out that many patient-education interventions exert their effects without support or even knowledge of the clinician (Wagner et al., 1996).

There are also precedents for patient-centered collaboration in managing chronic *mental* illnesses, despite the possibility that insight and decision making may be impaired for patients at times. Not surprisingly, much of the self-management intervention RCT work, to date, for mental illness has focused on extensive, multimodal interventions (reviewed in Burns & Santos, 1995; Mueser et al., 2002). There is an additional modest but rapidly growing literature on multimodal treatment of patients with depression in primary care (e.g., Katon et al., 1995; Wells, 1999; Wells et al., 2002; Simon, Von Korff, Rutter, & Wagner, 2000; see also Bauer, 2002).

Compared to the literature on multimodal interventions, the literature on patient-centered interventions for mental illness is smaller. For instance, the Cochrane review of 10 controlled trials of patient-plus-family education regarding schizophrenia (Pekkala & Merinder, 2003) found that psychoeducational interventions significantly reduced relapse or readmission rates (RR) at 9–18 months (RR = 0.8, 95%; CI [confidence interval] = 0.7–0.9), and that there appeared to be significant positive effects on patient well-being. There is also preliminary data that the community-developed and consumer-led National Alliance for the Mentally Ill (NAMI) Family-to-Family education program may increase family empowerment, self-care, and illness information and reduce perceived family burden (Dixon et al., 2002).

Various formal psychotherapies for manic–depressive disorder are reviewed in Chapter 11 (this volume). It is interesting that content analysis of these major manual-based psychotherapies (e.g., cognitive-behavioral [e.g., Lam et al., 2000], interpersonal and social rhythms [e.g., Frank et al., 1999], family [e.g., Miklowitz et al., 2000], and psychoeducational [Perry, Tarrier, Morriss, McCarthy, & Limb, 1999]) indicates that, despite their dissimilar forms, they share a disease self-management core similar to each other and to the Life Goals Program (Bauer, 2001a). Similarly, for chronic medical disease self-management, "The method of delivering the intervention—whether by class, one-on-one counseling, or computer program—may be less important than its ability to identify and respond to the individual needs and priorities of patients" (Wagner et al., 1996, p. 523).

THE STRUCTURE OF THE LIFE GOALS PROGRAM

The goals of the Life Goals Program are twofold:

1. The first goal is to improve clinical outcome by improving illness management skills, which facilitates the group member's participation in medical model treatment; improved disease-specific outcome is anticipated to have beneficial effects on both functional outcome and direct and indirect illness costs.
2. However, improvements in disease outcome alone do not necessarily lead to improvements in functional outcome (Vignette 10.1). Thus, the second goal is to improve functional outcome directly by assisting individuals in achieving the social, occupational, and quality-of-life goals they have identified and which they have not been able to attain due to illness.

Accordingly, the program is structured in two sequential Phases. In each phase, nonspecialist therapists lead groups of 5–10 patients. We have successfully trained master's level social workers, registered nurses, clinical specialists, psychologists, and physicians to provide the intervention (Bauer, McBride, Chase, Sachs, & Shea, 1998). Group sessions are 60–75 minutes in length and occur weekly. Specific components of Phases 1 and 2 are listed in Table 10.1.

In the original version (Bauer & McBride, 1996) Phase 1 included five sessions: one on basic information about the disorder and its neurobiological underpinnings, two on mania, and two on depression. Sessions on depression and mania cover a similar agenda with a similar orientation. The therapist and group members first discuss symptoms and impact of the illness in general, nonpersonalized terms—that is, what they may have heard or read about the disorder. The discussion then focuses on helping members develop a personal symptom profile for their own episodes of depression and mania. Members then identify their early warning signs of impending episodes from among these symptoms. Next, they identify their symptom triggers and their adaptive as well as maladaptive coping responses. Important related topics, such as suicidality and substance use, also are emphasized. In this exercise patients assess their responses using a personal cost–benefit analysis of their various coping responses, and they develop an action plan for responding to symptoms that emphasizes beneficial coping resources.

The revised version (Bauer & McBride, 2003) has been expanded to six sessions, based on patient and therapist feedback, to allow additional time to address the issue of stigma more explicitly, to discuss medications issues, and to formulate a more extensive action plan. An example of an exhibit for Phase 1 is shown in Figure 10.1.

TABLE 10.1. Components of the Life Goals Program

Structural component	Life Goals tasks	Main interventions
Phase 1		
Session 1: Orientation and illness overview Session 2: Mania Session 3: Mania Session 4: Depression Session 5: Depression Session 6: Treatments and treatment planning	• Understand illness basics • Develop personal illness profile for mania, depression • Identify triggers • Conduct personal cost–benefit analysis to identify and shift to optimal coping strategies for symptoms, triggers • Construct personal action plan • Construct overall care plan	• Education • Personal profiles • Personal cost–benefit analysis • Interpersonal group (secondary)
Phase 2		
Agenda-driven, open-ended sessions (median time to first goal attainment: 7 months [95% CI, 5.1–12.3 months])	• Identify goals • Break goals into realistic subgoals • Break subgoals into attainable behavioral steps • Remove roadblocks	• Behavioral strategies to develop plan • Personal cost–benefit analysis iteratively to develop plan and address roadblocks • Cognitive and behavioral strategies to address roadblocks • Interpersonal group strategies to address roadblocks

The concept of the *personal cost–benefit analysis* is critical to understanding the method; it is outlined in the next section. Throughout both Phase 1 and Phase 2, the group member is assumed to act always in his or her perceived best self-interest, which the Life Goals Program helps the member to clarify and modify to support improved illness management.

Phase 2 is open-ended and goal-driven, whereas Phase 1 is agenda-driven. The focus of Phase 2 is to (1) assist group members in identifying self-defined functional goals that they were not able to meet in life because of the illness, (2) help them to cast these goals in objective and feasible terms, and (3) take a predominantly behavioral approach to assist them in meeting these goals. Group members initially discuss various ways in which manic–depressive disorder has impacted their lives. In doing so, they identify areas in which they feel they have not achieved their potential because of the illness (i.e., areas of functional morbidity). The therapist helps them to articulate these goals in explicit behavioral terms. For instance, a member may be dissatisfied with his or her social life; the therapist helps this person to construct a goal related specifically to dating or other social activities. This goal is then broken down into identifiable subgoals (e.g., dating at least twice a month) and behavioral steps (e.g., ways to improve personal hygiene, putting him- or herself into situations where he or she is likely to meet people).

The emphasis is on (1) constructing *manageable* subgoals and behavioral steps that support "setting yourself up for success," and (2) articulating explicit behavioral goals so that the member can see when he or she has achieved the goal. During subsequent sessions, the therapist uses behavioral, cognitive, and supportive group techniques to help members address roadblocks to progress. Members share experiences and problem-solving efforts and provide mutual support. When an initial goal has been reached, the member may choose to leave the group or to continue to work on another goal.

In the second edition of the manual, Phase 2 has changed little, although a structured kick-off session has been added that recapitulates disease self-management issues and orients members to the procedures for this second Phase. In addition, throughout this Phase, more recognition has been placed on the importance of members continuing to practice the illness self-management skills learned in Phase 1.

In Phase 2, the therapist helps the member reformat goals according to four key behavioral principles:

1. The goals must be chosen by the individual and be important to his or her quality of life.
2. The goals must be measurable.
3. Achieving the goals must depend primarily on the actions of the individual him- or herself and not the cooperation of another person.
4. The goals must be broken down into a series of small, realistically attainable steps.

Examples

Spend money, use charge cards

Stop sleeping

Drive fast

Lots of projects (working, writing)

Use alcohol and street drugs

Make up for lost time from depression

Gamble

Travel

Pick fights

More relationships, less judgment

Stop medications

Drop out of treatment

Meditate

Stop listening to people's feedback

Retreat to a tranquil environment

Response:	
Good Effects: (Pro health, good for you)	**Bad Effects:** (More problems caused)
Response:	
Good Effects:	**Bad Effects:**

FIGURE 10.1. Sample worksheet: Costs and benefits of responses to a manic episode.

There are always roadblocks to success due to daily life problems, cognitive distortions, demoralization, feeling stigmatized, and lack of opportunity for learning from peers. Cognitive and interpersonal techniques are used to address and minimize these respective types of roadblocks.

Phase 2 does not have the same degree of a priori structure as Phase 1. Rather, duration of treatment and pace of therapeutic work are member-specific, dictated by progress toward identified goals. As identified goals are reached, the member either terminates the group or cycles back through another round of goal identification, subgoal construction, and work/monitoring. Median time to first goal attainment is 7 months (95% CI; 5.1–12.3; Bauer et al., 1998). Thus, Phase 1 is typically structured as a closed group, and Phase 2 is open-ended and can accommodate individuals joining at various stages.

KEY CONCEPTS FOR PHASE 1

A broad spectrum of theories has been applied to various aspects of health behavior, including how individuals participate in treatment (see, e.g., Glanz, Lewis, & Rimer, 1997). A number of aspects of the Life Goals Program resembles those found in widely disseminated health behavior interventions; for instance, the personal cost–benefit approach to understanding and improving treatment decisions resembles the "decisional balance" approach found in motivational interviewing (e.g., Miller & Rollnick, 2002). Similarities also exist between the approach to functional goals in Phase 2 and the approach used in problem-solving therapy for depression (e.g., Dowrick et al., 2000; Mynors-Wallis, Gath, Day, & Baker, 2000). Overall, we have been impressed with the relevance of Bandura's concepts of social cognitive theory to the Life Goals concepts and interventions (e.g., Bandura, 1992, 2001; Baranowski, Perry, & Parcel, 1997). In particular, Bandura's focus on agency and the effects that an individual has on his or her environment, and vice versa, is consistent with the focus of the Life Goals Program on assisting patients to move from the perceived position of passive victim to one of actively managing their illness and their lives. It is reasonable to distill from these various sources three major concepts that underlie the approach used: host factors in disease outcome, illness management skills, and the personal cost–benefit analysis.

Host Factors in Disease Outcome

We conceptualize outcome in manic–depressive disorder—and in *all* chronic illnesses—not only as a function of the disease process but also as a function of *host factors* (see Figure 10.2). Host factors may be broadly defined as those characteristics of the person that can be separately measured from his or her biologically determined manic–depressive disorder. For example, if the individual does not seek treatment, then the illness does not get treated (Vignette 10.2). We consider such host factors to be of two types: comorbid disorders (not dealt with further here) and illness management skills.

Illness Management Skills

Illness management skills can be defined as the ability to cope with the symptoms of illness and participate actively in treatment. As yet, there is little consensus on how to conceptualize these illness management skills, let alone how to identify and measure them. As detailed in Chapter 6 of Bauer and McBride (2003), each of the many theoretical and methodological approaches leads to a different conceptualization as to why individuals manage their illnesses in a particular manner. For example, in assessing the unwillingness of a person with manic–depressive disorder to accept medication treatment, a cultural approach might focus on the religious orientation that leads the individual to cast his or her abnormal thoughts, feelings, and behavior as a moral issue to be addressed by dint of will or grace rather than by succumbing to the weakness of taking a pill. A psychoanalytic approach might understand this unwillingness as a narcissistic defense against a defect for which the individual must rely on outside assistance. A cognitive approach might focus on cognitive distortions, particularly those underlying hopelessness, guilt, and dealing with uncertainty. An economic approach might emphasize the reluctance to assume the cost of medication treatment in terms of both monetary and personal time. Each of these approaches derives from a particular theory; these facets of understanding treatment behavior are neither mutually exclusive nor explicitly related; in some ways, they may be usefully complementary.

Finally, life would be simple if the causal relationship of illness management skills to outcome were simply unidirectional, as illustrated in Figure 10.2. In reality, this is not the likely case (Vignette 10.3). Outcomes themselves, particularly clinical and functional outcomes, affect host factors, which in turn affect participation in treatment. Thus, interventions to improve illness management skills must parallel medication management

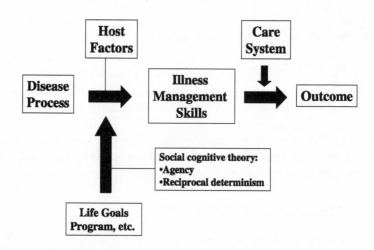

FIGURE 10.2. A model for chronic care interventions.

Vignette 10.1: Clinical Outcome ≠ Functional Outcome

Ms. A is a 37-year-old divorcée who has had manic–depressive disorder type I with psychotic mania since she was 18 years old. She has had three episodes of mania and severe depressive episodes every 1 to 2 years. However, she continues to work full-time as a secretary, at times working when mildly psychotic and always working despite severe depressive episodes. "How could I not work?" she says, when queried. "How would I eat?"

Mr. B is a 30-year-old single man who has had manic–depressive disorder type II since he was 25 years old. He has had hypomanic episodes twice per year, followed by depressive episodes. However, he abuses alcohol and is only intermittently compliant with his medications. He has been hospitalized four times for depression. He has not worked since his second depressive episode and is on disability.

---

targeted at symptoms, and must be iterative, often covering the same issues in many different guises and settings.

The Personal Cost–Benefit Analysis

A key assumption underlying the Life Goals Program, in both phases, is that individuals act in their own *perceived* best self-interest, consistent with the hedonic principle of outcome expectancies (i.e., incentives), as applied by social cognitive theory (Baranowski et al., 1997). Whether or not an individual's perception of his or her own best interest matches the clinician's, one can assume that the individual will tend to act in a manner that, *as best as the individual can tell*, helps him or her adapt successfully. In reality, individuals with an illness and their treating clinicians often differ in what they see as adaptive. One of the critical components of successful treatment—a successful treatment alliance—is a consensus on more (vs. less) adaptive coping strategies. To accomplish this consensus, the clinician must understand how an individual chooses and discards various options, both in managing his or her disease and in managing his or her life with the disorder. We refer to this process as a *personal cost–benefit analysis* (Vignette 10.4).

Two aspects of the personal cost–benefit analysis should be underscored. First, every treatment option has both benefits *and* costs, however purely "good" or "bad" the option may appear. Second, the metric applied to "balance" the benefits and costs is specific to the patient and is made according to his or her own internal value scheme.

Thus, if we listen to our patients, it is easy to see that there is a *logic* to illness management behavior, including noncompliant behavior. The goal of improved illness management skills is not served by convincing the person in treatment that taking a particular medication is the best option for him or her, but rather to understand the person's implicit cost–benefit analysis and to search for acceptable treatment alternatives. This aspect of cost–benefit analysis is the basis of the psychoeducational component of the Life Goals Program that seeks to improve illness management skills in Phase 1. The cost–benefit approach also underlies the therapist's work with individuals in their functional goal attainment efforts in Phase 2.

In summary, the person's choice of strategies for illness management as well as coping behavior in goal attainment can be considered a function of cost–benefit analyses conducted, on some level, by the individual him- or herself. Key concepts to keep in mind include:

- There are always both positive and negative aspects (costs and benefits) to each strategy.
- These calculations reduce diverse aspects of the decision to a common metric that produces a yes or no decision.
- The individual is the one who creates and implements this metric.
- The analyses are often only partially conscious to the individual, but they are always made on the basis of his or her attempt to adapt with the greatest benefit or least harm to self.

KEY CONCEPTS FOR PHASE 2

Medical-model treatment alone is not sufficient to ensure optimal outcome for manic–depressive disorder, because functional outcome is not simply

---

Vignette 10.2: Host Factors Drive Treatment Behavior

Ms. C is a 45-year-old married female who is a member of a fundamentalist religion and has had manic–depressive disorder type II. Despite crippling depressive episodes, she has refused medication or psychiatric referral from her primary care physician. She says, "If I were not a sinner, God would not have me suffer like this. He will guide me through."

Dr. D is a 55-year-old university professor with manic–depressive disorder type I. Although in danger of being placed in early retirement because of his symptoms, he continues to comply only intermittently with prescribed medications and psychiatrist appointments. He reports several reasons for his noncompliance, including not having the time to make appointments, go to laboratory tests, or pick up prescriptions; not liking the "feeling of being on medications"; and a preference to use "natural remedies," about which he reads assiduously and which he gets from a "nutrition counselor" at a local health foods emporium.

Vignette 10.3: Illness and Illness Management Skills—
A Bidirectional Relationship

Ms. E is a 25-year-old single nurse who has had manic–depressive disorder type I since she was 18 years old. She had been compliant with all medications and had developed a solid working relationship with her psychiatrist until last year, when she experienced a severe manic episode in the wake of the breakup of a romantic relationship, during which she lost her job and her insurance benefits. Since these crises, she has been unable to work and has applied for disability. She complains of low-grade depression that becomes severe at times. However, she is no longer able to see her psychiatrist as frequently or to afford the medications prescribed. She also has not used the referral for a psychotherapist, provided by her psychiatrist, because of the cost.

---

driven by clinical outcome (reviewed in detail in Bauer & McBride, 2003, Ch. 2). Optimal medication management, or even psychotherapy, aimed at reducing symptoms in no way guarantees an impact on functional outcome. These findings are predicted by Engel's (1977) biopsychosocial model of illness and its treatment. If improved functional outcome is a goal, then therapeutic interventions must be targeted directly at that goal. This improved functional outcome is the goal of Phase 2. The major conceptual bases for Phase 2 are derived from behavioral theory, cognitive theory, and interpersonal group therapy. The emphasis on personal cost–benefit ratios continues as members generate multitudinous functional goal attainment strategies.

Behavioral Elements

Several theorists have utilized behavioral concepts to attempt to understand and treat depression (e.g., Ferster, 1974; Lewinsohn, 1974; Peterson & Seligman, 1984; Rehm, 1985). The common theme among these diverse behavioral conceptualizations appears to be that depression is characterized by a perceived reduction in positive reinforcement, for which individuals perceive themselves to be responsible. To address this lacuna of positive life experience, the Life Goals Program focuses on identifying potential sources of positive reinforcement that are meaningful to group members—the goals. The therapist works with members to develop strategies that will maximize the chance of success in pursuing their goals. Phase 2 takes what appears to be very complex and overwhelming goals for group members and breaks the goals down into manageable steps. The point of this "breakdown" is to increase the probability of success at each step (Vignette 10.5). Consistent with the behavioral approach, Phase 2 relies almost exclusively on positive reinforcement for goals achieved, rather than negative reinforcement. Overall, then, the approach is to develop strategies that make goals attainable and increase the probability of success, thus maximizing positive reinforcement in this group in which demoralization and failure are endemic.

Cognitive Elements

Classic cognitive therapy (Beck, Rush, Shaw, & Emery, 1979; see also Chapter 7, this volume) developed with a focus on depressive symptoms. Our interest in cognitive therapy was that it also might be relevant in understanding and clarifying long-term coping strategies—that is, coping with chronic disease—rather than primarily in improving depressive symptoms. Support for this conceptualization comes from evidence that dysfunctional attitudes are likely not limited to depressive disorders but may be an important part of coping strategies for persons in many walks of life faced with varied demands (e.g., Carver & Scheier, 2001; Colligan, Offord, Malinchoc, Schulman, & Seligman, 1994; Kamen-Seigel, Rodin, Seligman, & Dwyer, 1991; Peterson & Seligman, 1987; Seligman, Nolen-Hoeksema, Thornton, & Thornton, 1990; Zullow & Seligman, 1990; Zullow, Oettingen, Peterson, & Seligman, 1988). The Life Goals Program does not attempt formal cognitive restructuring but rather uses cognitive techniques to challenge maladaptive cognitions and test negative attributions about events, most specifically outcomes of an individual's goal attainment strategies.

Vignette 10.4: The Personal Cost–Benefit Analysis

When Mr. F experiences a depressive episode, he misses work and secludes himself from his wife, children, and friends, who typically get frustrated with his behavior. When queried, he responds, "When I'm depressed, I get so damn irritable. I know I'm gonna bite someone's head off. It's better for my wife and my kids if I leave them the hell alone till it passes." At times he drinks two to three bourbons at bedtime, and sometimes during the day, to "zone out when I just can't take it anymore."

Ms. G is a violin teacher whose severe manic episodes and crippling depressions have been eradicated by lithium. However, she has been intermittently noncompliant despite this good effect. When discussing the reasons for her noncompliance, she focuses on what appears to her psychiatrist to be an almost invisible tremor, saying, "I prefer to supply my own vibrato, thank you very much." She went on to discuss how this apparently minor side effect impacted her teaching, her performance, and, ultimately, her income and her self-esteem.

Vignette 10.5: Behavior Plans Require Manageable Steps

Mr. G, who had been socially reclusive despite reasonably well-controlled symptoms, entered Phase 2 with the goal of "getting married." Working with the therapist, he reformatted this goal to one that was more modest and depended on his actions rather than on the actions of some unpredictable "other." He chose the goal, "asking women out." This primary goal was broken down into specific subgoals and behavioral steps that included some social skills work aimed at hygiene and social interactions, researching possible activities where he would meet appropriate women, identifying possible activities he would like to participate in, and attending the activities.

Interpersonal Group Elements

The above therapeutic orientations comprise the backbone or skeleton of the Life Goals Program, particularly Phase 2. However, to run an effective group, there must be a significant amount of interpersonal group "meat" on those bones. Interpersonal group strategies are applied in Phase 1 as well as Phase 2, though they are evident to a lesser degree in the former because of the greater structure of Phase 1 groups.

Interpersonal group theory and techniques (not to be confused with Klerman and Weismann's interpersonal therapy; Klerman et al., 1984) are less explicitly defined and operationalized than behavioral or cognitive techniques. However, giving attention to seemingly subjective yet critical aspects of the person's experience, such as a sense of stigma and isolation, can be of great importance in achieving therapeutic gains even in an expressly behavioral program. It is primarily the interpersonal, rather than the behavioral, aspects of the group that address these issues.

The key adaptation that differentiates the Life Goals Program from traditional interpersonal groups is that the therapist advocates the selective modulation of intensive interpersonal stimulation and changes the role of interpersonal techniques in treatment. These techniques are not seen as the major curative factors, but rather as adjuncts to the main task of behavioral change. They specifically target the demoralization, isolation, stigmatization, shame, and simple lack of peer behavior modeling that are commonly experienced by individuals with manic–depressive disorder (Vignette 10.6). This approach leads to judicious and limited use of the interpersonal techniques, primarily in Phase 2, that address these issues (Vignette 10.7).

DATA AND DISSEMINATION: CURRENT STATUS

The Life Goals Program has been studied as a stand-alone therapy added on to usual care in an open trial, and as a part of a multimodal intervention

---

Vignette 10.6: Stigma and Demoralization: The Rule,
Not the Exception

Ms. H had chosen the goal of "Finishing my bachelor's degree."
However, she dropped out of college during a depressive episode
because of inability to concentrate, poor energy, and hopelessness.
Although the episode remitted, she hesitated to sign up for classes for
the following semester, saying, "I just can't trust myself. What if it
happens again? That will be my second failure. What will my friends and
family think? Think of how much money it will cost."

---

in one open and several randomized controlled trials. In the open feasibility
trial we addressed two questions:

1. Can the program be exported to other therapists and sites with
   good adherence?
2. Is there evidence that the program can improve disease self-management
   skills and help patients improve function (Bauer et al., 1998)?

The program was taught to four therapists (one nurse, one MSW, one
psychiatry resident, and one junior attending psychiatrist) across two sites,
the Providence Veterans Affairs Medical Center (VAMC) and the Massachusetts General Hospital. Therapist adherence ratings for process and
content measures averaged 90–96%, indicating that the program could be
readily exported to other therapists and sites.

Utilizing the groups conducted at the Providence VAMC, we studied
29 members, (96% male) entering Phase 1 with evidence of significant clinical impairment, including 59% with a history of psychosis, 64% with a
history of suicide attempts, 33% meeting DSM-IV criteria for current
comorbid alcohol dependence, and 19% meeting DSM-IV criteria for current comorbid drug dependence. Analysis of Phase 1 data indicated that 20
subjects (69%) completed Phase 1, and those who remained showed good
to excellent indices of active group participation. There were no significant
predictors of dropout, such as current hypomania, psychosis, comorbid
substance dependence, or rapid cycling, indicating that subjects could participate despite the presence of common exclusionary conditions for efficacy clinical trials for manic–depressive disorder. In terms of intermediate
outcome variables, mean knowledge base showed modest but significant
increases, indicating that the group could reach its stated goal of increasing
knowledge about the disorder and its treatment. Analysis of Phase 2 experience indicated that 70% of members achieved stated goals. Median time to
goal attainment was 7 months (95% CI, 5.1–12.3 months).

The first study of the Life Goals Program as part of a multimodal intervention was described above (see above, "Our Initial Forays" (p. 204); Bauer et al., 1997). A sample of 103 veterans with manic–depressive disorder participated in this tripartite intervention, which demonstrated clear improvements in quality of care compared to preprogram levels. This sample was 94% male and also had evidence of significant clinical impairment, including 64% with a history of psychosis, 53% with prior suicide attempts, and 92% with prior psychiatric hospitalizations. Seventy percent had a lifetime history of alcohol dependence, and fully 22% met criteria for current dependence at the time of study intake; drug dependence rates were, respectively, 22% and 10%. Compared to preprogram levels, at the end of 1 year of follow-up, the intensity of pharmacotherapy delivered significantly increased, as did patient satisfaction. Direct mental health treatment costs for patients hospitalized in the prior year were significantly reduced to less than 67% of baseline. Because of the mirror-image design, convincing measures of change in disease status were not feasible, but we reasoned that, given high retention in the program plus reductions in use of the high-acuity services (i.e., hospital days and ER visits), clinical status of the sample likely did not worsen and may have improved.

The Life Goals Program is also an integral part of disease management programs being tested in two federally funded randomized controlled clinical trials (Bauer et al., 2001; Simon, Ludman, Unutzer, & Bauer, 2002a). The former study, an 11-site randomized controlled VA Cooperative Study, is ongoing, utilizing the tripartite intervention developed at the Providence VAMC. Three-year follow-up for all participants will be completed at the end of 2003.

The latter study involves four sites in the large staff-model health maintenance organization, the Group Health Cooperative of Puget Sound.

Vignette 10.7: Combatting Stigma and Demoralization: Interpersonal Techniques at Work

Mr. I had several goals during Phase 2. Currently he was working on "Telling my boss about my disorder." He had been a good worker at the plant for years. He was good friends with his boss, and their relationship meant a great deal to him. His boss knew that he didn't drink after work but thought that was because he was "an ex-alkie." Mr. I was concerned that telling his boss that he had a mental illness like manic–depressive disorder would compromise their friendship and maybe even their work relationship. Prior to beginning the program, Mr. I had never met another person with manic–depressive disorder. He was able to discuss his concerns with other group members. They in turn told him of their own experiences, the strategies they used to discuss this subject with people they were close to, and provided moral support as the time approached for him to tell his boss.

The intervention used by Simon and coworkers is similar in orientation and employs the Life Goals Program as the patient education program that complements nurse-based outreach and information management support for physicians. Two-year follow-up has been completed, and 1-year data have been reported (Simon, Ludman, Unutzer, & Bauer, 2002b), indicating significant effects on mania for the entire 12-month period and a greater decline in depression over the 12 months compared to control.

In addition, the Life Goals Program is being tested as a stand-alone treatment in two funded randomized controlled trials, one in a multisite Canadian trial (Principal Investigator: Sagar Parikh, Toronto) and one in a U.S. community mental health center (Principal Investigator: Martha Sajatovic, Cleveland). The program also has been adapted to an Internet-based version that is being tested as part of a randomized controlled trial in a large staff model health maintenance organization (Principal Investigator: Enid Hunkeler, Oakland) funded by Kaiser of Northern California and Lilly Pharmaceuticals.

A French-language version of the first edition has been published (Aubrey, 2001). An as-yet unpublished Spanish-language version is also available (author: Xochitl Alvarez Pulido, Mexico City).

ACKNOWLEDGMENT

Portions of this chapter were adapted from Bauer and McBride (2003). Copyright 2003 by Springer Publishing Company, Inc., New York 10012. Adapted by permission. Specific topics summarized here can be found in greater detail in this reference.

REFERENCES

Aubrey, J. M. (Trans). (2001). *Thérapie de groupe pour le trouble bipolaire: Un approche structurée.* Geneva, Switzerland: Éditions Médecine et Hygiene.

Bandura, A. (1992). Exercise of agency through the self-efficacy mechanism. In R. Schwarzer (Ed.), *Self-efficacy: Thought control of action* (pp. 3–38). Washington, DC: Hemisphere.

Bandura, A. (2001). Social cognitive theory: An agentic perspective. *Annual Review of Psychology, 52,* 1–26.

Baranowski, T., Perry, C. L., & Parcel, G. S. (1997). How individuals, environments, and health behavior interact: Social cognitive theory. In K. Glanz, F. M. Lewis, & B. K. Rimer (Eds.), *Health behavior and health education: Theory, research, and practice* (2nd ed., pp. 153–178). San Francisco: Jossey-Bass.

Bauer, M. S. (2001a). An evidence-based review of psychosocial interventions for bipolar disorder. *Psychopharmacology Bulletin, 35,* 109–134.

Bauer, M. S. (2001b). The collaborative practice model in bipolar disorder: Design and implementation in a multi-site randomized controlled trial. *Bipolar Disorders, 3,* 33–44.

Bauer, M. S. (2002). Quantitative adherence studies of mental health clinical practice guidelines. *Harvard Review of Psychiatry, 10,* 138–153.

Bauer, M. S. (2003a). *Field guide to psychiatric assessment and treatment.* Philadelphia: Lippincott Williams & Wilkins.

Bauer, M. S. (2003b). Bipolar (manic–depressive) disorder. In A. Tasman, J. Kay, & J. Lieberman (Eds.), *Psychiatry* (2nd ed., pp. 1237–1270). Philadelphia: Saunders.

Bauer, M. S., Callahan, A., Jampala, C., Petty, F., Sajatovic, M., Schaefer, V., Wittlin, B., & Powell, B. (1999). Clinical practice guidelines for bipolar disorder from the Department of Veteran's Affairs. *Journal of Clinical Psychiatry, 60,* 9–21.

Bauer, M. S., & McBride, L. (1996). *Structured group psychotherapy for bipolar disorder: The Life Goals Program.* New York: Springer.

Bauer, M. S., & McBride, L. (2003). *Structured group psychotherapy for bipolar disorder: The Life Goals Program* (2nd ed.). New York: Springer.

Bauer, M. S., McBride, L., Chase, C., Sachs, G., & Shea, N. (1998). Manual-based group psychotherapy for bipolar disorder: A feasibility study. *Journal of Clinical Psychiatry, 59,* 449–455.

Bauer, M. S., McBride, L., Shea, N., Gavin, C., Holden, F., & Kendall S. (1997). Impact of an easy-access clinic-based program for bipolar disorder: Quantitative analysis of a demonstration project. *Psychiatric Services, 48,* 491–496.

Bauer, M. S., Williford, W., Dawson, E., Akiskal, H., Altshuler, L., Fye, C., Gelenberg, A., Glick, H., Kinosian, B., & Sajatovic M. (2001). Principles of effectiveness trials and their implementation in VA Cooperative Study #430: "Reducing the efficacy–effectiveness gap in bipolar disorder." *Journal of Affective Disorders, 67,* 61–78.

Bayer Institute for Health Care Communication. (1996–2000). *Choices and changes: Clinician influence and patient action; annotated bibliography for references in clinician–patient communication to enhance health outcomes; annotated bibliography: Improving communications in oncology.* West Haven, CT: Bayer Institute for Health Care Communication.

Beck, A. T., Rush, A. J., Shaw, B., & Emery, G. (1979). *Cognitive therapy of depression.* New York: Guilford Press.

Beisecker, A. E. (1990). Patient power in doctor–patient communication: What do we know? *Health Communications, 2,* 105–122.

Braddock, C. H., III., Edwards, K. A., Hasenberg, N. M., Laidley, T. L., & Levinson, L. (1999). Informed decision making in outpatient practice: Time to get back to the basics. *Journal of the American Medical Association, 282,* 2313–2320.

Burns, B., & Santos, A. (1995). Assertive community treatment: An update of randomized trials. *Psychiatric Services, 46,* 669–676.

Carver, C. S., & Scheier, M.F. (2001). Optimism, pessimism, and self-regulation. In E.C. Chang (Ed.), *Optimism and pessimism: Implications for theory, research, and practice* (pp. 31–51). Washington, DC: American Psychological Association.

Center for the Advancement of Health. (1996) *An indexed bibliography on self-management for people with chronic disease.* Washington, DC: Author.

Ciechanowski, P. S., Katon, W. J., Russo, J. E., & Walker, E. A. (2001). The patient–provider relationship: Attachment theory and adherence to treatment in diabetes. *American Journal of Psychiatry, 158,* 29–35.

Colligan, R., Offord, K., Malinchoc, M., Schulman, P., & Seligman M. (1994). CAVing the MMPI for an Optimism–Pessimism Scale: Seligman's attributional model and the assessment of explanatory style. *Journal of Clinical Psychology, 50,* 71–95.

Cooper-Patrick, L., Gallow, J. J., Gonzales, J. J., Vu, H. T., Powe, N. R., Nelson, C., & Ford, D. E. (1999). Race, gender, and partnership in the patient–physician relationship. *Journal of the American Medical Association, 282,* 583–589.

Dixon, L., Burland, J., Lucksted, A., Stewart, B., Postrado, L., & Hoffman, M. (2002). *Effectiveness of the NAMI Family to Family education program.* Paper presented at the NIMH 15th Biennial International Conference on Mental Health Services Research, Washington, DC.

Dowrick, C., Dunn, G., Ayuso-Mateos, J. L., Dalgard, O. S., Page, H., Lehtinen, V., Casey, P., Wilkinson, C., Vazquez-Barquero, J. L., Wilkinson, G., & the Outcomes of Depression International Network (ODIN) Group. (2000). Problem solving treatment and group psychoeducation for depression: Multicentre randomized controlled trial. *British Medical Journal, 321,* 1–6.

Engel, G. L. (1977). The need for a new medical model: A challenge for biomedicine. *Science, 196,* 129–136.

Estroff, S. E. (1981). *Making it crazy: An ethnography of psychiatric clients in the community.* Berkeley, CA: University of California Press.

Ferster, C. (1974). Behavioral approaches to depression. In R. Friedman, M. Rand, & M. Katz (Eds.), *The psychology of depression: Contemporary theory and research* (pp. 29–53). New York: Wiley.

Frank, E., Swartz, H., Mallinger, A., Thase, M., Weaver, E., & Kupfer D. (1999). Adjunctive psychotherapy for bipolar disorder: Effects of changing treatment modality. *Journal of Abnormal Psychology, 108,* 579–587.

Glanz, K., Lewis, F. M., & Rimer, B. K. (Eds.). (1997). *Health behavior and health education: Theory, research, and practice* (2nd ed.). San Francisco: Jossey-Bass.

Greenfield, S., Kaplan, S., & Ware, J. E. (1985). Expanding patient involvement in care: Effects on patient outcomes. *Annals of Internal Medicine, 102,* 520–528.

Greenfield, S., Kaplan, S. H., Ware, J. E., Yano, E. M., & Frank, J. J. (1988). Patients' participation in medical care: Effects on blood sugar control and quality of life in diabetes. *Journal of General Internal Medicine, 3,* 448–457.

Institute of Medicine. (1985). *Assessing medical technologies.* Washington, DC: National Academy Press.

Inui, T. S., Jared, R. A., Carter, W. B., Plorde, D. S., Pecoraro, R. E., Chen, M. S., & Dohan, J. J. (1979). Effects of a self-administered health history on new-patient visits in a general medical clinic. *Medical Care, 17,* 1221–1228.

Kamen-Seigel, L., Rodin, J., Seligman, M., & Dwyer, J. (1991). Explanatory style and cell-mediated immunity in elderly men and women. *Health Psychology, 10,* 229–235.

Kaplan, S. H., Gandek, B., Greenfield, S., Rogers, W., & Ware, J. E. (1995). Patient and visit characteristics related to physicians' participatory decision-making style: Results from the Medical Outcomes Study. *Medical Care, 33,* 1176–1187.

Kaplan, S. H., Greenfield, S., Gandek, B., Rogers, W. H., & Ware, J. E. (1996). Characteristics of physicians with participatory decision-making styles. *Annals of Internal Medicine, 124,* 497–504.

Karp, D. A. (1996). *Speaking of sadness: Depression, disconnection, and the meaning of illness.* New York: Oxford University Press.

Katon, W., Von Korff, M., Lin, E., Walker, E., Simon, G., Bush, T., Robinson, P., & Russo, J. (1995). Collaborative management to achieve treatment guidelines: Impact on depression in primary care. *Journal of the American Medical Association, 273,* 1026–1031.

Katz, J. (1984). *The silent world of doctor and patient.* New York: Free Press.

Klerman, G., Weissman, M. M., Rounsaville, B. J., & Chevron, E. S. (1984). *Interpersonal psychotherapy of depression.* New York: Basic Books.

Lam, D., Bright, J., Jones, S., Hayward, P., Schuck, N., Chisolm, D., & Sham, P. (2000). Cognitive therapy for bipolar illness: A pilot study of relapse prevention. *Cognitive Therapy and Research, 24,* 503–520.

Lazare, A., Eisenthal, S., & Wasserman, L. (1975). The customer approach to patienthood: Attending to patient requests at a walk-in clinic. *Archives of General Psychiatry, 32*, 553–558.

Levinson, D., Merrifield, J., & Berg K. (1967). Becoming a patient. *Archives of General Psychiatry, 17*, 385–406.

Lewinsohn, P. (1974). A behavioral approach to depression. In R. Friedman & M. Katz (Eds.), *The psychology of depression: Contemporary theory and research* (pp. 157–185). New York: Wiley.

Lidz, C., Meisel, A., & Zerubavel, E. (1984). *Informed consent: A study of decision making in psychiatry.* New York: Guilford Press.

Lish, J. D., Dime-Meenan, S., Whybrow, P. C., Price, R. A., & Hirschfeld, R. M. (1994). The National Depressive and Manic–Depressive Association survey of bipolar members. *Journal of Affective Disorders, 31*, 281–294.

Little, P., Everitt, H.,Williamson, I., Warner, G., Moore, M., Goulde, C., Ferrier, K., & Payne, S. (2001). Preferences of patients for patient-centred approach to consultation in primary care: Observational study. *British Medical Journal, 322*, 1–7.

Lorig, K. R., Mazonson, P. D., & Holman, H. R. (1993). Evidence suggesting that health education for self-management in patients with chronic arthritis has sustained health benefits while reducing health care costs. *Arthritis and Rheumetism, 36*, 439–446.

Lorig, K. R., Sobel, D. S., Stewart, A. L., Brown, B. W., Bandura, A., Ritter, P., Gonzalez, V. M., Laurent, D. D., & Holman, H. R. (1999). Evidence suggesting that a chronic disease self-management program can improve health status while reducing hospitalization: A randomized trial. *Medical Care, 37*, 5–14.

Miklowitz, D. J., Simoneau, T., George, E., Richards, J., Kalbag, A., Sachs-Ericsson, N., & Suddath, R. (2000). Family-focused treatment of bipolar disorder: 1-year effects of a psychoeducational program in conjunction with pharmacotherapy. *Biological Psychiatry, 48*, 582–592.

Miller, W. R., & Rollnick, S. (2002). *Motivational interviewing: Preparing people for change* (2nd ed.). New York: Guilford Press.

Montgomery, E. B., Jr., Lieberman, A., Singh, G., & Fries, J. F. (1994). Patient education and health promotion can be effective in Parkinson's disease: A randomized controlled trial. PROPATH Advisory Board. *American Journal of Medicine, 97*, 429–435.

Mueser, K. T., Corrigan, P. W., Hilton, D. W., Tanzman, B., Schaub, A., Gingerich, S., Essock S. M., Tarrier, N., Morey, B., Vogel-Scibilia, S., & Herz, M. I. (2002). Illness management and recovery: A review of the research. *Psychiatric Services, 53*, 1272–1284.

Mynors-Wallis, L. M., Gath, D. H., Day, A., & Baker, F. (2000). Randomised controlled trial of problem solving treatment, antidepressant medication, and combined treatment for major depression in primary care. *British Medical Journal, 320*, 26–30.

National Depressive and Manic–Depressive Association (NDMDA). (2001). *Living with bipolar disorder: How far have we really come?* Chicago: Author.

Ong, L. M., & DeHaes, J. C. (1995). Doctor–patient communication: A review of the literature. *Social Science and Medicine, 40*, 903–918.

Pekkala, E., & Merinder, L. (2003). Psychoeducation for schizophrenia (Cochrane Review). *The Cochrane Library, Issue 2*, Update Software, Oxford, UK.

Perry, A., Tarrier, N., Morriss, R., McCarthy, E., & Limb, K. (1999). Randomised controlled trial of efficacy of teaching patients with bipolar disorder to identify early symptoms of relapse and obtain treatment. *British Medical Journal, 318*, 149–153.

Peterson, C., & Seligman, M. (1984). Causal explanations as a risk factor for depression: Theory and evidence. *Psychological Review, 91,* 347–374.

Peterson, C., & Seligman, M. (1987). Explanatory style and illness. Special Issue: Personality and physical health. *Journal of Personality, 55,* 237–265.

Rehm, L. (1985). A self-management therapy program for depression. *International Journal of Mental Health, 13,* 34–53.

Reissman, F., & Banks, E. C. (2001). A marriage of opposites: Self-help and the health care system. *American Psychologist, 56,* 173–174.

Renders, C. M., Valk, G. D., Griffin, S., Wagner, E. H., Eijk, J. T., & Assendelft, W. J. (2003). Interventions to improve the management of diabetes mellitus in primary care, outpatient, and community settings (Cochrane Review). Update Software, Oxford, UK.

Roter, D. (1989). Which facets of communication have strong effects on outcome: A meta-analysis. In M. Stewart & D. Roter (Eds.), *Communicating with medical patients* (pp. 183–196). Newbury Park, CA: Sage.

Seligman, M., Nolen-Hoeksema, S., Thronton, N., & Thornton, K. (1990). Explanatory style as a mechanism of disappointing athletic performance. *Psychological Science, 1,* 143–146.

Shea, N., McBride, L., Gavin, C., & Bauer, M. S. (1997). Effects of an ambulatory collaborative practice model on process and outcome of care for bipolar disorder. *Journal of the American Psychiatric Nurses Association, 3,* 49–57.

Simon, G. E., Ludman, E. J., Unutzer, J., & Bauer, M. S. (2002a). Design and implementation of a randomized trial evaluating systematic care for bipolar disorder. *Bipolar Disorders, 4,* 226–236.

Simon, G. E., Ludman, E., Unutzer, J., & Bauer, M. S. (2002, April 1). *Randomized trial of systematic care for bipolar disorder.* Paper presented at the NIMH 15th Biennial International Conference on Mental Health Services Research, Washington, DC.

Simon, G. E., VonKorff, M., Rutter, C., & Wagner E. (2000). Randomised trial of monitoring, feedback, and management of care by telephone to improve treatment of depression in primary care. *British Medical Journal, 320,* 550–554.

Simpson, M., Buckman, R., Stewart, M., Maguire, P., Liipkin, M., Novack, D., & Till, J. (1991). Doctor–patient communication: The Toronto consensus statement. *British Medical Journal, 303,* 1385–1387.

Starfield, B., Wray, C., Hess, K., Gross, R., Birk, P. S., & D'Lugoff, B. C. (1981). The influences of patient–practitioner agreement on outcome of care. *American Journal of Public Health, 71,* 127–132.

Stewart, M. A. (1995). Effective physician–patient communication and health outcomes: A review. *Canadian Medical Association Journal, 152,* 1423–1433.

Stewart, M. A., McWhinney, I. R., & Buck, C. W. (1979). The doctor–patient relationship and its effect upon outcome. *Journal of the Royal College of General Practice, 29,* 77–82.

Von Korff, M., Gruman, J., Schaefer, J., Curry, S. J., & Wagner, E. H. (1997). Collaborative management of chronic illness. *Annals of Internal Medicine, 127,* 1097–1102.

Wagner, E. H., Austin, B. T., & Von Korff, M. (1996). Organizing care for patients with chronic illness. *Milbank Quarterly 74,* 511–544.

Wagner, E. H., Glasgow, R. E., Davis, C., Bonomi, A. E., Provost, L., McCulloch, D., Carver, P., & Sixta, C. (2001). Quality improvement in chronic illness care: A collaborative approach. *Journal of Quality Improvement, 27,* 63–80

Wells, K. B. (1999). The design of Partners in Care: Evaluating the cost-effectiveness of improving care for depression in primary care. *Social Psychiatry and Psychiatric Epidemiology, 34,* 20–29.

Wells, K. B., Miranda, J., Bauer, M. S., Bruce, M., Durham, M., Escobar, J., Ford, D., Gonzalez, J., Hoagwood, K., Horowitz, S. M., Lawson, W., Lewis, L., McGuire, T.,

Pincus, H., Scheffler, R., Smith, W. A., & Unutzer, J. (2002). Overcoming barriers to reducing the burden of affective disorders. *Biological Psychiatry, 52,* 655–675.

The Worthlin Group. (1995). *Communication and the physician/patient relationship: A physician and consumer communication survey.* West Haven, CT: Bayer Institute for Health Care Communication.

Zullow, H., Oettingen, G., Peterson, C., & Seligman, M. (1988). Pessimistic explanatory style in the historical record: CAVing LBJ, presidential candidates, and East versus West Berlin. *American Psychologist, 43,* 673–682.

Zullow, H., & Seligman, M. (1990). Pessimistic rumination predicts defeat of presidential candidates, 1900 to 1984. *Psychological Inquiry, 1,* 52–61.

CHAPTER ELEVEN

TREATMENT OUTCOME STUDIES

JAN SCOTT

The basic aims of therapy for people with bipolar disorder are to alleviate acute symptoms, restore psychosocial functioning, and prevent relapse and recurrence. The mainstay of treatment has been, and currently remains, pharmacotherapy. However, the use of antipsychotic medications to stabilize or reduce the symptoms of mania can have significant side effects (particularly if used in conjunction with mood stabilizers), and the treatment of acute depressive episodes with antidepressant medications carries a small but significant risk of a switch into hypomania. Furthermore, there is a significant "efficacy–effectiveness" gap in the reported response rates to all mood stabilizers (Guscott & Taylor, 1994; Scott, 2001a; Scott & Pope, 2002). Even under optimal clinical conditions, prophylaxis protects fewer than 50% of individuals with bipolar disorder against further episodes (Dickson & Kendell, 1994). Given this scenario, the development of specific psychological therapies for bipolar disorder appears a necessary and welcome advance. However, progress in this area has been disappointingly slow.

Historically, individuals with bipolar disorder were not offered psychological therapies for three main reasons (Scott, 1995). First, etiological models highlighting genetic and biological factors in bipolar disorder have dominated the research agenda and largely dictated that medication was not just the primary but the *only* appropriate treatment. Second, there was a misconception that virtually all clients with bipolar disorder made a full interepisode recovery and returned to their premorbid level of functioning. Third, psychoanalysts historically expressed greater ambivalence about the suitability of psychotherapy for individuals with bipolar disorder than for those with other severe mental disorders. Fromm-Reichmann (1949) suggested that, in comparison to individuals with schizophrenia, clients with bipolar disorder were poor candidates for psychotherapy because they lacked introspection, were too dependent, and were likely to discover, and then play on, the therapist's "Achilles heel." Others—particularly clients and their significant others—argued strongly in favor of the use of psychological treatments (Goodwin & Jamison, 1990). However, the relative lack of empirical support (few randomized controlled trials have ever been published) meant that clinicians had few clear indicators on when or how to incorporate such approaches into day-to-day practice.

Over the last 20 years, two key aspects have changed. First, there is increasing acceptance of stress–vulnerability models that highlight the interplay between psychological, social, and biological factors in the maintenance or frequency of recurrence of severe mental disorders episodes. Second, evidence has accumulated from randomized controlled treatment trials regarding the benefits of psychological therapies as an adjunct to medication in treatment-resistant patients with schizophrenia and those with severe and chronic depressive disorders (Falloon, Boyd, McGill, & Fadden, 1985; Sensky et al., 2000; Thase, Greenhouse, & Frank, 1997; Paykel et al., 1999). Although there has been only limited research on the use of similar interventions in bipolar disorder, there are encouraging reports from research groups exploring the role of "manualized" therapies with this population (American Psychiatric Association, 1994). For persons with bipolar disorder who reported, about a quarter of a century ago, that psychotherapy could help them adjust to the disorder and overcome barriers to the acceptance of pharmacotherapy (Jamison, Garner, & Goodwin, 1979), these developments are long overdue.

This chapter briefly outlines the rationale for using psychological therapies in combination with medication in the treatment of adult clients with bipolar disorder. Outcome data from randomized controlled trials are reviewed, and the characteristics of therapies that are likely to be effective in bipolar disorder are highlighted.

THE RATIONALE FOR PSYCHOLOGICAL TREATMENTS

Other chapters in this book highlight the spectrum of psychosocial problems in bipolar disorder that may be addressed with adjunctive psychological and social therapies. However, there is a difference between the nonspecific benefits of combined pharmacotherapy and psychotherapy and the unique indications for psychosocial interventions.

For a specific psychological therapy to be *indicated* as an adjunct to medication for bipolar disorder it is necessary to identify a psychobiosocial model of relapse that does the following:

1. Describes how psychological and social factors may be associated with episode onset. For example, social rhythms disrupting life events may precipitate a bipolar relapse; therefore, stabilizing social rhythms is a key additional element in interpersonal therapy as applied in bipolar disorder.
2. Provides a clear rationale for which interventions should be used in what particular set of circumstances. For example, the use of family-focused therapy (FFT) is supported by research demonstrating that a negative affective style of interaction and high levels of expressed emotion in a family are associated with an increased risk of relapse in an individual with bipolar disorder.

Systematic research is currently underway, exploring cognitive, behavioral, emotional, and interpersonal aspects of bipolar disorder. These psychosocial models can be integrated with the "instability model of bipolar disorder relapse" proposed by Ehlers and colleagues (Ehlers, Frank, & Kupfer, 1988) and promoted by Goodwin and Jamison (1990). Briefly stated, the instability model identifies that, in individuals with biological vulnerability to bipolar disorder, there are four basic mechanisms of relapse, and each mechanism is associated with biological dysregulation (neurotransmitter or neuroendocrine disturbances), and each mechanism is hypothesized to act through the final common pathway of sleep disruption. As shown in Figure 11.1 (working from left to right), an individual may experience internal change in biological functioning that leads to the development of the early "prodromal" symptoms of relapse. Second, medication nonadherence may destabilize his or her physical state. Third, disruption to regular social routines (alterations to mealtimes, erratic weekly schedules, changes to the sleep–wake cycle) may produce circadian rhythm dysregulation, leading to relapse. Fourth, life events with specific personal meaning for that individual (as described in Beck's cognitive model) may lead to stress, which ultimately leads to biological dysregulation. Obviously, family attitudes and interactions can "stress" the individual's biological system via any of the last three pathways described. Likewise, an individual may engage in substance misuse as a consequence of specific beliefs and attitudes (pathway 4), or the impact of substance misuse may be directly via the third pathway.

Although this brief description is an oversimplification, the instability model is helpful when considering the potential use of psychological treatments. For example, where no external stressor is identified, it may still be possible to teach the individual to recognize the key early warning signs (such as sleep disruption) of episode onset and instigate a cognitive-behavioral

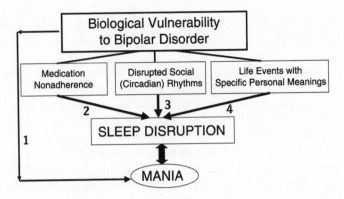

FIGURE 11.1. The instability model of bipolar relapse.

relapse prevention package (Perry, Tarrier, Morriss, McCarthy, & Limb, 1999). Psychoeducation and adherence therapy can be used to target the second pathway (Colom et al., 2001; Scott & Tacchi, 2003), and interpersonal social rhythms therapy (IPSRT) can be used to stabilize circadian rhythms (Frank et al., 1994), whereas cognitive therapy (CT) focuses mainly on the fourth pathway (Scott, Garland, & Moorhead, 2001; Lam et al., 2000). However, this is not to suggest that each therapy "maps" exclusively on to each pathway; the boundaries between therapies are flexible. For example, CT also addresses attitudes toward medication adherence and employs self-regulation techniques. Likewise, IPSRT explores an individuals' understanding of bipolar disorder and his or her beliefs about relationships or personal roles that may otherwise impair functioning. Family therapy also may target a number of pathways simultaneously (Miklowitz et al., 2000), including malevolent interpretations and attributions.

TREATMENT OUTCOME STUDIES

Early Treatment Studies

There is a large literature on the use of a variety of psychological therapies in individual case studies. The promising results described in these papers were followed by a number of open studies and case series. Between 1960 and 1998, there were 32 published papers describing the combined use of psychological and pharmacological treatments for bipolar disorder. However, the majority were small-scale studies, with an average sample size of about 25. The combined sample size for all studies was about 1,000 participants, of which about 75% received the experimental treatment ($n = 773$). The majority of the papers addressed group ($n = 14$) or family approaches

(n = 13), with only 15% of papers reporting on individual therapy. Furthermore, less than half of all studies (only 13) were randomized controlled trials.

The studies had many methodological limitations. However, there were clear trends that reached statistical significance in many studies for those receiving adjunctive psychological treatments: These subjects showed better subjective and objective clinical and social outcomes than those who received usual treatments (mainly comprised of mood stabilizers and outpatient support). These studies have been reviewed previously (e.g., Scott, 1995), so they will not be discussed again here, save to note that the encouraging results, such as reduced symptom levels and improvements in social functioning and sense of well-being, facilitated the development of more targeted interventions that focused on the particular issues related to bipolar relapse. The latter have since become the subject of specific randomized controlled trials.

In the last 5 years, the situation regarding psychosocial interventions in bipolar disorder has changed dramatically, with about 20 randomized controlled trials underway in the United States, the United Kingdom, and Europe. Given the current emphasis on the use of brief evidence-based therapies in clinical guidelines for the treatment of unipolar disorders, it is not surprising that the new treatment trials for bipolar disorder have focused on psychoeducational models, specifically on the three most well-researched manualized psychological approaches: IPSRT, CT, FFT, or techniques derived directly from these manualized therapies. The latter are used primarily to improve medication adherence or to teach recognition of prodromes and relapse prevention techniques. Core studies from each of these approaches are now reviewed.

Key Randomized Treatment Trials

Brief, Technique-Driven Interventions

Two randomized controlled trials administered brief (between six and 12 sessions) interventions, delivered on an individual basis to persons with bipolar disorder. Each study compared the experimental intervention to a treatment-as-usual condition (usually, medication plus outpatient support), and each study followed up participants for at least 12 months. Cochran (1984) undertook a small trial that compared 28 clients who were randomly assigned to standard clinical care alone or standard clinical care plus a six-session intervention that used cognitive-behavioral techniques to improve medication adherence. Following treatment, enhanced lithium adherence was reported in the intervention group, with only three patients (21%) discontinuing medication, compared to eight patients (57%) in the group receiving standard clinical care alone. There were also fewer hospitalizations in the group receiving CT (two vs. eight). Unfortunately, no information was available on the nature of any affective relapses.

Perry and colleagues (1999) recruited 69 participants at high risk of further relapse of bipolar disorder, who were in regular contact with mental health services in the United Kingdom. Individuals were randomly assigned to usual treatment or to usual treatment plus six to 12 sessions of cognitive and behavioral techniques that helped individuals to identify and manage early warning signs of relapse. The problem-solving strategies included identification of high-risk situations as well as prodromal symptoms (the relapse "signature") and taught clients to self-medicate and to access mental health professionals at the earliest possible time to try to avert the development of full-blown episodes. Over 18 months, the results demonstrated that, in comparison to the control group, the intervention group had significantly fewer manic relapses (27% vs. 57%), significantly fewer days in hospital, significantly longer time to first manic relapse (65 weeks vs. 17 weeks), and higher levels of social functioning and better work performance.

Group Psychoeducation

Van Gent and colleagues (Van Gent, Vida, & Zwart, 1988; Van Gent & Zwart, 1991, 1993) undertook two randomized trials using a group therapy format for individuals with bipolar disorder and one trial of psychoeducation for the partners of individuals with bipolar disorder. The first study (Van Gent et al., 1988) allocated 20 participants with bipolar disorder to four 90-minute sessions of group psychoeducation and 14 other participants to a waiting list control condition (usual treatment). Each group was followed for 15 months. Considerably more individuals in the intervention group (75%) than the control group (29%) reported significant subjective improvements in self-confidence, and those receiving psychoeducation also demonstrated significant improvements in behavior and social functioning. However, these between-group differences did not extend to mood, anxiety, or general symptom ratings.

In their second study, Van Gent and Zwart (1991) randomly assigned 15 participants to five sessions of psychoeducation and 20 participants to 10 sessions of psychoeducation plus psychotherapy. At the 15-month follow-up, both groups showed improved psychosocial functioning, and the only between-group difference was that those receiving the extended intervention demonstrated a greater improvement in their thinking and behavior, as measured on a general symptom checklist.

The last study by these researchers (Van Gent & Zwart, 1993) provided five structured group sessions for 14 partners of individuals with bipolar disorder and compared their knowledge of the disorder and its treatment and psychosocial management strategies over 6 months with 12 partners who were randomly allocated to a control condition. The study demonstrated that "partner only" education sessions led the experimental group to gain and sustain a significantly greater understanding of bipolar disorder than those allocated to the control group. However, perhaps the most significant finding was that the individuals with bipolar disorder became significantly more anxious after their partner attended the experimental group without them. This suggests that individuals with bipolar disorder may benefit from attending group psychoeducation sessions, but it may be more appropriate to use family sessions if the goal is for both the partner and the individual with bipolar disorder to benefit (see Chapter 9, this volume).

Colom et al. (2003) have undertaken the largest group therapy study so far. One hundred and twenty participants with bipolar disorder, who were euthymic and receiving medication and standard outpatient follow-up were randomly assigned to either 20 sessions of group psychoeducation (eight to 12 individuals per group) or to an unstructured support group. Sessions were 90 minutes in duration and were run by two experienced clinical psychologists. Manic relapses during the treatment phase were significantly lower in the intervention as compared to the control group (20% vs. 32%), with the same significant pattern apparent during the 24-month follow-up (48% vs. 72%). Depressive relapses showed the same significant differences between the psychoeducation group (12% treatment phase; 31% follow-up phase) and the control group (31% treatment phase; 71% follow-up phase). Furthermore, there were similar significant differences in relapse rates into mixed states.

Family or Couple Therapy

Four small randomized trials all identified that family therapy may be an important adjunct to pharmacotherapy for bipolar disorder. Honig, Hofman, Rozendaal, and Dingemans (1997) demonstrated that six sessions of a multifamily psychoeducational intervention (n = 23) produced a nonsignificantly greater reduction in expressed emotion in the experimental as compared to the waiting list control group (n = 23). Van Gent, Vogtlander, and Vrendendaal (1998) compared "couple psychoeducation" (n = 14) with usual treatment (n = 12) and found that those couples receiving the active intervention showed greater knowledge of bipolar disorder and its treatment and improved coping skills at the end of the psychoeducation sessions and at a 6-month follow-up.

Glick, Burti, Okonogi, and Sacks (1994) studied 50 inpatients, of whom 19 had been admitted following a bipolar relapse. They demonstrated that those randomly allocated to additional family therapy (n = 12) showed significant improvements in social and work functioning and family attitudes compared to those who received usual inpatient care alone (n =

7). These gains were particularly noticeable in females with bipolar disorder, and many of the immediate benefits associated with family therapy were maintained at an 18-month follow-up (Haas, Glick, & Clarkin, 1998).

Clarkin, Carpenter, Hull, Wilner, and Glick (1998) randomly assigned 42 outpatients to 11 months of standard treatment ($n = 23$) or standard treatment plus 25 sessions of "couple therapy" ($n = 19$). Unfortunately, the analysis was restricted to 33 treatment completers (couple therapy, 18; control treatment, 15). Participating in a course of couple therapy was associated with significantly higher levels of social adjustment and medication adherence compared to the control group, although there were no differences in overall symptom levels in the groups.

Miklowitz and colleagues (2000) undertook the largest trial of family therapy, using their 20-session FFT model. One hundred and one participants with bipolar disorder who were receiving usual treatment were randomly allocated to FFT ($n = 31$) or to case management ($n = 70$), which comprised two sessions of family psychoeducation and crisis intervention, as required. Over a 12-month period, individuals receiving FFT plus usual treatment, as compared to case management plus usual treatment, survived significantly longer in the community without relapsing (71% vs. 47%) and showed significantly greater reductions in symptom levels. However, further analysis demonstrated that these benefits were limited to depression; there was no specific reduction in manic relapses or symptoms. Overall, the benefits of FFT were most striking for individuals living in a high expressed-emotion environment.

IPSRT

The IPSRT intervention was one of the first systematic psychological therapies developed specifically for individuals with bipolar disorder. A randomized treatment trial with a 2-year follow-up is underway. Interim reports are available on 82 participants initially allocated to IPSRT or intensive clinical management. The trial has two phases: an acute treatment phase and a maintenance phase. Fifty percent of participants in each group remain in the same treatment arm throughout the study, whereas the remaining participants cross over to the other treatment arm (Frank et al., 1999). The key findings, so far, are that IPSRT does induce more stable social rhythms (Frank et al., 1999). There were no statistically significant treatment differences in time to remission, but those entering the trial in a major depressive episode showed a significantly shorter time to recovery with IPSRT, compared to intensive clinical management (21 weeks vs. 40 weeks; Hlastala et al., 1997). Interestingly, those receiving the same treatment throughout the acute and maintenance phases of the study showed greater reductions in symptoms, suicide attempts, and total number of relapses than those who were assigned to the crossover condition. This finding suggests that consistency in treatment was more important than type of treatment alone.

Cognitive Therapy

A study by Scott et al. (2001) examined the effect of 20 sessions of CT on 42 clients with bipolar disorder. Participants could enter the study during any phase of their disorder. Initially, clients were randomly allocated to the intervention group or to a waiting list control group, who then received CT after a 6-month delay. The randomized phase (6 months) allowed assessment of the effects of CT plus usual treatment, as compared with usual treatment alone. Individuals from both groups who received CT were then monitored for a further 12 months post-CT. At initial assessment, 30% of participants met criteria for an affective episode: 11 participants met diagnostic criteria for depressive disorder, three for rapid-cycling disorder, two for hypomania, and one for a mixed state. As is typical of this client population, 12 participants also met criteria for drug and/or alcohol problems or dependence, two met criteria for other Axis I disorders, and about 60% of the sample met criteria for personality disorder. The results of the randomized controlled phase demonstrated that, compared with participants receiving treatment as usual, those who received additional CT experienced statistically significant improvements in symptom levels, global functioning, and work and social adjustment. Data were available from 29 participants who received CT and were followed up for 12 months post-CT. These demonstrated a 60% reduction in relapse rates in the 18 months after commencing CT, as compared with the 18 months prior to receiving CT. Hospitalization rates showed parallel reductions. Scott et al. concluded that CT plus treatment as usual may offer some benefit and is a highly acceptable treatment intervention for about 70% of clients with bipolar disorder. This study was the forerunner of a large five-center trial of treatment as usual versus CT plus treatment as usual. The sample ($n = 250$) is the largest group on which a psychological therapy for bipolar disorder has been tested; results will be available in the near future.

Lam and colleagues (2000) followed up their pilot study (25 participants randomized to CT or to usual treatment) of 12–20 sessions of outpatient CT for patients with bipolar disorder with a large-scale randomized controlled trial (Lam et al., 2003). One hundred and three participants with bipolar disorder, who were currently euthymic, were randomly allocated to individual CT as an adjunct to mood-stabilizing medication or to usual treatment alone (i.e., mood stabilizers plus outpatient support). After controlling for gender and illness history, the intervention group had significantly fewer bipolar relapses (CT group = 43%; control group = 75%), psychiatric admissions (15% vs. 33%), or total days in episode (about 27 days vs. 88 days) over 12 months than the control group. The reduction in total number of episodes was comprised of significant reductions in major depressive (21% vs. 52%) and manic episodes (17% vs. 31%) but not mixed episodes. The intervention group also showed significantly greater improvements in social adjustment and better coping strategies for managing the prodromal symptoms of mania.

Similarities and Differences in Therapy Outcomes

As shown in Table 11.1, the use of adjunctive therapy leads to significant reductions in relapse rates and symptom levels and significant improvements in social functioning. A number of studies reported improvements in medication adherence in those receiving psychological therapy. However, this alone did not account for the improved outcomes of participants in the intervention group. Some studies also improved the understanding and attitudes of family members toward the individual with bipolar disorder and the treatment of the disorder.

It is noticeable that some therapies were most successful in reducing depressive rather than manic relapses. The reasons for this selective result are not entirely clear, but at least two hypotheses are reasonable. First, there may be different active ingredients in the therapy that more successfully tackle the syndrome of depression rather than mania. Alternatively, it should be noted that the symptoms of manic relapse are qualitatively different from day-to-day experiences, whereas depressive prodromes often represent quantitative variations of normal experience. Mania also has a longer prodrome than depression (median time approximately 3 weeks, compared to 2 weeks; Jackson, Cavanagh, & Scott, 2003). This means that interventions that focus primarily on teaching individuals to recognize early warning symptoms and to make effective interventions (e.g., behavior change or increases in medication) may prevent isolated manic symptoms from cascading into a full-blown manic relapse (see Jackson et al., 2003). However, interventions that tackle subsyndromal or acute bipolar depression often require complex, multifaceted approaches, such as those already known to be effective in unipolar depression.

In summary, although the randomized trials reviewed here are relatively small by comparison to medication trials, there is encouraging evidence for clinical effectiveness of each key approach. In addition, randomized trials of group therapies targeting comorbid bipolar disorder and substance misuse (Weiss, Kolodziej, Najavits, Greenfield, & Fucito, 2000) or using Bauer and colleagues' (1997) Life Goals Program are nearing completion. Importantly, large-scale studies are now underway on both sides of the Atlantic (the Medical Research Council study in the United Kingdom and the STEP-BD project in the United States). These trials are likely to an-

TABLE 11.1. Key Randomized Controlled Trials of Psychological Therapies of Bipolar Disorders

Key study	Sample size	Experimental intervention	Main differences in outcome between experimental and control treatments
Perry et al. (1999)	$n = 69$	Relapse prevention using cognitive and behavioral strategies	Reduced lengths of hospitalization. Increased time between episodes. More effective in preventing relapses into mania than depression.
Frank et al. (1999)	$n = 82$	Interpersonal and social rhythm therapy (IPSRT)	Increased stability of social rhythms. IPSRT more effective in depression than mania, with trend toward shorter time to recovery in depression.
Miklowitz et al. (2000)	$n = 101$	Family-focused therapy	Significantly fewer relapses, but FFT more effective in depression than mania. FFT particularly helpful in families with high levels of expressed emotion.
Lam et al. (2000)	$n = 103$	Cognitive therapy	Significantly fewer episodes of mania and depression. Improved social functioning. Greater awareness and better coping with manic prodromes.
Colom et al. (2001)	$n = 120$	Group psychoeducation	Significantly fewer bipolar episodes (manic, depressive, and mixed).

swer basic questions about the benefits and limitations of psychological therapies in the acute and maintenance treatment of bipolar disorder.

WHICH THERAPY SHOULD BE OFFERED?

There is no definitive evidence about which therapy a clinician should recommend for treating patients with bipolar disorder. However, this lack of such evidence should not disarm the clinician unduly, because there are a number of shared factors that characterize the brief, specific, "manualized" therapies, such as IPSRT, CT, and FFT, which have been tested in randomized trials. Scott (2001b) noted that each of these interventions assumes that cognitive, behavioral, emotional, and interpersonal domains are interrelated and, in interaction with biological factors, associated with the persistence or recurrence of affective symptoms. The therapies all regard these five domains as the key targets for change (see Figure 11.2), although the relative emphasis of each approach varies, giving clinicians some opportunity to select between approaches. For example, if the individual with bipolar disorder lives in an environment with high levels of expressed emotion, it may be most beneficial to use FFT.

Not only do the psychological interventions overlap in their objectives, but brief psychotherapies of proven effectiveness also demonstrate similarities in their core clinical characteristics (Teasdale, 1985; see Table 11.2). The therapies identify unique aspects of patients' reactions or adaptations to their illness and develop an individualized plan for treatment. By taking a collaborative and educational approach, the therapies allow the individuals (and their significant others, if appropriate) to be engaged as equal partners in the treatment process. There is also an emphasis on the development and independent maintenance of new coping skills and strategies.

The above characteristics are critical to the approach required for bipolar disorder. For example, many individuals with bipolar disorder would resist and challenge a more didactic approach to treatment (Scott, 1995). Because individuals with bipolar disorder, and sometimes significant others in their life, play an active role in formulating the problems, the interventions used then appear rational and logical, giving therapy a sense of coherence. The structured approach to each session, with agenda setting, prioritization of problems for discussion, and joint development of "homework" (i.e., in vivo) tasks, enables clients to retain their focus on the session even when hypomania leads to greater distractibility. The approaches also offer individuals with bipolar disorder respect, information, and choice. These features help increase their sense of self-efficacy, as they begin to learn to gain control over what they can realistically control and accept or acknowledge what they cannot. This learning may be particularly helpful to individuals who experience low self-esteem and perceive a loss of identity following repeated episodes of bipolar disorder.

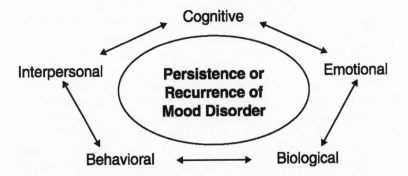

FIGURE 11.2. Biopsychosocial aspects of bipolar disorders: Key domains for intervention with cognitive therapy, interpersonal and social rhythm therapy, and family-focused therapy in bipolar disorders.

TABLE 11.2. Shared Characteristics of Effective Brief Therapies

1. The therapy offers a specific formulation that can be applied to the individuals' problems.
2. The model of therapy is shared openly with the client.
3. There is a clear rationale for the techniques used, and the techniques are applied in a logical sequence.
4. There is an emphasis on skill development and transfer of learning outside of therapy sessions.
5. Change is attributed to the client's rather than the therapist's efforts.
6. The client maintains the use of the techniques beyond the termination of therapy, thereby increasing the prospects that the benefits will endure.

CONCLUSIONS

This chapter highlights the point that psychosocial factors may be causes or consequences of bipolar episodes and that the instability model of relapse allows clinicians to recognize the potential mechanism by which psychological therapies may improve the prognosis of those at risk of persistent symptoms or frequent relapse. The three core manualized therapies (i.e., IPSRT, CT, and FFT) are all brief and have all developed specific models for use with patients with bipolar disorder. As such, the choice between the three individual approaches is more likely to be dictated by client choice or the availability of a trained therapist. The group psychoeducation model (Colom et al., 2003) appears to be a hybrid therapy that incorporates a number of key elements from each of the brief approaches, but it has the additional advantage of allowing individuals to share their views of bipolar disorder and learn adaptive coping strategies from other group members. Individuals who need help with more circumscribed problems, such as adapting to the disorder, adhering to medication, or identifying and self-managing early warning signs and symptoms of relapse, may benefit from more targeted interventions. Adherence therapy, relapse prevention training, or brief group psychoeducation sessions may be helpful in these circumstances.

The fundamental difference between these interventions and the specific models (i.e., IPSRT, CT, and FFT) is that the former is usually briefer than the specific therapies (about six sessions, compared to about 20 sessions) and usually offers a generic, fixed treatment package (a "one size fits all" approach) rather than an individualized, more flexible, formulation-based approach. However, these interventions appear to be potentially very useful in day-to-day clinical practice, and further randomized trials should be encouraged.

This chapter aims to give clinicians an overview of the empirically established importance of the psychological therapies that have been described in this book. The use of psychological therapy as an adjunct to medication is likely to be clinically beneficial and financially cost effective, as well as contributing to a significant improvement in the quality of life of individuals with bipolar disorder and, indirectly, their significant others. As such, brief evidence-based therapies represent an important component of good clinical practice in the management of bipolar disorder. Bauer, McBride, Chase, Sachs, and Shea (1998) also are involved in a multicenter study of a comprehensive "whole system" approach to the collaborative psychobiosocial management of bipolar disorder (described in Bauer et al., 1997). If this approach improves the quality and continuity of care for individuals with bipolar disorder, it will have implications for the future organization of health services. The number and variety of trials investigating psychosocial interventions are exciting for researchers and clinicians interested in bipolar disorder. However, for individuals with bipolar disorder and their significant others, this work is long overdue.

REFERENCES

American Psychiatric Association. (1994). Practice guidelines for the treatment of patients with bipolar disorders. *American Psychiatric Association, 151*(Suppl.), 1–36.

Bauer, M., McBride, L., Chase, C., Sachs, G., & Shea, N. (1998). Manual-based group psychotherapy for bipolar disorder: A feasibility study. *Journal of Clinical Psychiatry, 59*, 449–455.

Bauer, M., McBride, L., Shea, N., Gavin, C., Holden, F., & Kendall, S. (1997). Impact of easy access clinic based program for bipolar disorder: Quantitative analysis of a demonstration project. *Psychiatric Services, 44*, 159–168.

Clarkin, J., Carpenter, D., Hull, J., Wilner, P., & Glick, I. (1998). Effects of psychoeducation for married patients with bipolar disorder and their spouses. *Psychiatric Services, 49*, 531–533.

Cochran, S. (1984). Preventing medication non-compliance in the outpatient treatment of bipolar affective disorders. *Journal of Consulting and Clinical Psychology, 52*, 873–878.

Colom, F., Martinez-Aran, A., Reinares, M., Banabarre, A., Corbella, B., & Vieta E. (2001). Psychoeducation and prevention of relapse in bipolar disorders: Preliminary results. *Bipolar Disorders, 3*(Suppl.), 32.

Colom, F., Vieta, E., Martinez-Aran, A., Reinares, M., Goikolea, J. M., Benabarre, A., Torrent, C., Comes, M., Corbella, B., Parramon, G., & Corominas, J. (2003). A randomized trial on the efficacy of group psycho-education in the prophylaxis of recurrences in bipolar patients whose disease is in remission. *Archives of General Psychiatry, 60*, 402–407.

Dickson, W. E., & Kendell, R. E. (1994). Does maintenance lithium therapy prevent recurrences of mania under ordinary clinical conditions? *Psychological Medicine, 16*, 521–530.

Ehlers, C., Frank, E., & Kupfer, D. (1988). Social zeitgebers and biological rhythms: A unified approach to understanding the etiology of depression. *Archives of General Psychiatry, 45*, 948–952.

Falloon, I., Boyd, J., McGill, C., & Fadden, G. (1985). Family management in prevention of morbidity in schizophrenia: Clinical outcome of a two-year longitudinal study. *Archives of General Psychiatry, 42,* 887–896.

Frank, E., Hlastala, S., Ritenour, A., Houck, P., Tu, X., Monk, T., Mallinger, A., & Kupfer, D. (1994). Inducing lifestyle regularity in recovering bipolar patients: Results from the maintenance therapies in bipolar disorder protocol. *Biological Psychiatry, 41,* 1165–1173.

Frank, E., Swartz, H., Mallinger, A., Thase, M., Weaver, E., & Kupfer, D. (1999). Adjunctive psychotherapy for bipolar disorder: Effect of changing treatment modality. *Journal of Abnormal Psychology, 108,* 579–587.

Fromm-Reichmann, F. (1949). Intensive psychotherapy of manic–depressives: A preliminary report. *Confina Neurologica, 9,* 158–165.

Glick, I., Burti, L., Okonogi, K., & Sacks, M. (1994). Effectiveness in psychiatric care: Psychoeducationand outcome for patients with major affective disorder and their families. *British Journal of Psychiatry, 164,* 104–106.

Goodwin, F., & Jamison, K. R. (1990). *Manic–depressive illness.* Oxford: Oxford University Press.

Guscott, R., & Taylor, L. (1994). Lithium prophylaxis in recurrent affective illness: Efficacy, effectiveness and efficiency. *British Journal of Psychiatry, 164,* 741–746.

Haas, G., Glick, I., & Clarkin, J. (1988). Inpatient family intervention: A randomized clinical trial—results at hospital discharge. *Archives of General Psychiatry, 45,* 217–224.

Hlastala, S., Frank, E., Mallinger, A., Thase, M., Ritenour, A., & Kupfer, D. (1997). Bipolar depression: An underestimated treatment challenge. *Depression and Anxiety, 5,* 73–83.

Honig, A., Hofman, A., Rozendaal, N., & Dingemans, P. (1997). Psychoeducation in bipolar disorder: Effect on expressed emotion. *Psychiatry Research, 72,* 17–22.

Jackson, A., Cavanagh, J., & Scott, J. (2003). A systematic review of prodromal symptoms of mania and depression. *Journal of Affective Disorders, 74,* 209–217.

Jamison, K. R., Garner, R. H., & Goodwin, F. K. (1979). Patient and physician attitudes toward lithium. *Archives of General Psychiatry, 36,* 866–869.

Lam, D., Bright, J., Jones, S., Hayward, P., Schuck, N., Chisolm, D., & Sham, P. (2000). Cognitive therapy for bipolar illness: A pilot study of relapse prevention. *Cognitive Therapy and Research, 24,* 503–520.

Lam, D. H., Watkins, E. R., Hayward, P., Bright, J., Wright, K., Kerr, N., Parr-Davis, G., & Sham, P. (2003). A randomized controlled study of cognitive therapy for relapse prevention for bipolar affective disorder. *Archives of General Psychiatry, 60,* 145–152.

Miklowitz, D., Simoneau, T., George, E., Richards, J., Kalbag, A., Sachs-Ericsson, N., & Suddath, R. (2000). Family focused treatment of bipolar disorder: 1-year effects of a psychoeducational program in conjunction with pharmacotherapy. *Biological Psychiatry, 48,* 582–592.

Paykel, E., Scott, J., Teasdale, J., Johnson, A., Garland, A., Moore, R., Jenaway, A., Cornwall, P., Hayhurst, H., Abbott, R., & Pope, M. (1999). Prevention of relapse in residual depression by cognitive therapy: A controlled trial. *Archives of General Psychiatry, 56,* 829–835.

Perry, A., Tarrier, N., Morriss, R., McCarthy, E., Limb, K. (1999). Randomized controlled trial of efficacy of teaching patients with bipolar disorder to identify early symptoms of relapse and obtain treatment. *British Medical Journal, 318,* 149–153.

Scott, J. (1995). Psychotherapy for bipolar disorder: An unmet need? *British Journal of Psychiatry, 167,* 581–588.

Scott, J. (2001a). Cognitive therapy as an adjunct to medication in bipolar disorders. *British Journal of Psychiatry, 178*(Suppl.), S164–S168.

Scott, J. (2001b). Cognitive therapy for depression. *British Medical Bulletin, 57,* 101–113.

Scott, J., Garland, A., & Moorhead, S. (2001). A pilot study of cognitive therapy in bipolar disorder. *Psychological Medicine, 31,* 459–467.

Scott, J., & Pope, M. (2002). Non-adherence with mood-stabilizers: Prevalence and predictors. *Journal of Clinical Psychiatry, 65,* 384–390.

Scott, J., & Tacchi, M. J. (2003). A pilot study of concordance therapy for individuals with bipolar disorders who are non-adherent with lithium prophylaxis. *Bipolar Disorders, 4,* 386–392.

Sensky, T., Turkington, D., Kingdon, D., Scott, J., Scott, J., Siddle, R., O'Carroll, M., & Barnes T. (2000). A randomized controlled trial of cognitive behavioral therapy for persistent symptoms in schizophrenia resistant to medication. *Archives of General Psychiatry, 57,* 165–172.

Teasdale, J. (1985). Psychological treatments for depression: How do they work? *Behavior Research and Therapy, 23,* 157–165.

Thase, M. E., Greenhouse, J. B., & Frank, E. (1997). Treatment of major depression with psychotherapy or psychotherapy–pharmacotherapy combinations. *Archives of General Psychiatry, 54,* 109–115.

Van Gent, E., Vida, S., & Zwart, F. (1988). Group therapy in addition to lithium in patients with bipolar disorders. *Acta Psychiatrica Belgica, 88,* 405–418.

Van Gent, E., Vogtlander, L., & Vrendendaal, J. (1998, May). *Two group psychoeducation programs compared.* Paper presentation at the annual conference of the American Psychiatric Association, Toronto.

Van Gent, E., & Zwart, F. (1991). Psychoeducation of partners of bipolar manic patients. *Journal of Affective Disorders, 21,* 15–18.

Van Gent, E., & Zwart, F. (1993). Ultra-short versus short group therapy in addition to lithium. *Patient Education and Counseling, 21,* 135–141.

Weiss, R., Kolodziej, M., Najavits, L., Greenfield, S., & Fucito, L. (2000). Utilization of psychosocial treatments by patients diagnosed with bipolar disorder and substance misuse. *American Journal of Addictions, 9,* 314–320.

PART III

SPECIAL ISSUES
IN TREATMENT

CHAPTER TWELVE

TREATMENT COMPLIANCE

MONICA RAMIREZ BASCO
MEGAN MERLOCK
NOELLE MCDONALD

Every year new developments are made in the treatment of major psychiatric disorders, such as bipolar disorder. Newer medications have been developed with fewer side effects and more positive effects (e.g., Calabrese et al., 1999; Zarate, 2000), and psychotherapies that enhance outcomes show promise for helping people prevent relapse and adapt better to the limitations presented by their illnesses (e.g., Lam et al., 2003). Despite our greater understanding of the biopsychosocial mechanisms that underlie mental disorders, we are still left with the fundamental question of how to encourage patients to consistently utilize their pharmacological, psychosocial, and psychotherapeutic resources. Much has been learned about the treatment of bipolar disorder since the introduction of lithium in the early 1970s, yet only limited ground has been gained in improving treatment compliance rates. It is clear that degree of compliance with treatment is an important predictor of outcomes for patients with bipolar disorder (Craig, Fennig, Tanenberg-Karant, & Bromet, 2000; Kulhara, Basu, Mattoo, Sharan, & Chopra, 1999; Scott & Pope, 2002b; Tsai et al., 2001), with full compliance leading to the best overall outcomes.

Attempts to understand the nature of noncompliance have provided a few clues, which are discussed in this chapter, but no definitive answer has been found for resolving this perplexing problem. In general, it seems there are two requirements for compliance with treatment. First, patients must recall that a treatment-related behavior, such as taking a pill, is required, and second, they must make a decision to enact that treatment-related behavior. Many factors can interfere at either juncture, resulting in the patient's failure to enact the treatment behavior, intentionally or otherwise. The following summary of the literature on compliance with treatment in bipolar disorder attempts to elucidate the nature of the problem and suggest ways to maximize the likelihood that patients' self-care behaviors will match clinicians' recommendations.

• *Noncompliance is as much the norm as the exception.* Surveys of literature on medication compliance in psychiatric (Basco & Rush, 1995) and general medical populations (Meichenbaum & Turk, 1987) have found that most patients are either fully or partially noncompliant with treatment. Compliance is most likely to occur when treatment is short and health problems produce discomfort; compliance is least likely to occur for prophylactic treatment, when symptoms are in remission, or before significant complications have occurred (Meichenbaum & Turk, 1987). Among patients with bipolar disorder, estimates of noncompliance vary depending on the data collection method. For example, taking a global look at compliance, Svarstad, Shireman, and Sweeney (2001) examined Medicaid drug claims to assess the frequency with which medication prescriptions were filled by patients with severe mental illnesses over a 12-month period. They found that 33% of the 67 patients diagnosed with bipolar disorder irregularly filled their medication prescriptions. Keck and colleagues (1996) found that out of 101 patients hospitalized for mania, 64% had been noncompliant with pharmacotherapy in the month prior to admission. Basco and Rush (1995) found that across studies of patients with mood disorders, the probability of compliance varied from .53 to .63 for pharmacotherapy.

• *Compliance is not an all-or-nothing phenomenon.* Patients are often described clinically as compliant or noncompliant, as if it were a trait and not a behavior. Studies on compliance rates with pharmacotherapy show that most patients tend to miss some, but not all, doses of medication, whereas a smaller minority discontinue treatment altogether (Keck et al., 1996; Scott & Pope, 2002a). For example, Weiss and colleagues (1998) examined the compliance rates of 44 patients with bipolar disorder. Depending on the medication types, compliance rates for individual patients ranged from 66 to 100%. However, only 21% of patients taking lithium were completely adherent to treatment, and 13% of patients taking lithium and 8% of those taking valproate reported taking medication less than a third of the time.

The literature on patient factors that predict noncompliance with lithium and antidepressant medications has shed little light on the problem (Aagaard & Vestergaard, 1990; Connelly, Davenport, & Nurnberger, 1982; Danion, Neureuther, Krieger-Finance, Imbs, & Singer, 1987; Frank, Prien, Kupfer, & Alberts, 1985; Jacob et al., 1984). There does not appear to be a consistent association between compliance and illness characteristics, such as length of episode, age of onset, or polarity of episodes (e.g., Colom et al., 2000). However, greater psychiatric co-morbidity has been associated with lower compliance rates. In particular, patients treated for bipolar disorder who had substance abuse problems or personality disorders had more difficulty following treatment plans (Aagaard & Vestergaard, 1990; Colom et al., 2000; Danion et al., 1987; Jacob et al., 1984; Brown, Suppes, Adinoff, & Rajan, 2001). The varying rates of compliance across patients and the limited association with any predictors of compliance suggest that compliance may be more accurately viewed as a continuum of behavior, rather than a trait.

• *Compliance is more difficult than it looks.* The mental confusion and disorganization caused by depression, mania, and mixed states, as well as external distractions in the patients' environments, make compliance harder to accomplish than it might appear. Furthermore, patients are often requested to abide by complicated and expensive treatment recommendations that produce uncomfortable side effects and involve complicated dosing schedules.

Although physicians prescribe medications and therapists assign homework with the assumption that their directions will be followed, it is naive to assume that patients will adhere to a treatment plan just because clinicians say it will work. Acceptance of this fact will help clinicians lower their expectations to more realistic levels and plan ahead for noncompliance, rather than assume it will not occur or simply hoping for the best. Introducing patients to the complexities of compliance (e.g., "It is hard to stick with treatment for long periods of time") in a matter-of-fact discussion opens the door to frank discourse and proactive planning (e.g., "What do you think could interfere with you following this treatment plan?" "What could we do about that possibility?").

• *The best predictor of the future is the past.* Scott and Pope (2002a), in their examination of plasma blood levels of mood stabilizers in patients with bipolar disorder ($n = 78$) and major depressive disorder ($n = 20$), found that one of the best predictors of incomplete adherence to treatment was a prior history of noncompliance. Specifically, 84% of patients reporting a past history of noncompliance acknowledged that they had been only partially compliant with their medication in the month prior to evaluation, and 47% had been noncompliant within the week prior to the evaluation.

COMPLIANCE, DENIAL, AND ACCEPTANCE

Dell'Osso and colleagues (2002) found that inpatients with unipolar depression had more insight into their illness than did patients admitted for bipolar depression, mixed states, or manic episodes. Manic patients more often reported that medications are unlikely to help their symptoms subside, have less insight regarding the social consequences of bipolar disorder compared to patients with bipolar depressed and mixed episodes (Dell'Osso et al., 2000), and more often deny that their symptoms are a sign of mental illness (Swanson et al., 1995). This lack of insight appears to interfere with patients' engagement in the treatment process. For example, Lam and Wong (1997) found that level of insight and social functioning were both significantly correlated with the ability to detect depressive prodromes and to effectively cope with prodromal manic symptoms. Similarly, Ghaemi, Boiman, and Goodman (2000) found that lack of improvement in insight was associated with poorer outcome in patients with bipolar disorder.

A common clinical assumption is that patients who are not cooperative with treatment are in denial about their problems; therefore, the high noncompliance rates documented among patients with bipolar disorder could be considered evidence of their lack of acceptance of their illness. There is some empirical evidence that, in fact, noncompliance with treatment may be related to denial of illness in patients with bipolar disorder (Greenhouse, Meyer, & Johnson, 2000; Keck et al., 1996; Peralta & Cuesta, 1998; Scott & Pope, 2002a). For example, Keck et al. (1996) found that denial and poor insight were common factors associated with poor medication compliance among patients admitted for mania, and Greenhouse et al. (2000) found a curvilinear relationship, where high levels of denial were related to poorest compliance with treatment.

Although increasing insight can facilitate treatment compliance, it may come with a price. Williams and Collins (2002) found that patients with greater insight experienced more engulfment—that is, the extent to which patients identify with a sick role and feel damaged and deviant. A full awareness of the chronicity of bipolar disorder and its implications for future functioning, including the inevitable return of symptoms, can lead to sadness, despair, hopelessness, and suicidal ideation.

It should be pointed out that acceptance is not the absence of denial. In fact, the two are only moderately correlated (Greenhouse et al., 2000). Focusing merely on denial may oversimplify the process by which patients come to grips with their illnesses and begin to fully participate in, and cooperate with, treatment. Elisabeth Kübler-Ross (1970, 1974) proposed that denial and acceptance are the end points in a process of working through a significant sense of loss. Perhaps a broader model for understanding how people cope with a diagnosis of bipolar disorder is to conceptualize it as a process of grieving over the loss of the "normal" or "healthy" self. Using Kübler-Ross's description of the phases of grief, denial is but the first phase that people encounter when facing loss; denial is followed by anger, bargaining, hopelessness, and finally, acceptance. Although is it generally felt that people progress through these phases in this order, it is possible to regress to previous levels before finally achieving an acceptance of the loss of normalcy in mental health.

To determine a patient's progress through the stages of grief, it may be helpful to examine some behavioral or attitudinal indicators. The behaviors of interest are those related to participation in the treatment process—for instance, keeping appointments, taking medications, and modifying one's lifestyle to maximize adjustment to the illness (e.g., practicing good sleep hygiene). An example of the cognitive indicators might be the automatic thoughts verbalized by patients as they discuss their views of the disorder, treatment, or health care providers. Table 12.1 provides some examples of the negative automatic thoughts associated with each stage in the grieving process. As patients describe their views of their illness and treatment, these ideas can be compared to those in the table, or patients can be provided with the list and asked which best represents how they are feeling about their illness.

In patients with newly diagnosed bipolar disorder, acceptance of the initial diagnosis is dependent upon their conceptualization of the problem. Some suffer through several bouts of depression and mania before seeking

---

TABLE 12.1. Automatic Thoughts Associated with Stages of Grief over Illness

Denial

"I don't have it. The doctor made a mistake."
"It must be because I've been drinking too much."
"It will pass."

Anger

"It's not fair that I have this illness."
"I can't deal with this right now."
"Why me? What did I do to deserve this?"

Bargaining

"I'll clean up my act."
"I'll stop drinking, start waking up on time, start exercising, get a better job, and it will be OK."
"I'll make myself go on a diet, straighten out my sleep. It will get better."
"I'll try natural remedies. I don't really need medicine."

Depression

"I'll never have a normal life."
"No one will want me."
"I hate myself."

Acceptance

"I can work my way through this."
"It's not the end of the world."
"I don't have to give up everything just because I have to take medication."

treatment and find relief in the knowledge that what they have experienced can be diagnosed and treated. For those who have a family history of bipolar disorder, particularly in first-degree relatives, the diagnosis may not come as a surprise. These patients may forego denial if they have seen others suffer from similar symptoms and understand that there is a biological cause. Most others struggle with the idea that they have a chronic mental illness. They may intellectually comprehend the link between their genes, their biochemistry, and their mood symptoms, but their behavioral noncompliance with treatment suggests that they have not yet accepted the chronicity or severity of the disorder. Those in complete denial often are brought to treatment by family members or through law enforcement. They may be court ordered to receive care; once released, however, they are highly likely to discontinue their medications.

Understanding how compliance does or does not occur in children and adolescents requires consideration of special issues. For example, children's and teenagers' compliance with treatment is, to some extent, dependent upon the compliance of their caretakers in dispensing or supervising medication usage. Parents can bargain with or coerce their children to take medications, but they may not be able to force compliance with other self-management behaviors, such as going to sleep at a reasonable hour. Young adults who are no longer under parental control may demonstrate their inability or unwillingness to accept their diagnosis by ignoring symptoms, refusing medication, and "toughing out" the disruptions in their life. A 30-year-old high school teacher had suffered from bipolar disorder for 10 years but continued to refuse medication despite understanding the benefits. His illness had become rapid cycling over the course of time, but frequent symptom remissions reinforced his belief in his ability to handle the symptoms on his own.

Others have not suffered significant enough consequences of their illness to accept the notion that continuous treatment is necessary, particularly if supportive family members protected and aided the individual until the episode remitted. Colom et al. (2000) found the lowest compliance rates among people who had suffered relatively few episodes of depression and greater rates for those who had suffered through more episodes of illness. Early in the course, denial may be at its strongest, and acquiescence with family and doctor demands may only occur after life disruptions have become too severe or frequent to ignore.

COPING WITH DENIAL

Providing patients with a psychobiological conceptualization of bipolar disorder may be all that is needed for those ready and able to accept the diagnosis and treatment. However, for those in the denial phase, education about bipolar disorder is usually insufficient. The individual must first acknowledge the possibility of having a chronic mental illness before the educational material can be incorporated into his or her views of self and future. Socratic questioning is an effective cognitive therapy method for aiding patients in addressing issues of denial. The goal is for the patient to challenge his or her inaccurate views of bipolar disorder and replace them with a new perspective that will encourage self-care and compliance.

Below is an example of the use of Socratic questioning to explore the issue of denial in a patient with newly diagnosed bipolar disorder. Victor is a 26-year-old unmarried, Caucasian, computer programmer, who has been hospitalized twice for mania, the first time as a teenager. He has had one episode of depression, which lasted 2 years before his mother convinced him to seek treatment. Antidepressant therapy induced his second episode of mania. When he became psychotic, emergency treatment was arranged, followed by a 10-day hospitalization. Before discharge, the hospital staff, with assistance from Victor's mother, arranged a follow-up outpatient psychotherapy visit, despite his disinterest in attending. The following excerpt is from his first outpatient visit.

THERAPIST: Victor, your mom arranged this appointment for you. Do you know why you are here?

VICTOR: Not really. Well, I guess it's because my doctor thinks I need to see someone.

THERAPIST: How can I help?

VICTOR: You can tell my mother that I'm fine now and don't need anymore psychoanalyzing.

THERAPIST: So she brought you here for some psychoanalyzing?

VICTOR: Yeah. Sort of.

THERAPIST: What do you think you need?

VICTOR: I need to be left alone. I'm fine. I can take care of myself.

THERAPIST: Tell me about your stay in the hospital. Why were you there?

VICTOR: I freaked out one day and scared my mother. She thought I was going nuts and would hurt her or hurt myself. I don't remember exactly all that happened, but I ended up in the hospital. But I'm OK now.

THERAPIST: Tell me about freaking out.

VICTOR: I don't remember, but my mom said I was talking to myself and saying that I was God's prophet and that I was going to save the world. (*Laughs.*) Pretty weird, huh?

THERAPIST: How do you understand what happened to you?

VICTOR: The doctor says I have bipolar disorder, but I think he's just trying to cover up what really happened.

THERAPIST: And what really happened?

VICTOR: My mom thought I was depressed because I wasn't feeling well, and I was missing a lot of work. She took me to her doctor and he gave me what was supposed to be an antidepressant medication. Instead, it flipped me out. After about 2 days of the stuff, I was wired. I couldn't sleep. I was driving around all night, going to bars. My mom took me to the hospital, and they said I was manic. Now they tell me that I'm bipolar, and I have to take medications for the rest of my life. I don't buy it.

THERAPIST: I know quite a bit about bipolar disorder. I think that's why she brought you to see me. It sounds like you had depression and then something that looked like mania. Have you ever had times like this in the past?

VICTOR: When I was in high school I was drinking and smoking pot for a while. My parents got all worried because I had been out all night and was acting kind of weird, so they took me to my doctor. I got worse instead of better and got on that religious thing again. I wasn't making any sense to them, and they said I wouldn't shut up, so they took me to a psychiatrist that our neighbors knew, and he put me in the hospital.

THERAPIST: What do you know about bipolar disorder?

VICTOR: My uncle has it. You get depressed sometimes and you can get manic. He has rapid cycling, so he's always up or down. He takes a bunch of meds, but he still has problems.

THERAPIST: What makes your doctor think you have bipolar disorder?

VICTOR: I was acting manic after I took those pills.

THERAPIST: OK, and what else?

VICTOR: I guess I was depressed before that, and I might have been manic in high school.

THERAPIST: Do you know how a diagnosis of bipolar disorder is made?

VICTOR: Not really.

THERAPIST: To get a diagnosis of bipolar disorder, you must have had at least one episode of mania in your life. That's all. Mania is when your mood is either euphoric or very irritable, and you have other changes as well. For example, you can't sleep or don't feel like you need any, you talk a lot, perhaps too fast, and you jump around from subject to subject, making it hard for people to understand you. Sometimes you get some grand ideas that are not like your usual way of thinking, like thinking that God is sending you special messages or thinking that you have some other special ability that others do not have. So far, does this sound like you?

VICTOR: Yeah, from what I was told, but I don't really remember. I guess if everyone else thinks I'm manic, it must be true.

THERAPIST: But you don't buy it, right? (*Victor nods.*) Tell me what it would take to convince you that you have bipolar disorder.

VICTOR: I don't know.

THERAPIST: A second opinion? Reading about it? What about if someone you really trusted told you that you had it?

VICTOR: My uncle would tell me. He has it, so he would tell me the truth.

THERAPIST: Why don't you talk it over with him and then let's talk again. Do you think it would be helpful for you to read a description of what it's like to have bipolar disorder to see it if matches your experience?

VICTOR: Sure.

THERAPIST: Here is a book called *An Unquiet Mind*. It was written by a psychologist who has bipolar disorder. She does a good job of describing what it is like. Read as much as you can before we meet again.

In this example, the therapist does not try to convince the patient that he has bipolar disorder. Instead, the patient tells his story and information is gathered about the impressions that others have about the patient's experience. The patient is not pushed to accept the diagnosis; instead he is encouraged to explore the possibility that the diagnosis is correct. Consulting others and reading descriptions of the illness, even reading the DSM-IV criteria (American Psychiatric Association, 1994) can be useful as well.

Another strategy for coping with denial is to share with patients a list of common symptoms of mania and depression (see Tables 12.2 and 12.3), so that they can compare their subjective experience with what is commonly found in this disorder. It is more common for patients to recognize the most severe forms of the symptoms than the mild or moderate forms. However it is helpful for those unfamiliar with mania and depression to see how cognitive, behavioral, emotional, and physiological changes can progress from the normal range to the symptomatic range. Monitoring of the mild signs and symptoms of depression and mania can alert patients to recurrences of episodes while they are still at easily manageable levels.

Acknowledgment of a diagnosis of bipolar disorder does not necessarily open the door to compliance with treatment; it merely facilitates entering the adjustment process. Following agreement with a diagnosis, the individual can begin to consider how he or she will live with the illness. The early emotional reactions are usually anger or anxiety and rarely that of resignation or acceptance. When acceptance occurs too early in the adjustment process, it is likely that anger will reemerge at a later date, when the symptoms of the illness or inevitable life disruptions occur.

COPING WITH ANGER

Frustration and anger with the illness, its treatment, and care providers may surface when the patient confronts the physical, financial, and psychosocial consequences that ultimately result. There may be many medication trials before a combination is found that controls symptoms without intolerable side effects. In the process, patients become frustrated with the trial-and-error approach, the uncomfortable and unexpected side effects, and

TABLE 12.2. Common Symptoms of Mania

Mild form of symptom	Moderate form of symptom	Severe form of symptom
Everything seems like a hassle; impatient or anxious	More easily angered	Irritability
Happier than usual, positive outlook	Increased laughter and joking	Euphoria
More talkative; better sense of humor	In the mood to socialize and talk with others	Pressured or rapid speech
More thoughts; mentally sharp, quick; lose focus	Disorganized thinking, poor concentration	Racing thoughts
More self-confident than usual; less pessimistic	Feel smart; not afraid to try; overly optimistic	Grandiosity; delusions of grandeur
Creative ideas; new interests; change sounds good	Plan to make changes; disorganized in actions; drinking or smoking more	Disorganized activity; starting more things than finishing
Fidgety, nervous behaviors such as nail biting	Restless; preferring movement over sedentary activities	Psychomotor agitation; cannot sit still
Not as effective at work; having trouble keeping mind on tasks	Not completing tasks; late for work; annoying others	Cannot complete usual work or home activities
Uncomfortable with other people	Suspicious	Paranoia
More sexually interested	Sexual dreams; seeking out or noticing sexual stimulation	Increased sex drive—seeking out sexual activity; more promiscuous
Notice sounds and annoying people; lose train of thought	Noises seem louder; colors seem brighter; mind wanders easily; need quieter environment to focus thoughts	Distractibility—have to work hard to focus thoughts or cannot focus thoughts at all

the imposition the symptoms and treatment impose on their lives. They remember what it was like to feel normal and associate this normalcy with a time when they were not taking medications. The unfortunate conclusion drawn is that medication is the problem rather than the solution, and as a consequence, medication is taken less frequently. Clinicians often underestimate the patience it requires to tolerate the lengthy, costly, and uncomfortable treatment process. If this lack of empathy is communicated to the pa-

TABLE 12.3. Common Symptoms of Depression

Mild form of symptom	Moderate form of symptom	Severe form of symptom
Blue, down, or neutral mood	Cry more easily	Severe sadness
Not in the mood to socialize	Less involved with others	Lack of interest in usual activities
Usual activities are not as fun as expected	Has fun until activity is over	Decreased pleasure
Blame self more readily when things go wrong; sees own faults	Self-critical	Excessive and inappropriate guilt
Not as hungry as usual; can skip meals occasionally and not feel hungry	Eating brings less pleasure	Decreased appetite
Clothes fit slightly looser, but no big weight loss (e.g., 1–3 pounds)	Noticeable weight loss	Significant weight loss
Sleep seems less restful; ruminate at bedtime; falling asleep takes a little longer	Take much longer to fall asleep; wake up briefly during the night	Insomnia—cannot fall asleep easily; wake up during the night and stay awake
Lose interest in tasks such as reading; get frustrated with tasks that are lengthy	Must reread text; thoughts cannot be focused well	Impaired concentration
Feel as if moving slowly; not mentally sharp	Slowness in movement noticeable to others; long pauses before answering questions	Psychomotor retardation
Wish pain would go away; thoughts of running away; pessimistic	Thoughts that life may not be worth living; hopeless; can't imagine feeling better	Suicidal ideas or attempts; not caring about dying
Self-doubt; some self-criticism	Low self-esteem; dislike appearance; feel like a loser	Feelings of worthlessness

tient, it can cause a rift in the therapeutic alliance that results in resistance to clinician recommendations.

In response to patients' frustration and hopelessness about treatment, many clinicians instinctively provide encouragement and support, which might take the form of expressing confidence that therapy or medication will ultimately be successful and noting the improvement already achieved. Some patients might feel encouraged by such an assertion, whereas others may conclude that their provider cannot fully grasp the degree of dissatisfaction they feel with their care, thereby widening the rupture in the therapeutic alliance. An alternative, and perhaps more effective first-line response to patients' despair, is to validate their feelings rather than move too quickly to dispel them. Acknowledging their frustration and confiding your own feelings about the slow process, the less-than-perfect effectiveness of treatment, and the limited control over the symptoms will help to strengthen the alliance with the patient as a member of the treatment team.

Similarly, when patients voice their anger about having a mental illness, validating their feelings rather than quickly attempting to resolve the anger will allow them to work through the emotion. For example, the statement "I hate having this illness—it isn't fair" is best followed by an agreement, such as, "You are right. It does stink that you have this illness, and it isn't fair." Having empathized with the unfairness of life, the patient is then allowed ample time to feel outraged and to contemplate the meaning of having bipolar disorder before the therapist moves on to the resolution phase, saying, "So, what can we do about it?" To prompt discussion and resolution, the therapist may inquire about the impact of the illness on the patient's view of self, others, and his or her future. Standard logical analysis methods can be used to resolve any cognitive distortions.

BARGAINING FOR TREATMENT

As patients work through the adjustment process from denial to acceptance, they often engage in self-bargaining along the way. Although some will attempt to negotiate preferences with their psychiatrists concerning medication type and dose, hospitalization, or adjunctive outpatient treatment, many will hold an internal debate in which promises of improved self-care are made in exchange for reduction in need for formal treatments. Some might decide to reduce their alcohol consumption and improve sleep and eating habits with the hopes that their symptoms will improve. This type of bargain can be interpreted as acceptance of the illness without complete acceptance of the treatment. A patient might imagine that if he or she can manage the illness by making behavioral changes, then perhaps (1) the diagnosis is not entirely correct, (2) only a mild version of the disorder is present, or (3) mind can prevail over body. Each makes the case for reducing dependence on pharmacotherapy.

Bargaining also may take the form of self-designated adjustments to medication regimens, such as altering the timing or frequency of taking the medication according to an unsystematic algorithm created by the patient. This might include skipping medication doses, lengthening the interval between doses, or raising or lowering the dose to achieve a more complete remission. Some patients decide that discontinuation of some or all medications and replacement with "natural" methods of symptom control would be in their best interest. Others decide to suffer through an episode without any treatment, hoping the symptoms will remit on their own. The bargain made is usually to resume the prescribed medication regimen if they begin to feel worse. However, the desire to avoid medicine as much as possible can lead to underestimation of symptoms until they reach intolerable levels.

To address this bargaining behavior, it may be helpful to explain how this behavior may be a component of the adjustment process:

> "It seems like you may not be ready to accept that you have bipolar disorder and that it is going to require ongoing treatment. You are negotiating with yourself to make the whole thing seem more tolerable and less serious. This is part of your adjustment. You have to prove to yourself that medicine is really necessary. You would prefer to will it away, as do most people who struggle with this illness. I wish you could will it away too, but I know from experience with others that it is more complicated than that."

Another strategy is to respect patients' rights to try things their way. Rather than meet their resistance with more resistance, help them to plan a strategy for reducing dependency on medication, define criteria for success, and make a back-up plan should the strategy fail. It does not serve patients well to insist on compliance and ignore their concerns about treatment.

It is not unusual for patients to strongly express their displeasure with their drug therapy to a therapist but fail to offer any honest or direct feedback to the psychiatrist. This may be due to a lack of assertiveness, forgetfulness, poor planning in the patient, intimidation by the physician, or insufficient time during a medication visit. If you are the prescribing physician, ask patients how they have been taking their medication, inquire about any concerns, and if necessary, discuss the advantages and disadvantages of alternative strategies. If you are not the prescribing physician, help the patient to voice his or her concerns about treatment to the prescriber by practicing assertiveness through role-playing exercises. In some cases, it is helpful for therapists to contact prescribing physicians directly to discuss patients' difficulties with compliance, assuming patients have granted permission.

DEPRESSED ABOUT BEING ILL

As people progress through the stages of grief, working their way toward acceptance, they reach a point in which they become fully aware of the meaning and depth of the problem of bipolar disorder. Through education, observation, or experience, they realize the severity of the illness and its potential for disrupting their lives. They come to understand the necessity of pharmacotherapy and realize the cost and the discomforts they will be forced to endure. The weight of these realizations often leaves them feeling overwhelmed, distraught, and hopeless. They question their abilities to survive the process, to bear the financial burden, and to live independently. Sadness over being given a diagnosis of a chronic and incurable psychiatric illness is not a cognitive distortion requiring quick intervention, but a reasonable response to what often feels like a life sentence. The depression should be considered a necessary part of the grieving process and not dismissed or worked through too quickly.

Intervention is required if the depression prolongs or if patients' beliefs about their disorder become distorted. Catastrophizing, magnification, and fortune telling are the most common cognitive errors stimulated by distress over bipolar disorder. Patients can become overly negative and hopeless. Their imagination leaves them homeless, alone, and psychotic, wandering the streets in a mental fog. In these cases, cognitive restructuring can help patients to challenge their negative automatic thoughts and to set up experiments to test their assumptions about the future. Attendance at support groups, such as the Depression and Bipolar Support Alliance, can provide models of successful living with the illness, and numerous autobiographical books illustrate ways in which people have coped positively with bipolar disorder.

Self-esteem can be damaged by the realization of having a mental illness. To regain confidence, it may be necessary for people with bipolar disorder to revise their self-view to incorporate their premorbid strengths with the changes they have suffered as a result of their depression or mania. Some people see having bipolar disorder as a character flaw or a scar that everyone will notice. They underestimate their abilities to cope, often forget successful experiences from the past, and underestimate the capacities of others to be accepting and supportive. A therapist can help rebuild self-esteem by challenging patients to redefine themselves: "Who are you now? How are you different from before? In what ways are you just the same? Have you grown stronger than you were before?"

THE FANTASY OF ACCEPTANCE

Clinical lore suggests that once a person fully understands and accepts the conditions of his or her illness, he or she will eagerly cooperate with treatment. Acceptance consists of a shift in cognitive set toward a more realistic view of illness and its implications, accompanied by a sense of peacefulness or resignation. However, just as acceptance is not always a prerequisite for compliance, achieving acceptance does not always guarantee compliance. Even after psychological and emotional adjustments have resulted in acceptance, clinicians must tend to practical issues such as forgetfulness or lack of funds (Keck et al., 1996), intolerable medication side effects (Gitlin, Cochran, & Jamison, 1989; Keck et al., 1996; Nilson & Axelsson, 1989), discomfort with health care providers (Gitlin et al., 1989), and family discouragement of pharmacotherapy—all of which can interfere with even the best intentions to comply with treatment.

REMEDIES

Following the typical medication regimen for bipolar disorder requires several skills. These include organizational skills to seek help and acquire medication, normal memory functioning to take medication at the prescribed times, and self-discipline to set limits on sleep, alcohol consumption, overstimulation, and to make oneself stop and take medication when preferring to omit it altogether. When depression or mania interfere with cognitive processing, these tasks become more difficult at a time when strict compliance is needed the most. The implementation of some simple behavior management strategies can supplement existing skills to increase the chance that full adherence with treatment will occur.

Pillboxes

Pillboxes come in various shapes and sizes. The most helpful are those with slots for each day of the week and each time of the day that medications are taken. For example, medications can be stored in a two-by-seven box for twice-a-day dosing. Most pillboxes are clear plastic so that it is easy to verify whether medications have been taken. When forgetfulness occurs, the individual can verify whether the slot for the day is empty to avoid missing doses or double dosing. A clear plastic pillbox is particularly advantageous when the patient lives with others who monitor his or her medication intake. Placing the box in full view eliminates inquiries about compliance that can create tension between patients and family members. The date indicators on pillboxes begin with "S" for Sunday on the first slot and "S" for Saturday on the seventh slot. A routine should be established for refilling the boxes on Saturday, after the last dose is taken, or on Sunday, before the first weekly dose is taken.

Pair Medication with an Existing Activity

The goal of medication adherence is for the behavior of pill taking to become a habit—that is, an automatic response requiring little thought and no debate. Pairing pill taking with an existing habit makes it part of a well established response set. For example, the first dose of the day might be paired with morning coffee or teeth brushing, a midday dose paired with lunch, and an evening dose paired with bedtime activities. If a daily routine for taking other medications, such as vitamins or birth control pills, has been established, it is easiest to add psychotropic medications at the same time. Although it adds to the number of pills taken at a time, which patients often find objectionable, it reduces the number of times each day that the patient must remember to take medication. When designing the medication regimen, it would serve the process well to inquire about patients' daily routines, including work, social, meal, and sleep schedules. Compliance is more likely to occur if the regimen fits the patient's schedule rather than requiring the patient to change schedules to accommodate the medications.

Cues to Recall

Forgetfulness is a common obstacle to compliance, particularly after acute symptoms of depression or mania have remitted and therefore no longer serve as a cue to take the medication. Alarms on watches or pagers, reminder notes, computer or Personal Digital Assistant-generated messages, and placement of pill bottles on a nightstand or kitchen table can all cue a person to take medications. Particularly when developing a new routine for medications, recall cues, when strategically timed and placed, can help the patient remember the plan until it becomes a naturally occurring habit.

Family Support

Active family participation in treatment can be a tremendous resource for people suffering from bipolar disorder (see Chapter 9, this volume). For example, in Kim, Zisselman, and Pelchat's (1996) study of maintenance electroconvulsive therapy (ECT), patients who were most compliant with ECT were those who lived at home and/or whose families supported maintenance treatment. Unfortunately, family members also can interfere with treatment if they have misgivings about the diagnosis, health care providers, or the treatment. The social stigma attached to mental illness in family members can impede acceptance of treatment. Shame or guilt for passing on the genes for the illness, or negative family experiences with other relatives who have had bipolar disorder, can prime family members with discouragement regarding medication treatment and flat rejection of psychiatric diagnoses.

To preclude these obstacles to adherence, it can help to involve key family members in the patient's treatment. Education regarding the illness, diagnosis, and treatment options will help close the gaps in knowledge between care providers and family members. Misconceptions about the illness and treatment can be handled through discussion and provision of educational materials. Topics of discussion should include how to contact providers in the event of an emergency, how to recognize symptom relapse, and what to do when patient or family members have concerns about the treatment. After one or two initial visits with the patient and family members, individual treatment sessions can resume, with family sessions occurring on a monthly or bimonthly basis.

The Importance of Trust

When patients do not trust their therapists or psychiatrists, they are unlikely to follow treatment recommendations. Trust is formed through the demonstration of genuine concern, respect for the opinions of patients, and honesty. Small behaviors such as making eye contact with the patient during visits, recalling the discussions from the last visit, eliciting questions, and probing for concerns are the building blocks of trust. During a therapy session, one patient talked about her last visit with her psychiatrist, who had prescribed a new medication for insomnia. "I'm not going to take that medicine," she announced, "he was in such a hurry he didn't even take time to look me in the eye. He just looked at the chart, wrote a note, gave me a prescription, and left. He asked if I had any questions after opening the door and starting to walk out. I said no. Why bother? He didn't really care." In this example, the visit might have been efficient, but it served no real purpose, since the recommendations given were not going to be followed. It is easy to blame the patient for noncompliance in cases like this, but this problem was caused by a breakdown in the therapeutic alliance. A few more minutes of time spent in the visit might greatly increase trust and adherence to treatment and, in turn, prevent symptom exacerbations. In the long run, a small amount of attentiveness might prevent a great deal of patient misery and save the physician the time it takes to deal with crises.

Trust is particularly important when the provider, but not the patient, recognizes current manic symptoms. After a long period of depression, mania can feel like a welcomed relief, so some people downplay the signs and reject accusations that the changes in mood are pathological. When trust is present, patients can hear therapists' or psychiatrists' comments about emerging symptoms as evidence of concern for their well-being, especially if followed by acknowledgment of the frustration patients must feel when their relief from depression becomes as problematic as the depression itself.

Trust is also critical when a provider suggests changes in a patient's lifestyle, medication regimen, relationships, or ways of coping. Letting go of old patterns is difficult, even when they clearly create or exacerbate problems for the patient, and changing medications always runs the risk of making matters worse. Patients' cooperation in these times will depend upon trust in their providers' judgments. Eliciting patients' ideas for change, trying out their strategies rather than condemning them as useless, and asking their opinions about medication changes can strengthen trust. Willingness to "do it their way" some of the time will increase the odds that they will "do it your way" when you feel strongly that they do so.

Keeping a tab on the therapeutic alliance is the best preventative measure. Although a commonly suggested element of cognitive-behavioral therapy, clinicians often forget to elicit feedback from their patients on the progress of therapy, and psychopharmacologists are not trained to inquire regularly about the therapeutic relationship. Clinicians see dozens of patients in the time that intervenes between a given patient's treatment sessions, but the patient sees only one clinician. He or she remembers the last conversation, feels like the only person under care, and expects clinicians to feel the same. The relationship is an integral part of treatment, even with the most mechanistic approaches. Inquiry about and discussion of the relationship will allow rifts to be mended and problems to be avoided. Moreover, such discussion will communicate to patients that the relationship with them is important enough to take the time to maintain, despite a busy work schedule.

SUMMARY

Compliance is a behavior and not a character trait. Typically, people are compliant with treatment some of the time, for example, when symptoms are at their worst, but not all the time, such as when in remission. Usually, patients are moderately compliant most of the time, fully compliant a small percentage of the time, and completely noncompliant less often than most clinicians would predict. Noncompliance is the norm rather than the exception. Clinicians who can accept the inevitability of noncompliance can plan for it rather than feel betrayed when a patient fails to follow through on a procedure. Compliance is more difficult than it looks, particularly when medication regimens require multiple daily dosing or create uncomfortable side effects. The organizational skills, memory, and self-discipline needed to adhere consistently with treatment plans are compromised by the disorder.

Patient denial about having the illness is the reason posited most often by clinicians to explain noncompliance, but is only one step in the sequence of emotional adjustments made on the way to acceptance of their diagnosis and treatment. Patients mourn the loss of normalcy in a process similar to mourning the loss of a loved one. Denial is followed by anger about having the illness, bargaining with self and others about the medication regimen, depression about being ill, and finally acceptance of the fact that one must live with an illness. Even when acceptance is achieved, there are many other obstacles that can interfere with patients' best intentions to follow treatment. These include factors such as forgetfulness, breaches in the therapeutic alliance, family interference, and the complexity or discomforts associated with treatment. Interventions that move patients toward acceptance of the illness will ultimately aid the resolution of compliance problems. Continued discussion of the challenges of treatment compliance, including identification and resolution of the obstacles to full adherence with treatment, will increase acceptance of the challenges of living with this illness and, in turn, improve outcomes.

REFERENCES

Aagaard, J., & Vestergaard, P. (1990). Predictors of outcome in prophylactic lithium treatment: A 2-year prospective study. *Journal of Affective Disorders, 18,* 259–266.

American Psychiatric Association (1994). *Diagnostic and statistical manual of mental disorders* (4th ed.). Washington, DC: Author.

Basco, M. R., & Rush, A. J. (1995). Compliance with pharmacotherapy in mood disorders. *Psychiatry Annals, 25,* 78–82.

Brown, S., Suppes, T., Adinoff, B., & Rajan, T. N. (2001). Drug use and bipolar disorder: Comorbidity or misdiagnosis? *Journal of Affective Disorders, 65,* 105–115.

Calabrese, J. R., Bowden, C. L., Sachs, G. S., Ascher, J. A., Monaghan, E., & Rudd, G. D., for the Lamictal 602 Study Group. (1999). A double-blind placebo-controlled study of lamotrigine monotherapy in outpatients with bipolar I disorder. *Journal of Clinical Psychiatry, 60,* 79–88.

Colom, F., Vieta, E., Martinez-Aran, A., Reinares, M., Benabarre, A, & Gasto, C. (2000). Clinical factors associated with treatment noncompliance in euthymic bipolar patients. *Journal of Clinical Psychiatry, 61,* 549–555.

Connelly, C. E., Davenport, Y. B., & Nurnberger, J. I. (1982). Adherence to treatment regimen in a lithium carbonate clinic. *Archives of General Psychiatry, 39,* 585–588.

Craig, T. J., Fennig, S., Tanenberg-Karant, M., & Bromet, E. J. (2000). Rapid versus delayed readmission in first-admission psychosis: Quality indicators for managed care? *Annals of Clinical Psychiatry, 12,* 233–238.

Danion, J. M., Neureuther, C., Krieger-Finance, F., Imbs, J. L., & Singer, L. (1987). Compliance with long-term lithium treatment in major affective disorders. *Pharmacopsychiatry, 20,* 230–231.

Dell'Osso, L., Pini, S., Cassano, G. B., Mastrocinque C., Seckinger, R. A., Saettoni, M., Papasogli, A., Yale, S. A., & Amador, X. F. (2002). Insight into illness in patients with mania, mixed mania, bipolar depression and major depression with psychotic features. *Bipolar Disorders, 4,* 315–322.

Dell'Osso, L., Pini, S., Tundo, A., Sarno, N., Musetti, L., & Cassano, G. B. (2000). Clinical characteristics of mania, mixed mania, and bipolar depression with psychotic features. *Comprehensive Psychiatry, 41,* 242–247.

Frank, E., Prien, R. F., Kupfer, D. J., & Alberts, L. (1985). Implications of noncompliance on research in affective disorders. *Psychopharmacology Bulletin, 21,* 27–42.

Ghaemi, S. N., Boiman, E., & Goodwin, F. K. (2000). Insight and outcome in bipolar, unipolar, and anxiety disorders. *Comprehensive Psychiatry, 41,* 167–171.

Gitlin, M. J., Cochran, S. D., & Jamison, K. R. (1989). Maintenance lithium treatment: Side effects and compliance. *Journal of Clinical Psychiatry, 50,* 127–131.

Greenhouse, W. J., Meyer, B., & Johnson, S. L. (2000). Coping and medication adherence in bipolar disorder. *Journal of Affective Disorders, 59,* 237–241.

Jacob, M., Turner, L., Kupfer, D. J., Jarrett, D. B., Buzzinotti, E., & Bernstien, P. (1984). Attrition in maintenance therapy for recurrent depression. *Journal of Affective Disorders, 6,* 181–189.

Keck, P. E., McElroy, S. L., Strakowski, S. M., Stanton, S. P., Kizer, D. L., Balistreri, T. M., Bennett, J. A., Tugrul, K. C., & West, S. A. (1996). Factors associated with pharmacologic noncompliance in patients with mania. *Journal of Clinical Psychiatry, 57,* 292–297.

Kim, E., Zisselman, M. H., & Pelchat, R. (1996). Factors affecting compliance with maintenance electroconvulsive therapy: A preliminary study. *International Journal of Geriatric Psychiatry, 11,* 473–476.

Kübler-Ross, E. (1970). The care of the dying: Whose job is it? *Psychiatry in Medicine, 1,* 103–107.

Kübler-Ross, E. (1974). The languages of the dying patients. *Humanitas, 10,* 5–8.

Kulhara, P., Basu, D., Mattoo, S. K., Sharan, P., & Chopra, R. (1999). Lithium prophylaxis of recurrent bipolar affective disorder: Long-term outcome and its psychosocial correlates. *Journal of Affective Disorders, 54,* 87–96.

Lam, D. H., Watkins, E. R., Hayward, P., Bright, J., Wright, K., Kerr, N., Parr-Davis, G., & Sham, P. (2003). A randomized controlled study of cognitive therapy for relapse prevention for bipolar affective disorder: Outcome of the first year. *Archives of General Psychiatry, 60,* 145–152.

Lam, W., & Wong, G. (1997). Prodromes, coping strategies, insight and social functioning in bipolar affective disorders. *Psychological Medicine, 27,* 1091–1100.

Meichenbaum, D., & Turk, D. (1987). *Facilitating treatment adherence: A practitioner's guidebook.* New York: Plenum Press.

Nilson, A., & Axelsson, R. (1989). Factors associated with discontinuation of long-term lithium treatment. *Acta Psychiatrica Scandinavica, 80,* 221–230.

Peralta, V., & Cuesta, M. J. (1998). Lack of insight in mood disorders. *Journal of Affective Disorders, 49,* 55–58.

Scott, J. & Pope, M. (2002a). Nonadherence with mood stabilizers: Prevalence and predictors. *Journal of Clinical Psychiatry, 63*(5), 384–390.

Scott, J. & Pope, M. (2002b). Self-reported adherence to treatment with mood stabilizers, plasma levels, and psychiatric hospitalizations. *American Journal of Psychiatry, 159,* 1927–1929.

Svarstad, B. L., Shireman, T. I., & Sweeney, J. K. (2001). Using drug claims data to assess the relationship of medication adherence with hospitalization and costs. *Psychiatric Services, 52*(6), 805–811.

Swanson, C. L., Freudenreich, O., McEvoy, J. P., Nelson, L., Kamaraju, L., & Wilson, W. H. (1995). Insight in schizophrenia and mania. *Journal of Nervous and Mental Disease, 183,* 752–755.

Tsai, S. M., Chen, C., Kuo, C., Lee, J., Lee, H., & Strakowski, S. M. (2001). 15-year outcome of treated bipolar disorder. *Journal of Affective Disorders, 63,* 215–220.

Weiss, R. D., Greenfield, S. F., Najavits, L. M., Soto, J. A., Wyner, D., Tohen, M., & Griffin, M. L. (1998). Medication compliance among patients with bipolar disorder and substance abuse. *Journal of Clinical Psychiatry, 59,* 172–174.

Williams, C. C., & Collins, A. (2002). Factors associated with insight among outpatients with serious mental illness. *Psychiatric Services, 53,* 96–98.

Zarate, C. A. (2000). Antipsychotic drug side effect issues in bipolar manic patients. *Journal of Clinical Psychiatry, 61*(Suppl. 8), 52–61.

CHAPTER THIRTEEN

SUICIDALITY

Cory F. Newman

Suicide risk assessment and prevention are often prominent parts of the treatment of individuals with bipolar disorder. Conservative estimates of the lifetime likelihood of suicide for this population span from 15% (Simpson & Jamison, 1999) to 19% (Goodwin & Jamison, 1990), figures that include both those who do and do not receive treatment. It is likely that the impact of bipolar disorder on premature death may be even higher, as individuals with bipolar disorder incur a higher incidence of serious medical problems and auto accidents than the general population (Bowden, 1999). In a meta-analysis of 250 clinical studies, Harris and Barraclough (1997) determined that persons with bipolar disorder were 15 times more likely to kill themselves compared to the general population, a calculation that does not include the additive risk factor of alcohol and other substance abuse. Further, a review of 15 studies concluded that the prevalence of suicide attempts in bipolar patients approaches 50% (Goodwin & Jamison, 1990), a frighteningly high percentage that surpasses the rate for most other psychiatric populations (Lam, Jones, Hayward, & Bright, 1999). Indeed, therapists who treat patients with this spectrum of affective illness likely need to be vigilant for both the acute onset and chronic risk of suicidal crises in their patients.

Studying the course of bipolar illness reveals why so many of its sufferers fall prey, at some point, to thoughts of killing themselves. Simply put, bipolar disorder typically brings misery to those who have it, and—by extension—to those who care for them. The symptoms range from crushing depressions to reckless highs that alternately result in hopelessness and impulsive destructiveness. Cycles of these mood episodes can continue throughout sufferers' lives and wreak havoc on every aspect of their experience. Episodes of depressive withdrawal and manic highs frequently result in serious life consequences, including interruption or termination of interpersonal relationships, academic and vocational pursuits, financial health, and social standing in the community. It is particularly demoralizing when these individuals have to "pick up the pieces" and start again after a severe symptom episode has wrought such damage. When the cycle repeats itself—especially when the patients have earnestly tried to engage in the proper pharmacologic and psychosocial treatments—those with bipolar illness may begin to wonder if the struggle is worth continuing, and some may contemplate suicide.

The high comorbidity rate of alcohol and other drug abuse in this population (perhaps as high as 50%, the highest of any Axis I disorder [Sonne, Brady, & Morton, 1994]) also raises the risk, because impulsivity is exacerbated by intoxication. Patients who swear to their therapist, while they are sober, that they will not take action to harm themselves may become determined to commit suicide when they are inebriated. Psychoactive substances (both licit and illicit) are likely to interfere with proper pharmacotherapy and thereby add yet another obstacle to the patient's safety. As Jamison (1999) notes, "Substance abuse loads the cylinder with more bullets. By acting to disinhibit behavior, drugs and alcohol increase risk taking, violence, and impulsivity. For those who are suicidal or potentially so, this may be lethal" (p.127).

Suicide most often occurs when the person with bipolar illness is in the depressive phase of the illness (Jamison, 1999). However, this does not mean that patients are safe when they are manic. Mixed states of mania and agitated depression create times of high risk (Goldberg, Garno, Leon, Kocsis, & Portera, 1998; Dilsaver, Chen, Swann, Shoaib, & Krajewski, 1994), and depressive crashes can occur rather suddenly. As Jamison (1995) has noted, mania has a way of seducing individuals into believing that little can harm them; thus they engage in behaviors that result in severe, negative consequences. When such individuals lapse into depression, they are ill equipped to deal with the fallout; they often recognize the damage that has been caused but feel hopeless to correct it. In addition, their sense of public humiliation and loss of social support can increase the risk that they will look for the ultimate escape of suicide.

There is evidence that people with bipolar depression typically have more objective reasons to be unhappy than do their counterparts with unipolar depressive disorder. In a study from Finland, Isometsä, Heikkinen, Henriksson, Aro, & Lonnqvist (1995) retrospectively examined the lives of people who had committed suicide. They reduced and divided the sample into two groups: those who had had unipolar depression and those who had had bipolar depression. What these group members had in common were subjective reasons to want to kill themselves. However, when looking at the *objective* facts of their lives, those persons with bipolar depression had more serious problems with which to contend, including longer treatment histories, greater frequency of hospitalizations, and more divorces. In other words, patients with bipolar disorder who are depressed and suicidal often have truly problematic life conditions that might be daunting for anyone to face. Therapists, therefore, must be especially sensitive to this challenging state of affairs and not simply assume that the patients are magnifying their difficulties through the lens of cognitive distortions.

The typical cognitive therapy question, "What is the *evidence* for your negative thoughts," may be less helpful for such patients than the question, "What *constructive action* can I take to deal with this situation?" Therapists must be attuned to the all-too-real life circumstances of patients with bipolar disorder who are suicidal, and acknowledge their pain and suffering. At the same time, therapists have to find a way to encourage these patients not to give up and to maintain a determination to stick to a sensible treatment plan that gives them the best chance of normalizing their lives. In the process, therapists strive to equip their patients with as many psychological skills as possible, as an armamentarium against the changes in mood state. One of the most important of these skills is the ability to recognize early warning signs of an impending symptom episode, thus enabling patients to take steps to minimize risk, consolidate their support system, and shore up treatment (Lam et al., 2000; Lam & Wong, 1997; Perry, Tarrier, Morriss, McCarthy, & Limb, 1999). Additional skill areas include problem solving, communication, rational responding, and the effective management of time and activities.

One of the most striking hazards of bipolar disorder is that the subjective pain wrought by the illness and its objective consequences can conquer the will to live of even the most talented, successful, popular people. Many people with bipolar disorder are creative and accomplished individuals (Coryell et al., 1989; Jamison, 1993, 1999; Woodruff, Robins, Winokur, & Reich, 1971). Nevertheless, the emotional pain, real-life consequences, and sense of personal impairment caused by bipolar disorder can overshadow the positive aspects of their lives. Whereas it is important for therapists to turn their patients' focus to their strengths, as well as to the blessings and gifts in their lives, this alone may not suffice to reduce patients' risk for suicide. Therapists will also have to teach their patients a range of self-help techniques with which to mute, ride out, and otherwise combat the dark thoughts and moods that are associated with hopelessness and suicidality when they are at their worst.

SUICIDE RISK ASSESSMENT

It is customary for therapists to ask their prospective patients at intake about symptoms of suicidality, both past and present. Patients who have tried suicide in the past or who have thought extensively about the matter are often considered to be at risk in the future. Thus, therapists typically pay close attention to this subject and monitor their patients for suicidality throughout the course of treatment. Such an approach is especially relevant for patients with bipolar disorder, where mood shifts can be quite dramatic and highly frequent as well, as is the case with rapid-cycling bipolar disorder. The patient who is in good spirits in today's therapy session may well contemplate suicide before the next session. Therapists and patients alike have to monitor patients' moods and related suicidal ideation on a regular basis. When it comes to matters of life and death, it is prudent to be so cautious.

Therapists should bear in mind that patients who do not have a documented or self-reported history of suicidality may still be at risk for suicide. There is a subgroup of individuals who kill themselves on the first try (Kleepsies & Dettmer, 2000), as well as those who die by their own hand without ever receiving proper treatment. If a person with bipolar disorder arrives at a therapist's office, the therapist can legitimately state that the patient has survived the first hurdle—getting into treatment alive! Therapists need not worry that their questions about suicidality will put off these patients. Instead, therapists can explain that they take bipolar illness very seriously and appreciate the emotional pain and suffering it can cause. Thus, they are going to err on the side of caution by asking their patients about their suicidal thoughts, feelings, and actions *too often* rather than too little.

Combining Assessment Methods with Psychoeducation

Performing suicidality assessments—whether brief and informal, or extensive and structured (see Appendix 3)—gives the therapist the chance to provide simultaneous psychoeducation and therapeutic intervention. For example, the therapist can note that the patient's level of suicidal ideation, as indicated by the Beck Scale for Suicide Ideation (BSSI; Beck, Steer, & Ranieri, 1988), has fluctuated a great deal over the course of the past 6 months. This fact alone is instructive, as it points out how the patient can go from thinking that life is not worth preserving, to believing that life should go on, and back again. The implication is that *thinking* about suicide is transient and malleable. Unfortunately, the commission of suicide is a permanent condition that never allows the patient to return to a more hopeful state. Thus, any variability in suicidal symptoms is an inherent argument against the "validity" of suicide, which, by definition, is invariable and irreparable.

Each suicide assessment can lead to a discussion of the worthwhile and meaningful things that patients have experienced since their last suicidal crisis. None of these experiences would have occurred if the patients had succeeded in killing themselves. The therapist can then engage the patients in addressing the question, "What important experiences are awaiting you on the future side of *this* suicidal crisis, which you'll only have if you make the courageous decision to live?" As noted, therapists must be sensitive to patients' sense that they simply "do not care," during times when their present distress obliterates all other considerations in their thinking. This is when treatment and social support are most important.

When patients indicate that they do indeed have thoughts about suicide, it is customary for the therapist to ask questions regarding their level of intentions, their plans, means, opportunity, and other pertinent variables. However, it is also important to ask them *why* they feel suicidal. It is more empathic to inquire in this manner, rather than focusing only on the *how* and *what* questions about suicide risk. The therapeutic alliance is potentially strengthened when patients have the chance to express the reasons for their despair, rather than simply discussing the practical details of their ideation. Furthermore, the contents of patients' dysfunctional beliefs about themselves, their treatment, their future, and their lives as a whole can be assessed more thoroughly when the therapist listens to patients' entire stories about their suicidality.

Helplessness and Hopelessness

When patients talk about their suicidal ideation, they often reveal aspects of their thinking that will become prime targets for intervention in cognitive therapy. Commonly, they express views that reflect a sense of helplessness and hopelessness. *Helplessness* (Seligman, 1981) is revealed when they make statements such as "Nothing I do matters," or "When I feel so depressed [or high], I have no control over what I do." The therapist should identify these statements as problems unto themselves, as they oversimplify a situation that calls for complex interventions—not the simple "solution" of suicide. Although, admittedly, it is very difficult to perform self-monitoring and coping skills at times of extreme affect, it is possible to make some impact, especially if the skills are practiced frequently. In addition, though extreme dysphoria or euphoria are difficult to counteract quickly through cognitive-behavioral means, they can be ameliorated, over time, with diligent application of self-help skills—which also buys valuable time for making changes in pharmacotherapy in response to the suicidal crisis.

Hopelessness is highly associated with suicidal risk (Beck, Brown, Berchick, Stewart, & Steer, 1990; Beck, Steer, Beck, & Newman, 1993; Young et al., 1996). When patients speak of their thoughts of suicide, it is typical to hear statements such as "Nothing will ever work out for me," "My life is just going to get worse and worse," or "I have no future." These (and similar comments) should serve as red flags that patients may be considering cutting their losses by checking out of life altogether. An additional way to monitor thoughts of hopelessness is to ask patients to complete a brief, self-report inventory at each session—the Beck Hopelessness Scale

(BHS; Beck, Weissman, Lester, & Trexler, 1974). Scores at 9 or above on this 0–20 scale indicate heightened risk, though false positives are the norm (Beck et al., 1993; Beck, Steer, Kovacs, & Garrison, 1985). Aside from their assessment value, the endorsed items of the BHS suggest topics of discussion in session (e.g., when patients check "True" for the item "I might as well give up because there is nothing I can do to help myself").

Maladaptive Schemas, Bipolar Disorder, and Suicidality

Patients often demonstrate maladaptive beliefs about themselves. For example, they believe that they are defective, incompetent to deal with the demands of life, and unlovable. These are among the maladaptive schemas that have been described in the cognitive therapy literature on populations with chronic disorders (e.g., Beck, Freeman, & Associates, 1990; Layden, Newman, Freeman, & Morse, 1993; Young, 1999). Interestingly, when patients who maintain these types of schemas enter a manic state, they may act in ways that seem to reflect polar opposite beliefs of what their schemas would predict. For example, upon becoming manic, the person who typically believes he is defective may be particularly vehement about his normalcy while he accuses others of being "the real problems" in his life. Likewise, the individual who generally maintains an incompetency schema may go to great lengths, in a manic state, to prove that she is capable of great things; thus, she may overextend herself on projects and endeavors for which she is ill equipped. Similarly, people who ordinarily believe they are unlovable may try to have multiple sexual flings while manic, as if to prove their desirability. In cognitive terms, this dramatic shift may reflect the extreme pendulum swing in an all-or-none thinking process that is part and parcel of bipolar disorder. In the language of psychodynamic theory, this behavior can be conceptualized as reaction formation, whereby grandiosity is a defense mechanism against a true sense of vulnerability and low self-worth (see Alloy, Reilly-Harrington, Fresco, Whitehouse, & Zechmeister, 1999; Winters & Neale, 1985). In any event, the extremes of thinking are problems in and of themselves, more so than their valences per se. As is typical in the field of mental health, wellness lies somewhere in the middle range.

"Suicidogenic" Beliefs

Anecdotally, patients who are prone to suicidal ideation, intentions, and attempts have been found to endorse one or more beliefs that are specific to suicidality. The list in Table 13.1 does not represent an empirically validated identification of such beliefs, but rather serves as a starting point for hypothesis testing. Patients may endorse one or more of the beliefs at varying levels of strength. Needless to say, the more such beliefs are relevant to a particular patient's thinking style, and the more rigidly such beliefs are held, the more risk is involved, and the greater the need to address these beliefs as high-priority agenda items.

The first belief, "Suicide is the only way I can deal with my overwhelming problems," reflects a sense of being overpowered by life's difficulties, including those incurred directly as a result of the patient's behavior while previously manic. If this is the only belief on the list the patient endorses, it is a very good sign (relatively speaking), because a solid course of problem-solving can improve the patient's hopefulness and reduce the risk of suicide.

The second belief, "I am a burden to my loved ones, and they would be better off if I were dead," reflects extreme guilt and self-reproach. Although it is often true that the patient's condition and behaviors bring concern and stress to the lives of loved ones (Chakrabati, Kulhara, & Verma, 1992), these realities pale in comparison to the horror faced by survivors of a loved one's suicide. Intervening on this belief often means helping patients commit themselves fully to their treatment, so that their families can feel more secure about their condition. Furthermore, patients can work on being more helpful and collaborative with those closest to them, rather than distancing themselves in a dysfunctional manner—including via suicide.

The third belief, "I hate myself, and I deserve to die," is an indicator of marked shame. Often, a review of patients' histories shows that they have done things that they feel are inexcusable and unredeemable. Even when such events are objectively difficult to reframe more benignly, patients can still strive toward living their lives with more respect for self and others in the future. For those patients who are religious, the notion of performing "penitence" through good works and helping others can become an important goal in the future—something that can be achieved only if they remain alive. It is important to note that our identity is only

TABLE 13.1. "Suicidogenic" Beliefs

Belief 1:	"Suicide is the only way I can deal with my overwhelming problems."
Belief 2:	"I am a burden to my loved ones, and they would be better off if I were dead."
Belief 3:	"I hate myself, and I deserve to die."
Belief 4:	"The only way to alleviate my pain and suffering is by dying."
Belief 5:	"The only way to test whether my loved ones care about me is to try to kill myself and see if they come to my aid."
Belief 6:	"The best way to get back at others is to punish them for mistreating me by killing myself."

complete upon our death. The longer we stay alive, the greater chance we have of shaping our self-image in a more favorable way. Said another way, our identity—and our sense of how much we like or dislike ourselves—is comprised not only of who we are and who we have been, but also of everything we still can be in the future. Therapists must find a way to pique patients' curiosity about how they may yet be able to change themselves and their lives for the better.

The fourth belief, "The only way to alleviate my pain and suffering is by dying," signifies that patients have given up hope that their pain will ever lessen; they simply wish to cut their losses in life as soon as possible. Here, therapists are on notice that they must offer ways to help their patients find healthy respite from their emotional distress. Methods borrowed from behavioral pain management can be useful adjuncts (see Turk, Meichenbaum, & Genest, 1983; Dowd, 2000) to the most favorable combination of somatic treatments (e.g., pharmacotherapy, electroconvulsive treatment). Patients can also generate and practice a range of healthy, self-soothing techniques (i.e., *not* involving self-mutilation) to use in times of emotional crisis (see Layden et al., 1993).

The fifth and sixth beliefs are related indicators that communication has broken down between the patients and their important others. These beliefs—"The only way to test whether my loved ones care about me is to try to kill myself and see if they come to my aid," and "The best way to get back at others is to punish them for mistreating me by killing myself"—exemplify the phenomenon of "acting out." Here, patients have lost sight of the advantages of telling their loved ones verbally that they feel hurt, angry, misunderstood, neglected, and otherwise mistreated. Instead, they resort to threats or acts of suicidality to make their point, which results in increased discord in their relationships, at best, and death, at worst. Interventions in response to these beliefs involve reattribution of the behaviors of others and improved communication skills.

INTERVENTIONS

To maximize the chances that suicidal patients will be safe for the long run, therapists need to go beyond the case management interventions that are customarily used at times of acute suicidal crisis. Clinical responses such as increasing the frequency of sessions and phone contacts, involving patients' friends and family for at-home supervision, and facilitating hospitalization are vital in keeping patients alive for the short term (Bongar, 1991), but are insufficient for changing patients' basic beliefs about the value of continuing their lives.

To achieve a more comprehensive goal of long-term commitment to living, therapists help their patients with bipolar disorder learn the full range of cognitive therapy self-help skills, including self-monitoring, rational responding, and problem solving (Greenberger & Padesky, 1995). Furthermore, patients can engage in exercises and homework assignments that specifically focus their attention on the meaning and importance of their lives, including their interpersonal connections, personal goals, and basic self-respect. For example, Ellis and Newman (1996) recommend that suicidal patients take stock of all the people in their lives who have known and cared about them and painstakingly document events and other details about each relationship. In the same vein, patients are asked to identify and write about all of the "unfinished business" in their lives, and to make plans to address as many of these unresolved issues as possible as a prerequisite to considering their lives to be finished. When patients earnestly renew their investment in their problems and goals, their connection to life itself is strengthened.

Therapists who attempt to use some of the standard anti-suicide techniques soon find that patients with bipolar disorder have compelling reasons for doubting the efficacy or relevance of these techniques. To maintain an optimal therapeutic alliance—which, in itself, is a safeguard in keeping patients from leaving therapy, not to mention life itself (Bongar, 1991)—therapists must be willing to consider patients' complaints and doubts about the proposed interventions. For example, patients may give half-hearted responses to the intervention of listing the pros and cons, respectively, of committing to life and committing suicide. Therapists who notice this reaction should inquire about patients' thoughts regarding the intervention, which then can be discussed as clinical issues. Therapists can make alterations in the interventions that patients may find more to their liking. Additionally, therapists may be able to encourage or inspire their patients to engage in the intervention simply as a behavioral experiment in itself (e.g., "Let's try it and see what we come up with. I'm curious—how about you?").

Interventions Involving the Perception of Time

One way of construing suicidal thinking is that it is analogous to a "temporal black hole." To explain this metaphor, let us start by examining a counterpart to suicidal thinking—healthy, open-minded thinking—that takes into account all time frames: past, present, and future. This healthy line of thinking allows a person who is feeling dysphoric to reflect on all of his or her previous experiences, including those that have made life meaningful, those that have taught valuable lessons, and those that remind him or her that he or she is not alone, and to realize that even miserable feelings can be transient. Likewise, the healthy, constructive thinker looks to the future with hope and takes into account all of the possibilities for surprise, contentment, novelty, attachment, success, and the like. This temporal breadth of perception serves as a safeguard against taking the current moment of despair too seriously and disproportionately.

In contrast, acute suicidal thinking is often characterized by a temporal implosion. The past and all of its valuable lessons in survival are lost from view. The future, with all its unknowable possibilities, is not pondered. It is as if all thinking collapses to a point of inescapable, temporal *singularity*, not unlike a black hole. All that seems to matter is getting rid of the pain of the moment by any means possible, including suicide.

To intervene at such times, the therapist has to work diligently to focus the patient's attention on time frames other than the immediate present, which (clinically speaking) is now only important in terms of taking measures to protect the patient. The therapist can take patients on imaginal trips into the past, wherein they examine vignettes from their lives that have the potential to remind them of their self-worth, the positive regard of others, and their capacity for pleasure and mastery. When patients have difficulty in generating such memories, the therapist should proceed undeterred, explaining that such difficulty in conjuring up autobiographical recall is part and parcel of severely depressed states and can be overcome through perseverance, imagery exercises, journaling, and the like (Evans, Williams, O'Loughlin, & Howells, 1992; Newman, Leahy, Beck, Reilly-Harrington, & Gyulai, 2001; Williams & Scott, 1988).

It is also important to hypothesize about the future. Sometimes patients reject this idea because they believe that they "have no future" (but this is only true if they kill themselves), or that it is useless (and even dangerous) to raise their hopes. This is when therapists sometimes feel as if they have to be salespersons or stockbrokers and the commodity they are selling is *patient futures*. Yes, there is risk involved in "wagering" on better days ahead (see Leahy, 1997), but it can be very enlightening to consider the possible gains in betting on an improved state of mind, heart, and life in the months and years following a suicidal crisis.

The technique of *future imaging* asks patients to think extensively about how their lives could appear in the months and years ahead, by taking into account their current strengths, assets, and social support, combined with their hopes and goals. One of the rationales for this approach is to pry patients away from their excessive focus on current pain and suffering, and to envision something positive to anticipate. This future imaging also naturally leads to a problem-solving discussion, in which patients are asked to generate ideas about the steps they would need to take to increase the probability of achieving these imagined goals. This method is intended to increase patients' sense of hope, as if to say to them, "Even if you cannot see the reasons for living today, there are reasons for living tomorrow; but you can only see for yourself if you *get there*, which means you have to live." Individuals who have experienced the extreme, all-encompassing symptom episodes of bipolar disorder often retort that it is foolish to plan a future, because their mental illness can interrupt and sabotage all such plans at any time. One patient described his dreams as a "house of cards" that was difficult to construct but easy to collapse. Another likened herself to the mythological character Sisyphus, whose efforts at rolling the boulder up the hill were a repeated act of futility, as the rock would roll back down every time, again and again, into perpetuity. Thus, patients may view the technique of future imaging as an invitation to tantalize themselves with hopes that can never come to pass, or cannot last. The sentiment can be summed up by the plea, "Don't make me get my hopes up—it's too risky and hurtful!"

Therapists can acknowledge that bipolar illness has indeed been known to dash people's positive plans for their lives. Thus, it is understandable that patients would be hesitant to hope, dream, and plan once again. However, there are things patients can do to reduce the risk, minimize the potential damage, and increase the probability of some success. Note that the above sentence is couched in terms that are antithetical to a depressive, hopeless, all-or-none view. The question is not *whether or not* it is worth trying to create a better future. The question is *how to increase the likelihood* that life can improve, in spite of the bipolar illness. Answering this question requires a willingness to postpone suicide indefinitely, while simultaneously investing in the most positive habits of behavior and thought as a way of life. No guarantees can be offered, but if patients can "procrastinate suicide" (Ellis & Newman, 1996) and instead engage in life-affirming activities, they will increase their chances of improvement in spite of the bipolar disorder.

Increasing Security and Empowerment through Recognition of Prodromes

Patients sometimes retort that they have tried to be positive and hopeful, but that the specter of mania frightens them away. They begin to doubt their own reality, as if to ask themselves, "Are my positive thoughts accurate or just the manifestation of an impending manic episode?" When one is waging a war against dysfunctional moods on not one but *two* fronts, such a question has stark relevance. In response, the therapist can invite patients to work on learning to recognize the prodromal signs of oncoming symptom episodes. Recent studies suggest that patients who learn this skill can reduce the severity and duration of their mood swings, increase the length of their interepisode periods of wellness, reduce the likelihood of the need for hospitalization, and generally improve their general adaptive functioning (Lam et al., 2000; Perry et al., 1999). That these improvements are significant is self-evident. Less obvious but just as important is the confidence and sense of security gained when patients learn to trust their optimism and goal-directed behaviors without fearing they are manifestations of hypomania or mania. Hope is generated in this scenario, and hope is one of the natural enemies of suicidality.

Reducing Suicidal Ideation as a "Habit"

It goes without saying that therapists are invested in helping their patients to stay alive and to eliminate all self-harming behaviors. However, it is also important to help patients manage and minimize their suicidal *ideation* as well, regardless of whether or not it ever translates into suicidal behavior. The reasons go beyond the obvious goal of reducing the risk of suicide completion. Patients who frequently dwell on thoughts about suicide are apt to experience significant interruptions in their lives, including hospitalizations. Such individuals also suffer strained interpersonal relationships that stem from the stress that friends, family, and other loved ones incur as they worry about the risk of the patient's suicide. Furthermore, a person who regularly experiences suicidal ideation suffers the repeated reinforcement of a self-image as a damaged person who is perpetually in no-man's land between thoughts of living and dying. These conditions are antithetical to striving for maximal functioning, improved social support, and a more fulfilling future.

Granted, it is generally unrealistic to instruct patients simply *not to think* about something, especially something as conspicuous and perhaps as habitual as thoughts about wanting to die. However, it is possible to work with patients to assist them in changing their "relationship" with their most problematic thoughts (Teasdale et al., 2002; Wells, 2000), such that they view their thoughts not as inducements to suicide, but rather as a barometer of their level of general distress. This is both a cognitive distancing technique as well as a mindfulness exercise, in which patients observe their own thoughts and feelings without judgment, and instead try to understand their experience in a safe, accepting way. As one patient noted, her suicidal thoughts had become a "habit"; they entered her mind whenever she encountered adversity—a "conditioned cognitive response," if you will. This patient learned to take such self-destructive thoughts with a grain of salt, did not worry that she would actually harm herself, and mobilized her coping skills and social support network. She was also now less likely to escalate her suicidal thinking through worrying that the thoughts would necessarily lead her to harm herself. Instead, she kept the thoughts isolated, viewing them as a stray mental event signifying that she felt stressed.

Life-Affirming Views about Taking Medications

When patients with bipolar disorder constructively take part in their pharmacotherapy, they have a better chance of achieving therapeutic gains than they would if they were less inclined to participate optimally. By extension, the risk of suicide can be lessened if the therapist can help patients with bipolar disorder "make peace" with the need for ongoing medications (Newman et al., 2001). For example, there is a body of literature that suggests that lithium has powerful protective value against the threat of suicide (Isometsä & Lonnqvist, 1998; Nilsson, 1999; Tondo, Jamison, & Baldessarini, 1997). Thus, patients' adherence with medication literally can make the difference between life and death. Cognitive therapists can play an important role in addressing these patients' excessively negative beliefs about their medications—the sort of beliefs that might otherwise convince them to discontinue their regimens.

For example, one patient explained his suicidal thoughts as resulting from the idea that "No matter what happens, I will no longer have my life as I want it, so I might as well control the situation and die by my choice." When questioned further about this dark, foreboding belief, he stated that if he did not take his medications, his illness would worsen and would rob him of ever having a functional life; however, if he took his medication, it would change his personality and thus would steal away his identity. By looking at the medication as having the capacity to take away his "true self," the patient set himself up to feel trapped, hopeless, and suicidal. The therapist helped the patient examine this harmful belief from a number of different angles. For example, a plausible, alternative viewpoint was that by taking lithium, the patient would actually *restore* his personality to what it would have been had he never had to bear the brunt of the effects of the bipolar disorder. In this reframe, the lithium would help the patient reacquaint himself with the best aspects of his own functioning, albeit with some physical side effects that were a tolerable price to pay for recouping his sense of self. Such a viewpoint removed the feeling of entrapment, in that now the medication could be viewed as the path to life, rather than simply another route toward demise.

Overcoming Shame, Isolation, and Stigma

An important factor in the course of bipolar depression is social support. By and large, the data on bipolar illness indicate that those individuals with more and better ties to others have a better chance of managing their dysphoric states than those without such interpersonal attachments (Johnson, Meyer, Winett, & Small, 2000; Johnson, Winett, Meyer, Greenhouse, & Miller, 1999). Taking this thread of logic further, it is reasonable to hypothesize that social support is a safeguarding factor against suicide. However, many patients who suffer from bipolar disorder often find themselves isolated when they are deeply depressed, partly as a function of damaged relationships from mania, partly as a result of their poor responsiveness to those who reach out to help, and sometimes as a reaction to their own sense of stigma that keeps them hiding from the world.

At times, patients also avoid going to their therapy sessions, because they believe that nobody can help them, and they believe that all they will experience is the pity or scorn of others, including their therapist. When a patient does not show up for sessions, the therapist is advised to try to contact the patient promptly and invite him or her to return for an appointment as soon as possible. At the very least, this phone call will demonstrate that the therapist cares, and that the patient's whereabouts and well-being matter. It may not be possible to reengage with a deeply dysphoric patient who is staying away from therapy now, but it is important to make a conspicuous effort to encourage the patient to return for help, because he or she may decide to return at a later point.

Patients who are present in session but express doubts about why the therapist would want to help are signaling a high-priority item for therapy. Not only is it vital to give to the patient tangible evidence of the therapist's involvement and interest, it is also critical to explore how the patient similarly isolates him- or herself from others in everyday life. Sometimes patients claim that they have no interest in socializing with others, but further probing often reveals that the picture is not so simple and straightforward. Rather, these patients maintain certain negative schemas about themselves (see Young, 1999)—for example, that they are defective and unlovable—and thus they avoid putting themselves in a position where they believe they will experience social ostracism or shunning. By remaining isolated, these patients lose the opportunity to test their self-derogating hypotheses and hence remain stuck in a state of lonely despair. This grim state heightens the risk of suicide; therefore, the issue must be addressed.

To facilitate patients' acquisition of social support—and thus providing them with a buffer against the risk of suicide—there are at least three areas of intervention: (1) using the therapeutic relationship, (2) facilitating patients' bonds with available friends and family, and (3) encouraging patients to take part in support groups (such as those sponsored by the National Alliance for the Mentally Ill and the National Depressive and Manic–Depressive Association).

The Therapeutic Relationship

When patients report that they have little meaningful contact with people, their sessions with their therapists take on added significance. The therapist's office may be the only place they feel listened to, comforted, or encouraged. Ideally, this positive perception will translate into the patient's being open and honest about harboring any suicidal thoughts or intentions, so that the therapist can provide help in a prompt fashion when a clinical crisis occurs. Although a positive therapeutic alliance does not guarantee that patients will collaborate fully in treatment or will disavow suicide as an option once and for all, it is a factor that promotes safety. However, the therapist cannot be the patient's only source of support; a therapist is not a substitute for a network of family and friends, and he or she cannot serve as patients' guardian angels and "be there" for them all the time (Ellis & Newman, 1996). Therapists have to help their isolated patients make appropriate connections with others—and, in the process, to make more connections with life itself.

The Patients' Friends and Family

In an ideal world, patients' family members all would be healthy, present, supportive, and effective in dealing with their psychiatrically ill next of kin. Patients would never threaten suicide in response to family conflict and discord, and family members would never feel manipulated by such threats. In the real world, the picture is often fraught with difficulties. The relationships between persons with bipolar disorder and their families can become quite contentious, as the former try to assert their autonomy and avert criticism, while the latter worry about disaster and try desperately to control the situation through any means (Miklowitz & Goldstein, 1997; Miklowitz, Wendel, & Simoneau, 1998). The risk of suicide aggravates the situation, because patients feel rejected and abandoned by their families and may wish to express their anger by hurting themselves to punish their loved ones. Meanwhile, the family members struggle with guilt and fear, on the one hand, and anger and resentment, on the other.

Family sessions (which are not always so easily arranged) can go a long way toward reducing the suicide risk for the "identified patient." Not only do such sessions allow for problem solving regarding family conflicts, but they open up a vital line of communication between the therapist and the patient's closest others. At those times when the patient may be actively suicidal, the therapist and the patient's family may be in an improved position to communicate and coordinate the proper emergency response when it is most needed.

For patients and their families to help each other through the ongoing hardship of bipolar illness, they need to have compassion for each other's position. Patients need to understand how their families may be frightened by their suicidal or overexuberant behavior, and how they may show this concern by being critical or restrictive. The family would do well do appreciate the patient's sense of shame about being monitored and mistrusted, and to learn to demonstrate empathy for the patient's sense of despair, while at the same time encouraging him or her to make the best use of treatment (see Chapter 9, this volume).

Support Groups

Support groups are especially important when patients feel alone, misunderstood, and perhaps even forgotten. There are times when patients may not feel they can talk to their family or friends for support. At such times, their best source of support and understanding may be a support group. Unfortunately, patients may sometimes shun this potential lifeline, perhaps out of a sense of shame and stigma. Although it is inadvisable for therapists to try to force their patients to attend a support group, the matter should not be dropped so easily. Instead, it is important to assess the patient's negative beliefs about attending. Typical negative assumptions include: (1) the group experience would further demoralize the patient, (2) the patient would silently judge or be judged by the other group members, and (3) the meetings themselves would have no redeeming value. These pessimistic viewpoints are reflective of more overarching feelings of hopelessness and stigmatization—issues that need to be addressed in their own right, whether or not patients actually attend support group meetings (see Chapter 14, this volume).

Perhaps therapists can gently persuade their patients with bipolar disorder to go to one or two meetings as a behavioral experiment to see for themselves what may be learned and gained—or not. For example, one patient noted that he was surprised at the diversity in the group. As he put it, some people clearly were "low functioning," but others looked like "Joe Anybody" off the street. The patient was surprised at how easily he could converse with at least some of the other members, and this social ease made it worthwhile to go. In the meantime, the patient's social support system doubled—literally, in one evening—and this steady source of support weighed against his occasional bouts of suicidal ideation.

Anti-Suicide Contracts

Regardless of patients' official diagnosis, therapists often make use of "anti-suicide contracts" with patients who are at risk. Though empirical data on the preventative efficacy of such contracts are lacking (Kleepsies & Dettmer, 2000; Silverman, Berman, Bongar, Litman, & Maris, 1998), there is clinical consensus that it is wise to construct this type of agreement with patients who are plagued with suicidal ideation and intentions. From a clinical perspective, anti-suicide contracts allow patients and their therapists to address the relevant issues with thoroughness, sensitivity, and an air of enhanced collaboration as a team (Stanford, Goetz, & Bloom, 1994). When the stakes are as high as life or death, the parties need to know where each stands, so that appropriate action can be taken. From a legal standpoint, the courts often view anti-suicide contracts as a part of the "standard of care," a term that is familiar to therapists who are trying to minimize liability risks (Bongar, 1991).

To maximize the likelihood that patients will follow both the letter and the spirit of formal agreements to refrain from hurting themselves, it is vital that the therapist introduce and construct the contract collaboratively with patients. This collaboration, which is consistent with the way in which cognitive therapy is conducted across all populations, is intended to strengthen the therapeutic alliance and enhance adherence to treatment recommendations (Beck, Rush, Shaw, & Emery, 1979; Stanford et al., 1994). Ellis and Newman (1996) identify some of the qualities that create effective anti-suicide contracts, such as making the tone more affirmative than prohibitive, spelling out the responsibilities of both the therapist and the patient in crisis situations, and listing specific steps that the patient can take to cope and obtain social support while awaiting the next available professional intervention. A sample contract (adapted from Ellis & Newman, 1996) is illustrated in Figure 13.1.

An anti-suicide contract is just part of an overall approach to the management of patients who are at risk. The therapist should realize that the contracts, in and of themselves, are not sufficient as safeguards and that vigilance and a broad array of methods are needed to help keep patients safe. When the therapist learns that a patient has broken the contract (e.g., he or she is now in the hospital following a suicide attempt), it is not advis-

---

- I proclaim that my life is important, that it is worth preserving, and that I will maintain hope and work diligently in therapy to improve it.

- It is understandable that, at times, I may have thoughts or urges to harm myself; however, I will only document such occurrences in my therapy journal and discuss them with my therapist(s); I will bravely postpone acting on them in the meantime.

- If I should feel overwhelmed by my suicidal thoughts, feelings, or urges, I will make every effort to cope by reviewing my journal of meaningful memories and interpersonal connections, and by using self-soothing techniques such as playing my guitar, painting, washing my hair, and eating comfort food such as chicken soup.

- If I have given the above a fair try but I still feel suicidal, I will contact my support system, including "Aunt Sylvie" at 555-9323, my friend "Jill" at 555-2876, and my therapist(s) (or the therapist on call). Even if my personal support persons are not immediately available, I know that my therapist will make every effort to see me for an emergency session as soon as possible, and I will remain safe in the meantime.

- If I notice that I am experiencing helpless and hopeless thoughts, I will make the effort to write down these thoughts, and to respond with alternative viewpoints, so that I can remind myself that I do not have to buy into my seductive, dark, suicidal beliefs. My therapist will help me expound on this point at our next session.

- I will work with my therapist(s) as a team to help myself with my problems, and I will do everything in my power to stay on the team; I will not abandon my teammate(s) by killing myself. My therapist will not criticize me for feeling suicidal, but rather will be understanding and will try to help me utilize my coping skills.

- I will be faithful to the spirit of this contract, which is to be compassionate and helpful to myself, without fail, and to trust that my therapist is on my side.

FiGURE 13.1. Sample anti-suicide contract. Based on Ellis and Newman (1996).

able to terminate treatment on the basis of this breach. The long-term safety of the patient is not furthered by such a draconian interpretation of the agreement. Rather, the therapist should make every reasonable effort to reengage the patient in treatment and to process thoroughly what went wrong and how the goals for safety can be strengthened in light of the recent breakdown of the process.

It can be hypothesized that patients with the greatest propensity for mood lability may experience the most difficulty adhering to a contract that stipulates no self-harm. This correlation has been observed (anecdotally) with patients who meet diagnostic criteria for borderline personality disorder (Layden et al., 1993), as well as those who suffer from bipolar disorder. This fact should not deter us from using contracts—rather, it is a reminder of their limitations. Jamison (1999) illustrates the fallibility of anti-suicide contracts quite dramatically when she recalls the personal agreement she struck with a friend. Their contract required that if either of them felt suicidal, he or she would give the other person the chance to pay a lengthy personal visit to talk the distressed person out of committing suicide. Unfortunately, Jamison later discovered that the friend had indeed killed himself without ever giving her the agreed-upon opportunity to come to help him in person. Such a situation may not be generalizable to clinical situations, where a patient regularly consults with his or her therapist, but Jamison's vignette highlights the lethal character of bipolar disorder. Clinicians must always maintain a begrudging respect for the negative power of the illness to overcome reason, hope, and interpersonal ties. On the other hand, therapists have to be their patients' best role models for persevering and maintaining optimism against the odds.

REFERENCES

Alloy, L. B., Reilly-Harrington, N. A., Fresco, D. M., Whitehouse, W. G., & Zechmeister, J. S. (1999). Cognitive styles and life events in subsyndromal unipolar and bipolar disorders: Stability and prospective prediction of depressive and hypomanic mood swings. *Journal of Cognitive Psychotherapy: An International Quarterly, 13,* 21–40.

Beck, A. T., Brown, G., Berchick, R. J., Stewart, B. L., & Steer, R. A. (1990). Relationship between hopelessness and ultimate suicide: A replication with psychiatric outpatients. *American Journal of Psychiatry, 147,* 190–195.

Beck, A. T., Freeman, A., & Associates (1990). *Cognitive therapy of personality disorders.* New York: Guilford Press.

Beck, A. T., Rush, A. J., Shaw, B. F., & Emery, G. (1979). *Cognitive therapy of depression.* New York: Guilford Press.

Beck, A. T., Steer, R. A., Beck, J. S., & Newman, C. F. (1993). Hopelessness, depression, suicidal ideation, and clinical diagnosis of depression. *Suicide and Life-Threatening Behavior, 23,* 139–145.

Beck, A. T., Steer, R. A., Kovacs, M., & Garrison, B. (1985). Hopelessness and eventual suicide: A 10-year prospective study of patients hospitalized with suicidal ideation. *American Journal of Psychiatry, 142,* 559–563.

Beck, A. T., Steer, R. A., & Ranieri, W. F. (1988). Scale for suicidal ideation: Psychometric properties of a self-report version. *Journal of Clinical Psychology, 44,* 499–505.

Beck, A. T., Weissman, A., Lester, D., & Trexler, L. (1974). The measurement of pessimism: The Hopelessness Scale. *Journal of Consulting and Clinical Psychology, 42,* 861–865.

Bongar, B. (1991). *The suicidal patient: Clinical and legal standards of care.* Washington, DC: American Psychological Association.

Bowden, C. L. (1999). Comparison of open versus blinded studies in bipolar disorder. In J. F. Goldberg & M. Harrow (Eds.), *Bipolar disorders: Clinical course and outcome* (pp.149–170). Washington, DC: American Psychiatric Press.

Chakrabati, S., Kulharfa, P., & Verma, S. K. (1992). Extent and determinants of burden among families of patients with affective disorders. *Acta Psychiatrica Scandinavica, 86,* 247–252.

Coryell, W., Endicott, J., Keller, M., Andreason, N., Groove, W., Hirschfeld, R. M. A., & Scheftner, W. (1989). Bipolar affective disorder and high achievement: A familiar association. *American Journal of Psychiatry, 146,* 983–988.

Dilsaver, S. C., Chen, Y.-W., Swann, A. C., Shoaib, A. M., & Krajewski, K. J. (1994). Suicidality in patients with pure and depressive mania. *American Journal of Psychiatry, 151,* 1312–1315.

Dowd, E. T. (2000). *Cognitive hypnotherapy.* Livingston, NJ: Aronson.

Ellis, T. E., & Newman, C. F. (1996). *Choosing to live: How to defeat suicide through cognitive therapy.* Oakland, CA: New Harbinger.

Evans, J., Williams, J., O'Laughlin, S., & Howells, K. (1992). Autobiographical memory and problem-solving strategies for parasuicide patients. *Psychological Medicine, 22,* 399–405.

Goldberg, J. F., Garno, J. L., Leon., A. C., Kocsis, J. H., & Portera, L. (1998). Association of recurrent suicidal ideation with nonremission from acute mixed mania. *American Journal of Psychiatry, 155,* 1753–1755.

Goodwin, F. K., & Jamison, K. R. (1990). *Manic–depressive illness.* New York: Oxford University Press.

Greenberger, D., & Padesky, C. A. (1995). *Mind over mood: A cognitive therapy treatment manual for clients.* New York: Guilford Press.

Harris, E. C., & Barraclough, B. (1997). Suicide as an outcome for mental disorders: A meta-analysis. *British Journal of Psychiatry, 170,* 205–228.

Isometsä, E., Heikkinen, M., Henriksson, M., Aro, H., & Lonnqvist, J. (1995). Recent life events and completed suicide in bipolar affective disorder: A comparison with major depressive suicides. *Journal of Affective Disorders, 33*(2), 99–106.

Isometsä, E., & Lonnqvist, J. (1998). Suicide attempts preceding completed suicide. *British Journal of Psychiatry, 173,* 531–535.

Jamison, K. R. (1993). *Touched with fire: Manic–depressive illness and the artistic temperament.* New York: Free Press.

Jamison, K. R. (1995). *An unquiet mind: A memoir of moods and madness.* New York: Knopf.

Jamison, K. R. (1999). *Night falls fast: Understanding suicide.* New York: Knopf.

Johnson, S. L., Meyer, B., Winett, C., & Small, J. (2000). Social support and self-esteem predict changes in bipolar depression but not mania. *Journal of Affective Disorders, 58,* 79–86.

Johnson, S. L., Winett, C., Meyer, B., Greenhouse, W., & Miller, I. (1999). Social support and the course of bipolar disorder. *Journal of Abnormal Psychology, 108,* 558–566.

Kleepsies, P. M., & Dettmer, E. L. (2000). An evidence-based approach to evaluating and managing suicidal emergencies. *Journal of Clinical Psychology, 56,* 1109–1130.

Lam, D. H., Bright, J., Jones, S., Hayward, P., Schuck, N., Chisholm, D., & Sham, P. (2000). Cognitive therapy for bipolar disorder: A pilot study of relapse prevention. *Cognitive Therapy and Research, 24,* 503–520.

Lam, D. H., Jones, S. H., Hayward, P., & Bright, J. A. (1999). *Cognitive therapy for bipolar disorder: A therapist's guide to concepts, methods, and practice.* Chichester, UK: Wiley.

Lam, D. H., & Wong, G. (1997). Prodromes, coping strategies, insight, and social functioning in bipolar affective disorders. *Psychological Medicine, 27,* 1091–1100.

Layden, M. A., Newman, C. F., Freeman, A., & Morse, S. B. (1993). *Cognitive therapy of borderline personality disorder.* Needham Heights, MA: Allyn & Bacon.

Leahy, R. L. (1997). An investment model of depressive resistance. *Journal of Cognitive Psychotherapy: An International Quarterly, 11,* 3–19.

Miklowitz, D. J., & Goldstein, M. J. (1997). *Bipolar disorder: A family-focused treatment approach.* New York: Guilford Press.

Miklowitz, D. J., Wendel, J. S., & Simoneau, T. L. (1998). Targeting dysfunctional family interactions and high expressed emotion in the psychosocial treatment of bipolar disorder. *In-Session: Psychotherapy in Practice, 4*(3), 25–38.

Newman, C. F., Leahy, R. L., Beck, A. T., Reilly-Harrington, & Gyulai, L. (2001). *Bipolar disorder: A cognitive therapy approach.* Washington, DC: American Psychological Association.

Nilsson, A. (1999). Lithium therapy and suicide risk. *Journal of Clinical Psychiatry, 60*(Suppl. 2), 85–88.

Perry, A., Tarrier, N., Morriss, R., McCarthy, E., & Limb, K. (1999). Randomised controlled trial of efficacy of teaching patients with bipolar disorder to identify early symptoms of relapse and obtain treatment. *British Medical Journal, 318,* 139–153.

Seligman, M. E. P. (1981). A learned helplessness point of view. In L. P. Rehm (Ed.), *Behavior therapy for depression* (pp. 123–141). New York: Academic Press.

Silverman, M., Berman, A., Bongar, B., Litman, R., & Maris, R. (1998). Inpatient standards of care and the suicidal patient: Part II. An investigation with clinical risk management. In B. Bongar, A. Berman, R. Maris, M. Silverman, E. Harris, & W. Packman, (Eds.), *Risk management with suicidal patients* (pp. 34–64). New York: Guilford Press.

Simpson, S. G., & Jamison, K. R. (1999). The risk of suicide in patients with bipolar disorder. *Journal of Clinical Psychology, 60*(Suppl. 2), 53–56.

Sonne, S. C., Brady, K. T., & Morton, W. A. (1994). Substance abuse and bipolar affective disorder. *Journal of Mental and Nervous Disease, 182,* 349–352.

Stanford, E., Goetz, R., & Bloom, J. (1994). The no harm contract in the emergency assessment of suicidal risk. *Journal of Clinical Psychiatry, 55,* 344–348.

Teasdale, J. D., Moore, R. G., Hayhurst, H., Pope, M., Williams, S., & Segal, Z. V. (2002). Metacognitive awareness and prevention of relapse in depression: Empirical evidence. *Journal of Consulting and Clinical Psychology, 70*(2), 275–286.

Tondo, L., Jamison, K. R., & Baldessarini, R. J. (1997). Effect of lithium maintenance on suicidal behavior in major mood disorders. *Annals of the Academy of Sciences, 836,* 339–351.

Turk, D. C., Meichenbaum, D., & Genest, M. (1983). *Pain and behavioral medicine: A cognitive-behavioral perspective.* New York: Guilford Press.

Wells, A. (2000). *Emotional disorders and metacognition: Innovative cognitive therapy.* New York: Wiley.

Williams, J. M. G., & Scott, J. (1988). Autobiographical memory in depression. *Psychological Medicine, 18,* 689–695.

Winters, K. C., & Neale, J. M. (1985). Mania and low self-esteem. *Journal of Abnormal Psychology, 94*, 282–290.

Woodruff, R. A., Robins, L. N., Winokur, G., & Reich, T. (1971). Manic–depressive illness and social achievement. *Acta Psychiatrica Scandinavica, 47*, 237–249.

Young, J. (1999). *Cognitive therapy for personality disorders: A schema-focused approach* (3rd ed.). Sarasota, FL: Professional Resource Exchange.

Young, M. A., Fogg, L. F., Scheftner, W., Fawcett, J., Akiskal, H., & Maser, J. (1996). Stable trait components of hopelessness: Baseline and sensitivity to depression. *Journal of Abnormal Psychology, 105*, 155–165.

CHAPTER FOURTEEN

CONSUMER ADVOCACY AND SELF-HELP

Interface with Professionals

HARRIET P. LEFLEY
SUZANNE VOGEL-SCIBILIA

Advocacy organizations in the mental health field typically combine self-help activities with political agendas to promote the funding of research, services, and legal protections for persons with mental illness. More specifically, through lobbying and legislative action, they are beginning to speed the pace of basic etiological research, alter the shape of mental health law, eliminate disparities in insurance coverage for psychiatric conditions, reduce stigma by improving media portrayals of people with mental illness, and expand the parameters of treatment systems. Advocacy organizations have had an impact on clinical training and have been instrumental in helping research studies, from providing participants to refining informed consent forms. Coexisting with the professional mental health system, advocacy movements also offer social support, meaningful roles, and an accepting, destigmatizing milieu for persons who may need more than pharmaceutical or psychotherapeutic interventions to cope with their disabilities.

The 1999 Report of the Surgeon General (U.S. Department of Health and Human Services, 1999) strongly recommended consumer participation in mental health services. For many years now, the Center for Mental Health Services (CMHS) of the Substance Abuse and Mental Health Services Administration (SAMHSA) has been funding demonstration projects that required public mental health agencies to hire and train former patients to deliver services. They also have funded self-help agencies that are managed and staffed by former patients. According to Segal, Hodges, and Hardiman (2002), these free-standing self-help agencies often serve as adjunct or referral sources for community mental health centers, and sometimes represent alternative service sites. A study by these authors compared the service selections of 673 new users of self-help and professionally staffed agencies in the same geographic area. They found that prospective mental health agency clients sought medications and counseling, whereas prospective peer agency clients sought self-help services, drop-in features, socialization, and above all, a guarantee against coerced treatment. Basically, the mental health agency was viewed as offering needed clinical services, whereas the self-help agency provided an ongoing social support system. The researchers noted that their results reflect a newly emerging cooperative division of labor between community mental health agencies and colocated self-help agencies.

Not all localities have self-help agencies, but many have support groups affiliated with consumer organizations. Consumer groups augment the mental health system with mental health education, social activities, encouragement for medication compliance, and increased social integration and support. They also serve as sources of reciprocal referrals to mental health professionals. Members with major depression, bipolar disorder, or schizophrenia, for example, are experts in knowing an area's specialists in these disorders. In turn, many practitioners are happy to learn of available resources for socialization and peer support for their patients.

Many individuals with bipolar disorder lose opportunities to participate fully in the workforce. An increasing number of consumer enterprises, particularly those funded by the CMHS, offer job training and a forum for developing work skills. Even if they do not focus on vocational recovery, self-help groups tend to offer their members a chance for productive organizational roles, and many offer training in political advocacy.

The psychological benefits of self-help groups can be extremely empowering. Their immediate benefit is empathic understanding of their members' narratives. But perhaps more important is their role-modeling function. The groups offer peers who have suffered similar symptoms and experiences in the mental health system and can relate to the loss of self-esteem that so often accompanies the status of being mentally ill. The redemptive power of role models is evident in the following letter. A woman involved with a self-help group wrote to thank a peer for her help in recovering from an episode of severe depression and despair:

We've all known so much pain and so many years of struggling, that I feel we share a bond the likes of which the so-called "normal" world will never know. I consider it a privilege to be associated with people who have survived, and survived, and survived again, but still have the courage, the compassion, and the humanity to keep on striving and caring about themselves and reaching out to touch others in trouble. Although the rest of the world perceives us as different and pretty much useless, I think we're about as special as you can get. (Deegan, 1994, p. 18)

This letter captures the basic therapeutic aspects of self-help—that is, the feeling of no longer being alone and bonding with others who have shared the same experience. But the writer also has learned to reassess her own potential strengths from people who have overcome the same kind of agony and then have reached out to help others. Given these examples of courage, this woman rejects the world's stigmatization of the mentally ill and reevaluates, with pride, her own identity. There is a new appreciation of herself as someone who is able to transcend the pain and emerge a survivor.

The world of consumer advocacy is much larger than that of local support groups and self-help services. In this chapter we describe the major advocacy organizations and their functions, including disparate philosophies among some of the groups. A brief historical overview is followed by a discussion of major contributions of the various groups, and how their organizational missions affect their relations with professionals. Concrete examples are given of advocates' contributions to training guidelines and practice, as well as political alliances that have generated desired legislation.

BRIEF OVERVIEW OF ADVOCACY MOVEMENTS

Mental health advocacy organizations are by no means homogeneous in their missions and interests. They can be roughly divided into at least three generic categories: omnibus advocacy organizations composed of citizens, family members, and consumers; protection and advocacy programs; and exclusively consumer groups. Major omnibus organizations are the National Alliance for the Mentally Ill (NAMI) and the National Mental Health Association (NMHA). NAMI is composed primarily of family members and consumers with serious psychiatric disorders. The NMHA is composed primarily of citizen advocates, along with some family members and consumers. Although it has always advocated for people with psychiatric disabilities, the NMHA has viewed its essential mission as prevention and has focused on a wide range of issues pertaining to mental health rather than mental illness. NAMI has focused on people with severe mental illness, with primary diagnoses of schizophrenia, depression, unipolar depression, bipolar disorder, other psychotic conditions, and more recently, anxiety and obsessive–compulsive disorders.

Other citizen advocacy organizations focus on protection of the rights of all persons with mental illness. The Judge David L. Bazelon Center for Mental Health Law, formerly the Mental Health Law Project, has a basic mission of protecting patients' civil liberties. Additionally, the center provides legal resources to (1) combat exclusionary zoning and rental policies; (2) promote patients' access to health care, social services, and income support; (3) reform state systems of care; and (4) help generate a continuum of community services for persons with psychiatric and developmental disabilities. Working in the courts and in legislative and policy arenas, the Bazelon Center offers legal assistance to consumers, other advocacy groups, and policy-makers.

Additional support for patients' rights is guaranteed by the federal Protection and Advocacy for Individuals with Mental Illness Act (Public Law 102-173). Each state is federally mandated and funded to have a Protection and Advocacy (P & A) Center. The function of these centers is to protect developmentally and psychiatrically disabled persons from neglect and abuse, and to protect their rights in institutional and community settings. Much of the work of the state P & A centers involves grievance casework for individuals, although they also initiate lawsuits to upgrade institutional conditions. All 50 states, the District of Columbia, and five territories have federally funded programs under this legislation.

CONSUMER ORGANIZATIONS

Persons with major mood disorders have been active throughout the various consumer movements, both as leaders and advocates. The consumer movement itself is divided philosophically and functionally. There are groups that advocate for more research and services and have a strong collaborative alliance with professionals, such as the Depression and Bipolar Support Alliance (DBSA). The DBSA, the major organization for persons with bipolar disorder, is described below. Other groups focus on self-determination and seek a separate consumer-run system of care. The terminology used by present or former service recipients also reflects these different orientations. Terms such as *survivor* or *person psychiatrically labeled* are usually preferred by individuals who feel they have been mistreated in the mental health system. The abbreviation c/s/x (consumer/survivor/expatient) is sometimes used to incorporate all identities. It is of great interest that a fall 2002 survey of members of the DBSA indicated that almost 60% pre-

ferred the term *patient* to any other term. This finding highlights the philo-
sophical distance of the members of this organization from those who tend
to reject diagnostic labels and professional care ("Survey reveals," 2002).

Today, the most commonly accepted term in the field is *consumer.* The
term covers all persons with a diagnosed mental illness but typically is
applied to those with a history of hospitalization, crisis intervention, or ongoing outpatient care who accept the need for psychiatric treatment. Most
states have a Consumer Affairs office that promotes consumer self-help organizations. Many of these states have networks of consumer-run drop-in
centers funded through their block grants from the federal government.
The centers' primary functions are to provide mutual help, social support,
education, and socialization. Most drop-in centers are supplemental to the
professional mental health system. Many, but not all, require that the members be currently in treatment.

Some rehabilitation centers have drop-in features and employees who
may be consumers or nonconsumers. The clubhouse model pioneered by
Fountain House in New York is one example of a recovery-oriented program that has professional and consumer staff but uses peer-counseling and
consumer decision making as its basic rehabilitative model.

Consumer organizations have been heavily promoted by the Community Support Program (CSP) of the CMHS and by the National Association
of State Mental Health Program Directors (NASMHPD). CMHS has supported an annual or biannual Alternatives conference that brings together
all local and state consumer groups for mutual education and capacity
building. These conferences also have emphasized political advocacy for a
greater consumer role in mental health services, policy planning, and governance. CMHS funds three major consumer-led technical assistance centers:
the National Mental Health Consumer Self-Help Clearinghouse in Pennsylvania, the National Empowerment Center in Massachusetts, and the Consumer Organization and Networking Technical Assistance Center in West
Virginia and Arizona. These centers work to build the capacity of local and
state consumer organizations nationwide, to teach organizational and business skills, and to help develop consumer-run enterprises ranging from resi-
dential development to job training and actual business services. They also
educate professional mental health staff on consumers' experience of mental illness. As an example, in an innovative Disability Awareness Workshop, mental health professionals are asked to wear headphones blaring
negative voices as they take a mental status examination, undergo psychological testing, or fill out a social security or job application. They are then
asked to assess the effects of stimulus bombardment and vocal interference
on task completion. CMHS also has provided scholarships for persons with
mood disorders to attend annual meetings of DBSA, and worked with the
organization to develop a training film for psychiatric residents called *Partners in Recovery.*

Specific Consumer Organizations for Mood Disorders

Depression and Bipolar Support Alliance (DBSA, formerly NDMDA)
http:// www.DBSAlliance.org

The National Depressive and Manic–Depressive Association (NDMDA) changed its name to DBSA in August 2002, reflecting an increasing emphasis of the membership on a more scientific description of their disorders. The DBSA has been termed "the nation's largest patient-directed illness-specific organization" (Charney, 2002, p. 262). The DBSA is exclusively devoted to consumers with major mood disorders. The following information is reported on the DBSA website:

The bylaws of national DBSA require that at least 51% of its board or directors be diagnosed with depression or bipolar depression. Incorporated in 1986 and based in Chicago, the organization's mission is "to educate patients, families, professionals and the public concerning the nature of depressive and manic–depressive illnesses as *treatable* medical diseases; to foster self-help for patients and families; to eliminate discrimination and stigma; to improve access to care; and to advocate for research toward the elimination of these illnesses."

The DBSA began as small local support groups and emerged as a national organization with the help of concerned professionals. National DBSA's prestigious 66-member Scientific Advisory Board (SAB) is comprised of leading researchers and clinicians in the field of mood disorders. The SAB was chaired in 2002 by Dennis Charney, MD, of the National Institute of Mental Health. SAB members review all national DBSA publications and programs for medical and scientific accuracy. In addition, SAB members present at national DBSA conferences, author peer-reviewed manuscripts on behalf of the organization, and represent national DBSA to the media.

The national DBSA website receives more than 35,000 unique visitors monthly. More than 5,000 calls per month are personally answered on the DBSA toll-free information and referral line. Each year the organization distributes more than 50,000 information packets free of charge to anyone requesting information about mood disorders.

National DBSA has a network of more than 1,000 patient-run support groups that hold regular meetings across the United States and Canada. More than 50,000 people attend meetings every year. Support groups play an important role in recovery; according to the DBSA website, more than 85% of support group members reported that their group helped them achieve treatment adherence. National DBSA has made it a recent priority to organize state chapters throughout the country that will offer local advocacy as well as support groups.

National DBSA publishes brochures, books, and videotapes about the treatment of mood disorders. Publications are reviewed by members of the Scientific Advisory Board and most informational booklets are free of charge. Examples are *Guide to Depression and Manic–Depression, Dealing Effectively with Depression and Manic–Depression, Finding Peace of Mind: Medication and Treatment Strategies for Bipolar Disorder,* and *Bipolar Disorder: Rapid Cycling and its Treatment.* The DBSA launched two new initiatives in 2002. The *Taking On (and Talking on) Bipolar Disorder kit* is available free to individuals with bipolar disorder and their families. The kit includes a mood-charting calendar, video, testimonials, and expert advice. It also includes information for families to help someone who may have bipolar illness get into treatment. *Taking Care of Both of You: Understanding Mood Changes after the Birth of Your Baby* is a brochure display being distributed free to thousands of obstetricians/gynecologists, pediatricians, and family practitioners.

National DBSA advocates in Washington, DC, on behalf of people living with mood disorders by providing congressional testimony and ensuring the voice of the consumer is heard. Local support groups often advocate in their state capitals as well. National DBSA hosts an annual conference for its constituents, hosts international scientific conferences on critical issues related to mood disorder research, and sponsors consumer surveys on issues of importance to those living with mood disorders.

The DBSA has a strong alliance with professionals and an influential role in developing practice guidelines and consensus statements on the treatment of patients with bipolar disorder. Consultants from the DBSA were involved in the *Practice Guidelines for the Treatment of Bipolar Disorder* (American Psychiatric Association, 2002). In a major undertaking, the organization convened mental health professionals, policy-makers, researchers, clinicians, patients, and families for a national conference to seek solutions for the undertreatment of depression. A consensus statement was published in *JAMA* (Hirschfeld et al., 1997). This venue made it available not only to the mental health community but to all physicians who might encounter the symptoms of mood disorders. More recently, the organization convened a large group of mood disorder researchers to discuss the use of placebos in clinical trials. The conference consisted of expert presentations on bioethics, biostatistics, unipolar depression, and bipolar disorder (see Rosack, 2002). The consensus statement, published in the *Archives of General Psychiatry,* underscored that patients' safety and well-being must come first but stressed the importance of placebo in developing new treatment options (Charney et al., 2002). In a press release the executive director of DBSA emphasized that an important safety measure is to shorten the length of a patient's exposure to placebo. She told the drug companies: "When patients in a trial respond exceptionally well to a trial drug, it should be made available at an affordable cost when they complete the study" (Rosack, 2002, p. 27). The DBSA's emphasis on informed consent, appropriate placebo usage, and responsibility of pharmaceutical companies implied that consumer groups might assume an active role to ensure informed participation in clinical trials and optimal availability of useful medications.

Child and Adolescent Bipolar Foundation (CABF)
http:// www.cabf.org

CABF is an organization that maintains an active website with constantly updated material on child and adolescent bipolar disorder. Like DBSA, this organization has a professional advisory council of prominent researchers, clinicians, and other experts who provide advice and review the content of materials for scientific accuracy. The CABF website offers full text and abstracts of relevant books and articles from the scientific literature, such as the NIMH Research Roundtable on Prepubertal Bipolar Disorder. They also have a section on brain images and graphics to educate the public on neurological substrates. The website offers national and local directories of professional members who specialize in treating bipolar disorder in children and adolescents. There are also directories of local support groups and suicide hot lines. Additionally, there is a wide pool of information on resources, including social security disability criteria and applications.

Families for Depression Awareness (FDA)
http://www.familyaware.org

Founded in January 2001, FDA helps family caregivers and friends to recognize and cope with unipolar depression and bipolar disorder in a loved one. The organization provides education, outreach, and advocacy, distributes a booklet ("Helping Someone Who Is Depressed"), and offers extensive resources on its website. The site offers a series of "family profiles" that report experiences and coping strategies of individuals with major mood disorders and their family members. Their essential mission seems to be to provide support and information to bewildered and suffering families, including those whose children have bipolar disorder. The organization partners with other organizations that have support groups, such as the DBSA and NAMI (see Bender, 2002a).

Depresson and Related Affective Disorders Association (DRADA)
http:// www.med.jhu.edu/drada

DRADA is an international organization with 82 affiliated groups in the mid-Atlantic area. Founded in 1986, DRADA offers peer support and assists self-help groups by providing education and information and supporting research. They also have a Young People's Outreach Project (White & Madara, 2002, p. 326).

Bipolar Consumer Websites and Information Sources

A number of important informational resources for consumers with bipolar disorder is offered on the web by well-educated consumers.

McMan's Web
http://www.mcmanweb.com

McMan's Depression and Bipolar Weekly
http://jmcnamanamy@snet.net

The McMan website abstracts a wealth of information on major depression and bipolar disorder from professional journals. The Weekly also surfs the information network for relevant legislation and public policy. A representative McMan Weekly (November 2002) provides an abstract of the state of the mental health system from the interim report of the President's Commission on Mental Health, offers a model curriculum for children with bipolar disorder from the Austin Harvard School, gives an update on FDA approval for relevant medications, and directs readers to the website and URL for the American Psychiatric Association's revised Practice Guidelines for the Treatment of Patients with Bipolar Disorder. The website also offers a bookstore, readers' forum, message boards, and other features.

Mary Ellen Copeland's website
http://www.mentalhealthrecovery.com

Mary Ellen Copeland, MS, MA, is author of six self-help books that SAMHSA recently made available through its website (*www.samhsa.org*). The booklets, produced as government-sponsored publications, cover the following topics: Building Self-esteem, Making and Keeping Friends, Dealing with the Effects of Trauma, Developing a Recovery and Wellness Lifestyle, Speaking Out for Yourself, Action Planning for Prevention and Recovery. Each booklet contains ideas and strategies that people from all over the country have found to be helpful in managing their own illnesses and services.

Mary Ellen Copeland's other publications include the Adolescent Depression Workbook; the Depression Workbook: A Guide to Living with Depression and Manic Depression; the Loneliness Workbook: Living without Depression and Manic Depression; and many others. She also has produced video- and audiotapes that are used in training staff members and mental health consumers, such as Strategies for Living with Depression and Manic Depression (video) and Winning Against Relapse Program (audio).

Walkers Web for Depression and Bipolar Disorder
http://www.walkers.org

Walkers Web started more than a decade ago, as a group of people with depression or bipolar disorder sending e-mail to each other. Walkers now has 16 message boards, including those for depression, bipolar disorder, PTSD, and panic disorder, as well as one addressed to teens and other special subjects. They also host four chat rooms and six mailing lists that serve 14,000 registered users. Trained volunteers put in 400 hours a week moderating discussions.

Bipolar Significant Others (BPSO) Bulletin Board
http://www.bpso.org

This is an online resource that provides support for families and friends of people with bipolar disorder. It offers an opportunity to communicate with others in similar situations (White & Madara, 2002, p. 327).

Omnibus Consumer Support Groups

There are many national self-help organizations comprised of present or former patients that, like DBSA, are diagnosis-specific. Examples are Schizophrenics Anonymous, Obsessive–Compulsive Anonymous, Anxiety Disorders Association of America, and Agoraphobics in Motion. The following organizations are examples of self-help groups that are open to persons with a variety of mental illnesses. People with bipolar disorder are frequently found in these more generic groups, which focus on emotional growth rather than education about a specific diagnosis. The following are three major organizations that serve this purpose.

> *GROW* (not an acronym) is an international organization founded in Australia in 1957. It has more than 143 groups in the United States, primarily located in Illinois, New Jersey, and Rhode Island. GROW offers a 12-step program to provide skills for avoiding and recovering from a breakdown, as well as a caring and sharing community to facilitate attainment of emotional maturity, personal responsibility, and recovery from mental illness. Leadership and training are offered to new groups.
>
> *Recovery Inc.*, founded in 1937, has 700 chapters nationally and offers "a self-help method of will training; a system of techniques for con-

trolling temperamental behavior and changing attitudes toward nervous symptoms, anxiety, depression, and fears. Program is based on a medical model and group principles parallel cognitive behavioral therapy" (White & Madara, 2002, p. 330)

Emotions Anonymous, with 1,100 national chapters, is described as a fellowship for people experiencing emotional difficulties. It uses a 12-step program to improve emotional health (White & Madara, 2002, p. 329).

MAJOR OMNIBUS ADVOCACY ORGANIZATIONS

The National Alliance for the Mentally Ill (NAMI)
http://www.nami.org

The organization of NAMI has been termed one of the most important events in the history of American psychiatry (Kaplan & Sadock, 1991). For the first time the major psychiatric disorders had their own important national presence, a grassroots constituency of families and consumers with a profound commitment to improving services, research, and public awareness and to reducing the stigma of mental illness. A scientific study of NAMI done by Johns Hopkins researchers indicated that the consumers represented by the organization are those with serious mental illness, with primary diagnoses of schizophrenia and major mood disorders (Skinner, Steinwachs, & Kasper, 1992).

Although local family support groups had been organized in the 1960s, it was not until 1979 that 284 family members convened at the University of Wisconsin, Madison, to form the national organization NAMI. Since that time NAMI has grown exponentially into a powerful movement. In 2002 NAMI reported 220,000 members and over 1,200 affiliates in all 50 states as well as Puerto Rico and the Virgin Islands. Today, there is a well functioning NAMI office in Arlington, Virginia, disseminating information and lobbying for research and services at the national level, as well as state-level NAMI organizations that work for improved services in their individual states. Specialized units in the national office include NAMI's Center for Research, Education, and Practice, NAMI's Multicultural and International Outreach Center, the National Center for Mental Health and Juvenile Justice, and the Treatment/Recovery Information and Advocacy Database.

Like most organizations that are formed by stakeholders rather than interested outsiders, NAMI merges self-help and advocacy. Thus, the basic armature in all localities is mutual support groups and membership education about all aspects of major mental illnesses. Most groups also engage in public education; resource development; antistigma campaigns; and service on mental health planning, policy, and governance boards at local and national levels. Consumers and family members are trained to become effective lobbyists and advocates for patients.

NAMI also has had an impact on clinical training. The NAMI Curriculum and Training Network focused on influencing mental health professionals to work with persons with severe mental illness, and on ensuring state-of-the-art education in clinical training programs from preservice to continuing education levels. Several national conferences cosponsored by NAMI and NIMH brought together leading clinical educators, researchers, and practitioners with family member-mental health professionals for concept development and curriculum planning in the core professions (Lefley & Johnson, 1990; National Institute of Mental Health, 1990).

A major phenomenon is NAMI's *Family-to-Family* program, developed by a psychologist-family member as a 12-week educational program on schizophrenia, bipolar disorder, and major depression (Burland, 1998). The program is carefully structured to train family members (many of whom are former teachers or mental health professionals) as educators. They provide some of the content of evidence-based family psychoeducation, such as state-of-the-art information on the illnesses and their treatments, problem-solving and communication skills, as well as understanding the patient's experience. The program also teaches families how to cope with family burden, avoid overinvolvement, set limits, and see to their own needs and those of other family members. The Family-to-Family program is available, free of charge, in numerous states, funded and sponsored by state mental health authorities. NAMI reports that Family-to-Family is taken by approximately 10,000 family members in 45 states annually.

NAMI also has a program for consumers, *Peer-to-Peer.* This 9-week course focuses on education, self-help, and recovery principles for people with a major mental illness. It is taught by three consumer-mentors who have received an intensive 3-day training class. As of December 2002, the newer NAMI signature program had in excess of 150 trained peer-teachers and had quickly expanded to 12 states and more than 40 local sites across the country.

Additionally, an antistigma public education program, *In Our Own Voice: Living with Mental Illness,* has received considerable community acclaim. Consumer speakers receive 2-day training and use a nationally produced video to inform the public about the human face of mental illness and the potential for recovery. Consumer feedback from these courses highlight self-determination and empowerment skills. This program grew from six states in 2001 to 25 by the end of 2002. Both of the consumer programs provide the presenters with a salary. For persons attempting to re-enter the traditional workforce, this position provides employment experience following a period of disability.

Additionally, NAMI has targeted educational activities for providers with the NAMI *Provider Education Course,* currently available in 17 states. This 12-week course uses a team of two family members, one consumer, and one professional to educate providers about the actual experience of mental illness. These educational programs, which offer a wealth of materials to participants, are usually funded through state mental health program offices.

On the national level, the family constituency has been powerfully influential in raising research dollars for mental illness. NAMI has successfully lobbied for substantial increases in congressional appropriations for NIMH research on the major psychiatric disorders and helped launch the National Schizophrenia and Brain Research campaign. NAMI cofounded the National Alliance for Research on Schizophrenia and Depression (NARSAD) in 1985 and has generated millions of dollars in research awards through the Ted and Vida Stanley Foundation. Because of its strong commitment to basic research on brain diseases, NAMI was an influential force in the return of NIMH to the National Institutes of Health.

NAMI research-based publications have had a substantial influence on mental health services. These have included *Care of the Seriously Mentally Ill: A Rating of State Programs* (Torrey, Wolfe, & Flynn, 1990) and *Criminalizing the Seriously Mentally Ill: The Abuse of Jails as Mental Hospitals* (Torrey, Wolfe, & Flynn, 1992).

With a major stake in legislative advocacy at the federal level, NAMI was active in promoting passage of Public Law 99-660, which required all 50 states to develop a comprehensive mental health plan, including provision of community care to persons with serious mental illness. This legislation required, for the first time, family and consumer participation on a state advisory council. Reauthorization language linked the approved state plans to the federal block grant, and local NAMI groups became active in monitoring their state's compliance with the plan's objectives. NAMI fought for the 1986 Protection and Advocacy for Individuals with Mental Illness legislation, and the organization was a vocal advocate for the Americans with Disabilities Act. NAMI has been actively working for mental health parity legislation. With a targeted grant from CMHS, NAMI disseminates materials for implementation of the Wisconsin Program for Assertive Community Treatment (PACT) program as evidence-based practice in all states. Furthermore, NAMI was actively involved in the dissemination of the findings of the Schizophrenia Patient Outcomes Research Team (PORT), which recommended specific parameters for prescribed antipsychotic medications (Lehman & Steinwachs, 1998). NAMI produced and distributed more than 50,000 brochures highlighting these recommendations. Additionally, NAMI was instrumental in helping develop the 1999 *Expert Consensus Treatment Guidelines for Schizophrenia* and has widely disseminated the "Guide for Patients and Families" appended to the guidelines (Weiden, Scheifler, McEvoy, & Frances, 1999).

The NAMI Consumer Council is a group of primary consumers who function as a separate interest group within NAMI and have a very substantial role in policy making. During the past several years at least one-quarter of the members of NAMI's board of directors have been consumers (Frese, 1998), and the few NAMI presidents elected for two terms have been consumers. Many consumer leaders in NAMI began their service to the national organization through participation in Consumer Council committees or as council state representatives. The Consumer Council provides leadership training and service opportunities for its members and a consumer-specific voice within the larger organization. Members of the NAMI Consumer Council generally support the NAMI agenda, but many have overlapping affiliations and common interests with other consumer groups. The Consumer Council has made it a recent priority to interface with other consumer organizations throughout the country.

National Mental Health Association (NMHA)
http://www.nmha.org

The National Mental Health Association (NMHA), with 340 affiliated mental health associations (MHAs), was the major advocacy group for persons with serious mental illness until NAMI was founded in 1979. Founded by a former mental hospital patient, Clifford Beers, the NMHA has always advocated for persons with serious mental illness. However, the NMHA's mission has been primarily aimed at improving mental health in the population at large, with a strong emphasis on primary prevention. Examples of activities sponsored by local branches include conferences on sexuality, police training to deal with interethnic conflict, support groups for at-risk groups (e.g., newly widowed persons), and training volunteers to befriend troubled schoolchildren or work with victims of natural disasters. The MHA groups also have served as an education and referral resource for persons needing psychiatric help. In 1987, the Mental Health Information Center was developed as the NMHA clearinghouse to answer personal inquiries and disseminate publications on mental illness and mental health topics.

In most areas, the local MHA branch has been the major umbrella organization linking professionals with interested citizens, facilitating joint advocacy efforts, and providing mental health education for the public. Mental health professionals have been actively involved in governance boards of the lay organization, and there are friendly, affiliative relationships with professional societies. In contrast to self-help groups, Mental Health Association support groups traditionally were led by volunteer professionals, and persons needing further help were urged to use the mental health system.

Today many more MHA affiliates are offering space and resources for peer-led groups that function independently of the host organization. NMHA has taken increasing interest in consumer groups and currently has a CMHS-funded National Consumer Supporter Technical Assistance Center. The center works to strengthen consumer and consumer-supporter networking partnerships at local and state levels. They provide technical assistance in the form of research, information, and financial aid. NMHA has an active partnership with the National Consumer Self-Help Clearinghouse.

Private Research Foundations and Media Organizations

The growth of consumer advocacy groups has brought an increasing focus on research together with the organization of privately funded foundations to supplement the work of the National Institute of Mental Health. The *National Alliance for Research on Schizophrenia and Depression (NARSAD)* was organized through the combined efforts of NAMI, NMHA, DBSA, and the American Schizophrenia Foundation. NARSAD is a major nongovernmental source of support for research on bipolar disorder. The foundation has progressed from awarding $250,000 to 10 researchers in 1987 to more than $20 million to 598 scientists in 2002 (Bender, 2002b).

The *Stanley Medical Research Institute,* according to a report of the Treatment Advocacy Center (2002), has been termed "the largest private provider of research on schizophrenia and bipolar disorder in the United States. It funds approximately half of all U.S. research on bipolar disorder and approximately one quarter of the research on schizophrenia" (p. 2).

Another private organization, the *Mental Illness Education Project, Inc.* in Brookline Village, Massachusetts, produces books and videotapes on the experiences of persons with mental illness and their family members. They have issued a three-part videotape series called The Creating Wellness Series, developed by consumer Mary Ellen Copeland as a self-help model for recovery.

DESTIGMATIZATION THROUGH SELF-DISCLOSURE

For many years persons with mental illness hid their condition from others on the realistic basis that disclosure might harm their chances for marriage, insurance, employment, housing, or higher education. On public records or job applications long periods of a person's life might be shrouded in darkness. In writing *A Beautiful Mind,* the biography of Nobel Prize winner John Nash, author Sylvia Nasar described to a reporter her difficulties in finding material after Nash had developed schizophrenia.

> I knew that Nash had formulated the equilibrium theory but I hadn't known he was this great mathematician because every fact of his life had

been obliterated. The Nobel committee, when they were preparing the prize, had no facts about him. They had to turn to someone at Princeton who spent six weeks gathering, I think, something like 12 little lines of bio figuring out, like, where was he born? What positions had he held? What were his publications? It has all been erased because of what had happened to him. (quoted in Fichtner, 2002, p. 2M)

Although some consumers had previously written about their experiences, in the last two decades there have been numerous autobiographies of prominent persons with mental illness. Books by Kay Jamison, Martha Manning, William Styron, and Patty Duke are a few that have dealt with depression or bipolar disorder. Special television programs have featured prominent people talking about their coping with a major mood disorder. Kay Jamison (1993) has explored the relationship between creativity and bipolar disorder, highlighting the many prominent artists, writers, and composers who have suffered from this illness. Meanwhile, NAMI and other national consumer organizations have conducted militant antistigma campaigns, including targeting advertisers and companies that stigmatize persons with mental illness through the way they advertise or name their products (e.g., Certifiably Nuts, Psycho Joe, and the like).

CONCLUSIONS

Consumer advocacy organizations offer education, peer counseling, self-help enterprises, and ongoing mutual support systems to persons with serious mental illnesses. In addition, these organizations also have affected the course of knowledge development and the form of services in mental health systems, both in general and with specific relevance to depression and bipolar disorder. They promote funding for research and services, insurance parity, protection of patients' rights, antistigma campaigns, and knowledge dissemination. In educating and providing support systems for their members, in advocacy and resource development, consumer groups supplement professional interventions and offer clients an improved quality of life.

What is the interface of consumer organizations and professionals? We have noted reciprocal referrals with practitioners at the local level. At the national level, NAMI and DBSA have collaborated with mental health professionals in developing and disseminating treatment and research guidelines published in the scientific press. Increasingly, family members and consumers participate as members on governance and advisory boards of service providers and on state mental health planning councils. Family members and consumers have been asked to give lectures on the experience of mental illness in clinical training programs and have made presentations at local and national meetings of professional associations. Moreover, they have been encouraged to enter professional training programs through various NIMH training initiatives.

The rise of consumerism also has generated a new emphasis on consumer roles in research. The Boston University Center for Psychiatric Rehabilitation and the University of Illinois at Chicago Center for Research on Psychiatric Disability are among several academic institutions that emphasize hiring consumers as staff to provide research ideas, design, interviewing, and data analysis. Many of these participants are highly functional individuals, self-identified as suffering from bipolar disorder. Currently there is a consumer emphasis on positive prognoses and recovery. William Anthony, Director of the Boston University Center, called recovery "the guiding vision of the mental health systems of the 1990's" (Anthony, 1993, p. 17). Consumers remain conflicted about how to conceptualize and operationalize recovery, although almost all agree this term does not imply return to a premorbid state (Frese, 1998). Rather, most seem to agree that recovery connotes improvement in self-efficacy and quality of life. There are also divisions of opinion about the relative value of evidence-based practices, which are professionally driven and based on quantitative research, compared to the value of consumer-driven practices and qualitative research (Frese, Stanley, Kress, & Vogel-Scibilia, 2001).

Research findings have begun to accumulate on the efficacy of self-help enterprises. A 1-year prospective cohort study of Internet support groups for depression (n = 103) found that users who had high depression scores on the CES-D and were socially isolated perceived considerable benefit from the Internet group. During follow-up, 81% were still receiving face-to-face professional care, but 73% still participated in the online group, and 38% preferred online communication to face-to-face counseling (Houston, Cooper, & Ford, 2002).

Studies of self-help groups for consumers with psychiatric diagnoses and substance abuse problems show increased adherence to medication regimens (Magura, Laudet, Mahmood, Rosenblum, & Knight, 2002). In self-help agencies that use consumer-providers, there is an increased sense of personal empowerment provided by opportunities for clients to participate meaningfully in decisions about their care (Segal & Silverman, 2002). Peer-providers also benefit from their role as helpers, building knowledge and skills, and facilitating their own recovery through their ability to help others (Salzer & Shear, 2002).

Consumer advocacy is now highly valued when professional organizations seek increased funding for research and services. At an annual meeting of the National Association of Psychiatric Health Systems, the *Psychiatric News* reported the following message from former American Psychiatric Association president Paul Fink:

> Not too many years ago, patient advocacy was an unknown for most therapists or one they chose to ignore. Now nobody "in their right mind" would

make major policy decisions or testify before governmental bodies without including patients or their advocates in the process. (Alliances, 1994)

The consumer movements, however, provide far more than an enhanced capability for political lobbying. For individuals suffering from some of the most devastating human disorders, they are a community of peers offering socialization, skill development, empowerment, and renewed self-esteem. Ongoing research on these movements may tell us much about the mechanisms of therapeutic growth.

REFERENCES

Alliances with advocacy groups urged as psychiatrists try to shape health care reform. (1994, February 7). *Psychiatric News, 29*, p. 8.

American Psychiatric Association. (2002). Practice guidelines for the treatment of patients with bipolar disorder (rev.). *American Journal of Psychiatry, 159*(Suppl. 4), 1–50.

Anthony, W. A. (1993). Recovery from mental illness: The guiding vision of the mental health service system in the 1990's. *Innovations and Research, 2*(3), 17–24.

Bender, E. (2002a, October 18). Advocates ease depression's toll on family members. *Psychiatric News, 37*, pp. 20, 45.

Bender, E. (2002b, November 1). An advocate's journey started at home. *Psychiatric News, 37*, 11–12.

Burland, J, (1998). Family-to-Family: A trauma and recovery model of family education. *New Directions for Mental Health Services, 77*, 33–41.

Charney, D. S., Nemeroff, C. B., Lewis, L., Laden, S. K., Gorman, J. M., Laska, E. M., et al. (2002). National Depressive and Manic–Depressive Association consensus statement on the use of placebo in clinical trials of mood disorders. *Archives of General Psychiatry, 59*, 262–270.

Deegan, P. (1994). A letter to my friend who is giving up. *Journal of the California Alliance for the Mentally III, 5*(3), 18–20.

Fichtner, M. (2002, April 14). "Beautiful" spotlight on Nash shifts toward his biographer. *Miami Herald*, p. 2M.

Frese, F. J. (1998). Advocacy, recovery, and the challenges for consumerism for schizophrenia. *Psychiatric Clinics of North America, 21*, 233–249.

Frese, F. J., Stanley, J., Kress, K., & Vogel-Scibilia, S. (2001). Integrating evidence-based practices and the recovery model. *Psychiatric Services, 52*, 1462–1468.

Hirschfeld, R. M. A., Keller, M. B., Panico, S., Arons, B. S., Barlow, D., Davidoff, F., et al. (1997). The National Depressive and Manic–Depressive Association consensus statement on the undertreatment of depression. *JAMA, 277*, 333–340.

Houston, T. K., Cooper, L. A., & Ford, D. E. (2002). Internet support groups for depression: A 1-year prospective cohort study. *American Journal of Psychiatry, 159*, 2062–2068.

Jamison, K. (1993). *Touched with fire: Manic–depressive illness and the artistic temperament*. New York: Free Press.

Kaplan, H. I., & Sadock, B. J. (1991). *Synopsis of psychiatry* (6th ed., rev.). Baltimore, MD: Williams & Wilkins.

Lefley, H. P., & Johnson, D. L. (Eds.) (1990). *Families as allies in treatment of the mentally ill: New directions for mental health professionals*. Washington, DC: American Psychiatric Press.

Lehman, A. F., & Steinwachs, D. M. (1998). Translating research into practice: The Schizophrenia Patient Outcomes Research Team (PORT) treatment recommendations. *Schizophrenia Bulletin, 24,* 1–10.

Magura, S., Laudet, A.B., Mahmood, D., Rosenblum, A., & Knight, E. (2002). Adherence to medication regimens and participation in dual-focus self-help groups. *Psychiatric Services, 53,* 310–315.

National Institute of Mental Health. (1990). H. P. Lefley, Ed. *Clinical training in serious mental illness.* U.S. Department of Health and Human Services publication (ADM) 90–1679. Washington, DC: U.S. Government Printing Office.

Rosack, J. (2002, May 17). Mood-disorder experts give qualified nod to placebo trials. *Psychiatric News, 37,* 27.

Salzer, M. S., & Shear, S. L. (2002). Identifying consumer-provider benefits in evaluations of consumer-delivered services. *Psychiatric Rehabilitation Journal, 25,* 282–288.

Segal, S. P., Hodges, J. Q., & Hardiman, E. R. (2002). Factors in decisions to seek help from self-help and co-located community mental health agencies. *American Journal of Orthopsychiatry, 72,* 241–249.

Segal, S. P., & Silverman, C. (2002). Determinants of client outcomes in self-help agencies. *Psychiatric Services, 53,* 304–309.

Skinner, E. A., Steinwachs, D. M., & Kasper, J. D. (1992). Family perspectives on the service needs of people with serious and persistent mental illness. *Innovations and Research, 1,* 23–30.

Survey reveals vast preference for the term "patient." (2002, Fall). *Outreach: Newsletter of the Depression and Bipolar Support Alliance* (DBSA), p. 1.

Torrey, E. F., Wolfe, S. M, & Flynn, L. M. (1990). *Care of the seriously mentally ill: A rating of state programs* (3rd ed.). Arlington, VA: Public Citizens Health Research Group and National Alliance for the Mentally Ill.

Torrey, E. F., Wolfe, S. M., & Flynn, L. M. (1992). *Criminalizing the seriously mentally ill: The abuse of jails as mental hospitals.* Arlington, VA: Public Citizens Health Research Group and National Alliance for the Mentally Ill.

Treatment Advocacy Center. (2002, April 19). Message posted to *TAC@mh.databack.com,* p. 2.

U.S. Department of Health and Human Services. (1999). *Mental health: A report of the surgeon-general.* Rockville, MD. Author.

Weiden, P.J., Scheifler, P.L., McEvoy, J.P., & Frances, A. (1999). Expert consensus treatment guidelines for schizophrenia: A guide for patients and families. *Journal of Clinical Psychiatry, 60*(Suppl. 11), 73–80.

White, B. J., Madara, E. J. (Eds.). (2002). *The self-help group source book: Your guide to community and online support groups* (7th ed.). Denville, NJ: American Self-help Clearinghouse.

CHAPTER FIFTEEN

CONCLUSIONS

ROBERT L. LEAHY

When Kraepelin (1921) described the symptomatic profile and life course of manic–depressive illness, he reflected the common belief of many European psychiatrists a century ago. This was the assumption that psychiatry could contribute to our understanding of the diagnosis and prognosis of mental illnesses, but could do very little to change its course. Perhaps because of this assumption that little could be done to alter outcome, attention was focused on detailed descriptions of the patient's physical and mental state. Palliative treatments—rest, warm baths, and reduced stress—were the only interventions available.

Twenty years ago the clinical picture had changed for what is now called "bipolar disorder." The clinician, informed by a biological and genetic model of bipolar illness, could rely on the use of lithium and, in some cases, electroconvulsive treatment, for the alleviation of severe mood episodes. The general rule was simply this: "If the patient has bipolar disorder, put him or her on lithium." Although clinicians today have a wide range of drug treatments available, there still is an assumption among many practicing clinicians that the only effective treatment is pharmacological.

The contributors to this volume provide substantial evidence that vulnerability to bipolar episodes is affected by biological predisposition, cognitive diathesis, psychosocial stressors, and expressed emotion. Although many clinicians claim that they adhere to a stress–diathesis model of psychiatric illness, much of conventional treatment has been based on the biological diathesis of the disorder, with an almost complete emphasis on medication. The contributors to this volume provide substantial evidence and strategies that argue in favor of a more integrative understanding and treatment of bipolar disorder.

EVALUATING BIPOLAR DISORDER

Experienced clinicians familiar with bipolar disorder often encounter individuals with bipolar disorder who have been treated by numerous clinicians, who have been prescribed a variety of antidepressant and anxiolytic medications, but who have never been diagnosed as bipolar. Altman's valuable contribution (Chapter 3), along with Youngstrom, Findling, & Feeny's description of bipolar disorder in children and adolescents (Chapter 4), demonstrate the complexity and finer points of differential diagnosis, as well as the importance of early diagnosis and prophylactic treatment. The various manifestations of bipolar disorder—bipolar I and II, rapid cycling, and cyclothymic disorder—as well as the existence of mixed states and hypomania, which are difficult to evaluate for many clinicians, often lead to incorrect diagnosis of unipolar depression, anxiety, or borderline personality. As a result, many bipolar patients are placed on antidepressants, without mood stabilizers, resulting in exacerbation of mood cycling.

Comorbidity with substance abuse often may mask proper diagnosis of bipolar disorder. Since a large percentage of these individuals abuse substances, the clinician may correctly (or incorrectly) attribute mood volatility to substance abuse, although substance abuse may be independent of manic episodes. Careful evaluations of mood variation—especially the existence of hypomania (which few patients view as a problem)—may help the clinician differentiate between mood variation attributable to substance-induced disorders and mood variation that is systemic, chronic, and reflecting the bipolar process.

My observation of many clinicians who have misdiagnosed bipolar disorder is that they often become overly committed to their earlier, incorrect diagnosis, very much like a cognitive dissonance process. The clinician who has falsely diagnosed a patient with unipolar depression is often reluctant to modify the evaluation to consider the possibility of bipolar disorder. Since many patients with bipolar disorder provide a complex clinical profile of comorbid personality and anxiety disorders, as well as substance abuse—and since manic symptoms are often expressed as mixed-state, agitated, or hypomanic symptoms—the diagnosis is often clouded. Seeking second opinions or reviewing the alternative diagnoses with the help of both patient and observant family members often may clarify the clinical picture and facilitate the appropriate modification in medication.

Are psychosocial factors related to the course of illness? Hammen and Cohen's review (Chapter 2) suggests that there are multiple impairments related to bipolar disorder, many of which are a consequence and some of which may be an added predisposing factor. Individuals with bipolar disorder have higher divorce rates, greater unemployment and poverty, impaired parental functioning, and more limited social functioning. Although we might be inclined to interpret these data as reflective of the consequences of bipolar illness, they also may reflect added sources of stress that are more likely to predispose the person to relapse. The skills deficits (or skill utilization deficits) and lack of emotional regulation characteristic of some of these individuals may lead to added social conflicts and daily hassles, contributing to the stress that adds fuel to the bipolar diathesis.

Johnson and Meyer provide an interesting review of the psychosocial predictors of illness outcome (Chapter 5). Expressed emotion (which also receives considerable attention in Chapter 9) has a significant impact on relapse risk. This expressed negative emotion may partly reflect the causal attributions of family members, who view the patient's symptoms as under his or her voluntary control, as opposed to viewing these symptoms as reflections of a biological illness. Of special significance is the fact that negative life events—especially interpersonal and more serious events—are predictive of vulnerability (see also Johnson & Roberts, 1995). Personality disorders or personality styles also are predictive of greater relapse potential. The evidence for cognitive style, or cognitive vulnerability, is somewhat mixed, with some data supportive of underlying differences between individuals with bipolar disorder and controls, whereas other studies report no differences. These mixed findings may reflect the question of whether euthymic cognitive style needs to be "primed" by mood induction in order to access latent vulnerability, as Ingram, Miranda, and Segal (1998) have proposed.

On the other hand, it may be that underlying attributional styles are not always accessible during a euthymic phase. Individuals may simply manifest mood-specific or symptomatic cognitive biases—that is, they evidence overly positive cognitions only when they are actually manic. This possibility would suggest that the vulnerability is in the dysregulation of mood, perhaps reflecting the strong biological diathesis. What is needed—and currently lacking—are more longitudinal data on the effects of attributional *training* as an inoculation against episodic relapse. The question would be, "Can attempts to modify attributional style during the euthymic phase result in improvements (i.e., less relapse) in the course of the illness?"

TREATMENTS ARE EFFECTIVE—BUT WHY?

As pointed out by Scott (Chapter 11), psychosocial treatments are faring better in influencing some outcomes than others. In particular, early evidence suggests that these treatments are most helpful in improving medication adherence and in alleviating symptoms of depression. So far, it has been harder to influence the course of mania with adjunctive psychotherapy (see Johnson, 2002, for more discussion of this issue). It may be that

mania, as a more biologically driven phenomenon, is more purely responsive to medications. On the other hand, it may be that once the mania has
emerged, the patient lacks the insight and the motivation to utilize psychotherapeutic support. In this case, approaches that emphasize education
regarding symptoms and monitoring will be most helpful. It also remains
possible that advances in our understanding of how to conduct psychotherapy specifically to help prevent manic symptoms as our psychosocial models of mania become more sophisticated.

It is not entirely clear why cognitive-behavioral interventions, family-
focused treatment, or IPSRT treatment works with bipolar disorder. What
are the mechanisms of change? Do these treatments increase medication
compliance, improve interpersonal functioning, modify illness attributions
by family members, decrease emotional expression in the family, stabilize
biological rhythms, modify cognitive style, improve problem-solving skills,
increase a sense of self-efficacy, or decrease the likelihood of stressful life
events? Which treatment works through which mechanisms?

Perhaps clinicians care less about the mechanisms of change and are
more enthusiastic about the *fact* that something positive can be done.
Moreover, clinicians are likely to integrate elements from each of these
approaches, paying less heed to theoretical purity and more attention to fit-
ting the treatment to the individual patient. But mechanisms of change will
have clinical relevance—if we can identify these mechanisms. Just as we
know that there are numerous effective treatments for unipolar depression
(i.e., cognitive, behavioral, interpersonal, marital, pharmacological), we
know that there are different effective treatments for bipolar disorder.
Would dismantling studies assist us in finding the "essential" ingredient?
Or should we go the other way and develop a "grand theoretical model"
that incorporates all of these approaches? I discuss some of these common
elements below, but I believe that clinicians are likely to want to use something from each. Consequently, "all deserve prizes."

Scott's review of the outcome studies, as well as evidence provided by
both Miklowitz (Chapter 9) and Bauer (Chapter 10) for their respective
treatment modalities, are encouraging. There can be no doubt that psychosocial treatments significantly improve the functioning of individuals with
bipolar disorder. Indeed, we can now argue that failing to provide adjunctive psychosocial treatment is to underserve the patient with bipolar
disorder.

WHY NOT USE EVERYTHING?

Clinical researchers are fond of their unique perspective and contribution—as
they should be. However, those who see patients with bipolar disorder
every day and must deal with the complexity of their lives may feel—as I

do—"Why not use everything?" Psychosocial treatments include interventions that modify or attempt to improve interpersonal functioning, diurnal rhythms, expressed emotion, problem-solving abilities, and cognitive, behavioral, and family communication patterns. My experience is that patients generally come in with almost all of these areas needing to be addressed. For example, even though I identify myself as a cognitive-behavioral therapist, I utilize many of the ideas represented by interpersonal and social rhythm therapy, family therapy, the life goals approach, consumer or self-help groups, and, of course, pharmacotherapy. Moreover, since a majority of patients with bipolar disorder will, at some time, abuse drugs and alcohol, motivational interviewing, relapse prevention, harm reduction, 12-step programs, identifying the triggers and facilitative cognitions of substance abuse, and providing alternatives are often part of the treatment. It is for these reasons that I am convinced that the treatment of bipolar illness—more than in any other psychiatric disorder—requires the integration of techniques and interventions from numerous modalities.

Unlike Kraepelin, who was limited to providing detailed descriptions of his patients and who could only recommend warm baths, numerous biological treatments are available to us today. As Goldberg indicates (Chapter 6), the physician can now utilize anticonvulsants, antipsychotics, thyroid medications, and antidepressants, depending on the specific kind of bipolar disorder that is being treated. Nonmedical therapists working with patients who have bipolar disorder will find Goldberg's detailed description of the advantages and disadvantages of various pharmacological treatments to be invaluable. Many patients with bipolar disorder may become discouraged with medication, partly because mood instability is not entirely controlled, partly because of the risk of breakout episodes of mania or depression, and often because of the untoward side effects. Referring to Table 6.1 in Goldberg's chapter, which lists the psychotropic medications commonly used in the treatment of bipolar disorder, the clinician can counsel the patient about the common side effects and the specific applications of these medications. As indicated, some medications help stabilize manic episodes but offer little added benefit for stabilizing depressive episodes. The clinician will need to consider the tradeoffs of augmenting the usual mood stabilizers with antidepressant medication by evaluating the added risk of kindling effects pursuant to antidepressant use. Goldberg observes correctly that the use of antidepressants must be weighed against the risk of increasing rapid cycling or manic symptoms. Moreover, electroconvulsive therapy (ECT) is an effective treatment for reversing severe and often intractable mood episodes and should be considered as a possible alternative.

Psychosocial treatments augment medication and, in fact, can increase compliance with medication treatment. Indeed, it may be that one of the major contributions of psychosocial treatments is to increase medication compliance. Individuals with bipolar disorder understandably may have some reluctance to take medications that have uncomfortable side effects. As noted in Goldberg's review, numerous alternatives are now available, some with fewer side effects.

Autonomous or even rebellious attitudes characteristic of the manic state may interfere with medication compliance. Individuals with mania often believe that the medication slows them down and inhibits their unlimited potential. Alternatively, depressed individuals may believe that their hopelessness is realistic and that medication is just another pointless dead end. The clinician who is able to integrate the various psychosocial treatment models presented in this volume will be more effective in implementing medication compliance. Providing psychoeducation for the patient and significant family members will assure greater alliance in the support of biological treatment and in early detection of significant mood shifts. Helping patients during the euthymic period recognize how manic or depressed mood will later interfere with medication compliance can help "inoculate" them against later tendencies toward nonadherence. Providing patients with information and ongoing support through advocacy and group discussions with other individuals who have bipolar disorder further supports the medical treatment of the illness. Indeed, by coordinating the use of each of these psychosocial approaches, the clinician may add considerable resources toward ensuring the effectiveness of the treatment.

In my chapter on cognitive therapy (Chapter 7), I identify some of the typical thought patterns that foster manic risk behavior or that contribute to the depressive regret, self-criticism, and hopelessness. Self-monitoring of mood—an intervention recommended by all the treatments represented here—provides the patient and clinician with an early warning system that can identify mood dysregulation and activate changes in medication, reduction of opportunities for risky manic behavior, involvement of family members in a supportive role, and utilization of self-instructional scripts to address depressive and manic thinking and behavior. I recently spoke with the patient whose experiences are described in my chapter. She indicated to me that she still keeps a laminated copy of her mood-check chart on her wall—even though her moods have been stabilized successfully for years. Indeed, her experience in treatment—and her continued good functioning—attests to the value of integrating all of these modalities.

The family therapy perspective that Miklowitz provides (Chapter 9) indicates how important it is to view psychiatric illness within a social context. Bipolar illness is episodic and lifelong; individuals with bipolar disorder often return to family environments. The old behavioral maxim—gain as much control over the environment—is best exemplified by addressing the family context, as Miklowitz does. There is considerable support for the view that psychosocial stressors add to risk of relapse (see Chapter 5, this volume) and that expressed (negative) emotion in the family is a risk factor.

There are a number of features common to each psychosocial approach:

1. Providing psychoeducation about the illness.
2. Addressing medication compliance.
3. Involvement of significant others or family.
4. Identifying symptoms that are an early sign of episodes.
5. Improving problem-solving skills.
6. Encouraging the use of support or advocacy groups.

In addition to the commonalities of these psychosocial treatments are important differences in which area domain is stressed. The cognitive-behavioral approach emphasizes rational disputation or testing of negative or overly positive (manic) thoughts and utilizes activity scheduling, graded task assignments, and other behavioral interventions. The family-focused approach stresses the enhancement of communication patterns and support within the family context, including modifying illness conceptualization and attribution of behavior by family members, and improving listening skills and communication without criticism of the patient. Other approaches to improving the interpersonal environment are reviewed by Frank and Swartz in their chapter on IPSRT (Chapter 8).

Bauer's Life Goals Program (Chapter 10) emphasizes both illness management skills (coping with symptoms) and attainment of life goals. The phase of treatment focused on attaining life goals stresses a problem-solving model that identifies behavioral goals, strategies, alternatives, and roadblocks. Both aspects of therapy include behavioral and cognitive interventions, with the focus on action plans and problem solving. The Life Goals Program is based on practical interventions that can be implemented readily.

Several of the treatments described in this book aim to improve the social worlds of individuals with bipolar disorder; Bauer's approach also places a primary focus on social functioning. Given that psychosocial problems are well documented as both predictors and sequelae of this disorder, these approaches seem quite sound in their emphasis. However, it is worth noting that in the treatment of schizophrenia, much more intensive day hospital and occupational rehabilitation programs have received attention. It is striking that, despite the similar severity of bipolar disorder and schizophrenia, the treatments for bipolar disorder remain much more limited in intensity than some of the treatments used for schizophrenia.

Lefley and Vogel-Scibilia (Chapter 14) describe the use of consumer advocacy and/or support groups in the treatment of bipolar illness. Many patients are avid users of Internet sources and may be encouraged to utilize information resources, chat rooms, and other "consumer" resources available on the Internet. These groups are helpful in numerous ways: They destigmatize the illness, provide the patient with a sense of community with people who have similar problems, provide role models of coping with the illness, and are a source of creative ideas about how to handle specific problems. Many clinicians realize that advice or examples from someone who has a similar illness may be more compelling than advice from the "doctor." Chat rooms and group meetings enhance the regular and often immediate support that these people may need and allows them to feel that ongoing support is available, even after psychotherapy is "completed." The very nature of these advocacy groups helps focus the patient on practical, "here-and-now" strategies, further empowering the consumer. Moreover, many individuals with bipolar illness (or other psychiatric problems) become important advocates for the rights and needs of people similarly affected.

Consumer and support groups may provide both positive and negative experiences for some individuals. The positive aspect of these groups is the recognition that there are many others who have coped well and who understand the patient's experience. However, some patients may be alarmed to hear about the devastating effect of the illness on some. "Higher-functioning" patients, first learning of their diagnosis, may feel uncomfortable learning of the degree of impairment experienced by some people with bipolar illness. However, the clinician can make positive use of this information by describing the range of functioning people with bipolar disorder demonstrate (emphasizing the autobiographical work of Jamison), and by encouraging utilization of all available treatment resources, lest the severity of the illness unfolds.

In Chapter 13, Newman elucidates the most significant outcome—suicide. Close to 20% of patients affected with bipolar illness eventually kill themselves—a rate of mortality as high as many cancers. The clinician needs to understand how these individuals often may feel drawn to suicide as a "solution" to their lifelong struggle with this illness. Many patients on medication experience relapse, and there is often a severe negative impact of the illness on marriage, family life, work, and financial status. The depressive episodes are experienced as relentless and devastating. Clinicians need to place themselves in the shoes of these individuals to understand why suicide seems attractive.

Fortunately, as the contributors to this volume clearly indicate, the management of this illness is far more advanced today than ever before. First, patients are not limited to lithium and may benefit from multidrug treatment that can be modified for specific symptom profiles and specific mood. As indicated earlier, ECT and other biological treatments should be considered in refractory cases; significant and rapid improvement is often seen. Second, episodes are just that—*episodes*—they come to an end. Third, as Scott indicates in Chapter 11, the treatments described in this book have been proven to be highly effective in shortening the duration and decreasing the severity of episodes, increasing the time between episodes, and decreasing the number of days in the hospital. Fourth, the clinician might further enhance efficacy by utilizing something from each of these approaches—thereby getting the best of everything.

FINAL OVERVIEW

What can we conclude from these contributions that helps us understand the importance of psychosocial factors in the treatment of bipolar disorder? Let me summarize some of the main points.

1. There is a strong biological (and genetic) causality; the disorder is systemic and carries with it lifelong vulnerabilities (similar to diabetes and hypertension).
2. These vulnerabilities are exacerbated by stressors (life events).
3. The interaction between the biological domain and stressful events is moderated by psychological diathesis (e.g., attributional style, personality, neuroticism) and behavioral and social skills.
4. Substance abuse is both a consequence of attempts at self-management of mood and an added vulnerability to further relapse.
5. The likelihood of occurrence of symptomatic episodes is affected by interpersonal factors, such as expressed emotion in the family context, social support, and relationship conflicts and terminations.
6. The outcome (e.g., relapse, hospitalization, risk of suicide, etc.) can be affected by psychosocial therapies that address risk variables.
7. Psychosocial therapies assist the patient in coping with the symptoms of the illness (e.g., reducing risk behavior in mania).
8. Psychosocial treatments are often partly effective because they increase medication adherence as well as reduce the interaction between biological diathesis and the impact of stressors.

Is there reason for optimism? Many patients confronted with the diagnosis of "bipolar disorder" may feel demoralized—they now realize they have a lifelong "mental disease." It is one thing to recognize that your depression is due to a recent breakup in a relationship—you can hope that future relationships will be more stable or that you will learn to cope with breakups more effectively. It is quite another thing to recognize that you are vulnerable to considerable mood variation and recurrence of episodes even while you are taking prescribed medication.

But even with these apparently discouraging realities in mind, there is reason for measured optimism. First, there are numerous medications—and combinations of medication classes—that have fewer side effects and can be combined to address specific mood episodes or specific symptoms (e.g., increased anxiety or insomnia). Second, the clinician and patient can now work collaboratively, utilizing many of the strategies and interventions provided in this volume, to significantly increase the efficacy of medication and reduce the impact of the illness. Third, because of the strong emphasis on the psychoeducation component in each of these treatments, family members can become empowered as part of the treatment of their valued, but sometimes "ill," member. I believe that including significant others is an especially important and hopeful component of these adjunctive psychosocial treatments. Bipolar individuals live in a social context that can either help them or make life more difficult. Coordinating treatment with family members reduces the negative expressed emotions, modifies attributions about the illness, provides the patient with willing and caring observers of early warning signs, reduces relationship terminations, and reduces the feelings of helplessness in both patient and family members.

Yes, perhaps there is some reason to feel much more optimistic. We are no longer limited, as was Kraepelin, to detailed descriptions of debilitating illness, and we no longer need to stand by, passively waiting for the lithium to take effect. These psychosocial treatments, along with the growing advocacy and support movements, provide hope for lifelong support for an illness that, for many, has proved so overwhelming.

REFERENCES

Ingram, R. E., Miranda, J., & Segal, Z. V. (1998). *Cognitive vulnerability to depression.* New York: Guilford Press.

Johnson, S. L. (2002). Some unanswered questions regarding psychosocial treatments for bipolar disorder: Commentary on "Psychosocial Interventions for Bipolar Disorder" by Mark Bauer. In M. Maj, H. S. Akiskal, J. J. Lopez-Ibor, & N. Sartorius (Eds.), *Bipolar disorder* (World Psychiatric Association, Evidence and Experience in Psychiatry, Vol. 5, pp. 319–322). Chichester, UK: Wiley.

Johnson, S. L., & Roberts, J. R. (1995). Life events and bipolar disorder: Implications from biological theories. *Psychological Bulletin, 117,* 434–449.

Kraepelin, E. (1921). *Manic–depressive insanity and paranoia.* Edinburgh: Livingstone.

APPENDICES

GUIDELINES

Purpose

The ASRM may be used as a self-report instrument in either an inpatient or outpatient setting to screen for the severity of manic symptoms for clinical or research purposes. The time frame covered is generally the most recent week, although this may be lengthened or shortened if clinically necessary. Because the ASRM is compatible with DSM-IV criteria and correlates significantly with clinician-administered mania rating scales, it can be used as a screening instrument to facilitate diagnostic assessment in patients with manic symptoms. However, the ASRM should not be used solely as a diagnostic instrument. In outpatient settings, it may be used as a psychoeducational tool to help patients recognize and monitor their own symptoms. It also may be used as a measure of clinical treatment efficacy. Finally, it may be used in combination with depression scales to assess mixed states of mania and depression. It is not designed to assess psychotic symptoms.

Scoring

Items 1 through 5 should be summed. A cutoff score of 6 or higher indicates a high probability of a manic or hypomanic condition (based on a sensitivity rating of 85.5% and a specificity rating of 87.3%). A score of 5 or lower is less likely to be associated with significant symptoms of mania. A score of 6 or higher may indicate a need for treatment or a further diagnostic workup to confirm a diagnosis of mania or hypomania. As a measure of clinical efficacy, total scores before, during, and after treatment can be compared.

Name _____ Date _____ Score _____

INSTRUCTIONS

1. On this questionnaire are groups of five statements; read each group of statements carefully.
2. Choose the one statement in each group that best describes the way you have been feeling for the past week.
3. Circle the number next to the statement you picked.
4. *Please note:* The word "occasionally" when used here means once or twice; "often" means several times or more; "frequently" means most of the time.

1) 0 I do not feel happier or more cheerful than usual.
   1 I occasionally feel happier or more cheerful than usual.
   2 I often feel happier or more cheerful than usual.
   3 I feel happier or more cheerful than usual most of the time.
   4 I feel happier or more cheerful than usual all of the time.

2) 0 I do not feel more self-confident than usual.
   1 I occasionally feel more self-confident than usual.
   2 I often feel more self-confident than usual.
   3 I feel more self-confident than usual most of the time.
   4 I feel extremely self-confident all of the time.

3) 0 I do not need less sleep than usual.
   1 I occasionally need less sleep than usual.
   2 I often need less sleep than usual.
   3 I frequently need less sleep than usual.
   4 I can go all day and night without any sleep and still not feel tired.

4) 0 I do not talk more than usual.
   1 I occasionally talk more than usual.
   2 I often talk more than usual.
   3 I frequently talk more than usual.
   4 I talk constantly and cannot be interrupted.

5) 0 I have not been more active (either socially, sexually, at work, home, or school) than usual.
   1 I have occasionally been more active than usual.
   2 I have often been more active than usual.
   3 I have frequently been more active than usual.
   4 I am constantly active or on the go all the time.

APPENDIX 2. Mood Chart

Name _____

Mood Chart
Month/Year _____

MOOD
Rate with 2 marks each day to indicate best and worst (if applicable)

Elevated
- Severe — Significant Impairment NOT ABLE TO WORK
- Mod. — Significant Impairment ABLE TO WORK
- Mild — Without significant impairment

WNL
- MOOD NOT DEFINITELY ELEVATED OR DEPRESSED. NO SYMPTOMS
- Circle date to indicate Menses

Depressed
- Mild — Without significant impairment
- Mod. — Significant Impairment ABLE TO WORK
- Severe — Significant Impairment NOT ABLE TO WORK

Psychotic Symptoms
Strange Ideas, Hallucinations

Hours Slept Last Night

0 = none
1 = mild
2 = moderate
3 = severe

Anxiety

Irritability

Daily Notes

Weight: _____

1 2 3 4 5 6 7 8 9 10 11 12 13 14 15 16 17 18 19 20 21 22 23 24 25 26 27 28 29 30 31

TREATMENTS
(Enter number of tablets taken each day)

Verbal Therapy

Lithium ____mg

Benzodiazepine ____mg

Anticonvulsant (e.g., Depakote) ____mg

Antidepressant ____mg

____mg

Antipsychotic ____mg

WNL, within normal limits. Copyright 1993 by Gary Sachs, MD. (Reprinted in Miklowitz, D. J. [2002]. *The Bipolar Disorder Survival Guide.* New York: Guilford Press.

APPENDIX 3. **Evaluation of Suicidal Risk**

Patient's Name: _____ Today's Date: _____

Therapist's Name: _____

Evaluate for current suicidal ideation and behavior and for any past incidence of suicidal plans, intentions, or behavior.

Question	Current	Past
Do you have any thoughts of harming yourself? [If yes:] Describe.		
Have you ever felt indifferent about whether something dangerous would happen to you and you took a lot of risk—like you really didn't care if you died or hurt yourself? [If yes:] Describe.		
Have you ever threatened that you would hurt yourself? [If yes:] Whom did you say this to? Why?		
Have you ever tried to hurt yourself on purpose? [If no, go on to p. 3 of form]		
Exactly what did you do to try to hurt yourself?		

Question	Current	Past
How many times have you tried this? When? Describe.		
Did you tell anyone before or after your attempt? Had you threatened to hurt yourself or talked about it before? [If yes:] Describe.		
Had you planned to hurt yourself, or was it spontaneous?		
What was your state of mind when you attempted to hurt yourself? Were you depressed, spaced out, anxious, relieved, angry, excited? Were you using alcohol, medication, other drugs?		
Did you call someone at that time, or were you discovered by someone? What happened?		
Did you go to a doctor or to the hospital? [If yes:] Which doctor/ hospital? [Obtain release of information.]		

(continued)

Questions	Current	Past
Did you feel glad that you were alive? Embarrassed? Guilty? Sorry you didn't kill yourself?		
Did you want to hurt yourself soon after your attempt?		
Was there any event that triggered your attempt? [If yes:] Describe. [If no, go to next page of form]		
What were you thinking after this event that made you want to hurt yourself?		
If something like that happened again, how would you handle it?		
Has any family member or close friend ever hurt himself or herself?		
How would you describe your current [past] desire to live? None, weak, moderate, or strong?		

Questions	Current	Past
How would you describe your current [past] desire to die? None, weak, moderate, or strong?		
[If current or past desire to die:] What would be the reason for wanting to die or harm yourself? Hopelessness, depression, revenge, getting rid of anxiety, being with a lost loved one again, other reasons?		
[If current or past desire to die:] Have you ever planned to hurt yourself? What was that plan? Why did you [did you not] carry it out?		
Are there any reasons why you would not harm yourself? Explain.		
Do you have more reasons to live than reasons to die?		
[If not:] What would have to change so that you would want to live more?		
Do you own a weapon?		

(*continued*)

Question	Current	Past
Do you live on a high floor or near a high bridge?		
Are you saving medications for a future attempt to hurt yourself?		
Do you drive excessively fast?		
Do you ever space out, not knowing what is going on around you? [If yes:] Describe.		
Do you drink more than three glasses of liquor or beer a day? Do you use any medications? Other drugs? Do these substances affect your mood? [If yes:] How?		
Have you written a suicide note? Have you recently written out a will?		
Do you feel there is any hope that things can get better?		
What are the reasons why things could be hopeful?		

Questions	Current	Past
Why would things seem hopeless?		
Would you be willing to promise me that you would not do anything to harm yourself until you have called me and spoken with me?		
Is your promise a solemn promise that I can rely on, or do you have doubts about whether you can keep this promise? [If doubts:] What are these doubts?		
Can I speak with [loved ones or a close friend] to be sure that we have all the support that we need?		
[Does this patient need to be hospitalized? Increase frequency of treatment contact and level or type of medication? ECT?]		

(continued)

Therapist: Summarize dates, precipitating factors, and nature of the patient's previous suicide attempts, if any: _____

_____

_____

If the patient is willing to promise that he or she will contact and speak with the therapist before engaging in any self-harmful action, have him or her sign this statement:

I, _____, promise that I will not do anything to harm myself until I have called and spoken to you, my therapist. I also agree that you may speak with a loved one or close friend of mine to be sure that you and I have all the support we need.

_____

Patient's Signature

_____

Therapist's Signature

_____

Date

APPENDIX 4. Recommended Resources for Consumers and Their Families

WORKBOOKS AND PSYCHOEDUCATIONAL MATERIALS

Copeland, M. E. (2002). *The depression workbook (2nd ed.): A guide for living with depression and manic depression.* Oakland, CA: New Harbinger.

Fawcett, J., Golden, B., & Rosenfeld, N. (2000). *New hope for people with bipolar disorder.* Roseville, CA: Prima.

Miklowitz, D. J. (2002). *The bipolar disorder survival guide.* New York: Guilford Press.

Mondimore, F. M. (1999). *Bipolar disorder: A guide for patients and families.* Baltimore, MD: Johns Hopkins University Press.

Papolos, D. F., & Papolos, J. (1997). *Overcoming depression: The definitive resource for patients and families who live with depression and manic–depression* (3rd ed.). New York: Harper Collins.

Scott, J. (2001). *Overcoming mood swings: A self-help guide using cognitive behavioral techniques.* New York: New York University Press.

Torrey, E. F., & Knable, M. B. (2002). *Surviving manic depression: A manual on bipolar disorder for patients, families, and providers.* New York: Basic Books.

BOOKS SPECIFIC TO DEPRESSION

American Psychiatric Association. (2000). *Major depressive disorder: A patient and family guide.* Washington, DC: American Psychiatric Press.

Burns, D. D. (1989). *The feeling good handbook: Using the new mood therapy in everyday life.* New York: Morrow.

Gilbert, J. (2001). *Overcoming depression: A step-by-step guide to gaining control over depression.* New York: Oxford University Press.

Wright, J. H., & Basco, M. R. (2001). *Getting your life back: The complete guide to recovery from depression.* New York: Free Press.

AUTOBIOGRAPHIES AND BIOGRAPHIES

Duke, P., & Hochman, G. (1993). *A brilliant madness: Living with manic–depressive illness.* New York: Bantam Books.

Hinshaw, S. P. (2002). *The years of silence are past: My father's life with bipolar disorder.* New York: Cambridge University Press.

Jamison, K. R. (1997). *An unquiet mind.* New York: Random House.
Solomon, A. (2001). *The noonday demon: An atlas of depression.* New York: Scribner.
Styron, W. (1992). *Darkness visible: A memoir of madness.* New York: Vintage Books.

VIDEO

Living well with bipolar disorder: A new look. [VHS]. (2001). Monkey See Productions, NSW,
    Australia. Available in the United States from Guilford Publications, 72 Spring Street, New
    York, New York 10012.

APPENDIX 5. **Outline of Collaborative Disease Management Strategies**

PANEL 1: THE COLLABORATIVE DISEASE MANAGEMENT AGENDA FOR SUPPORTIVE PSYCHOTHERAPY

1. What is this disorder?
   a. What causes these symptoms?
   b. What treatments in general are used?
   c. What is the course and outcome with/without treatment?
2. What is *your* specific pattern of symptoms?
3. What are the most troublesome symptoms for you?
4. (for chronic illness): What are the Early Warning Signs for relapse?
5. What are your triggers that lead to new or worsening symptoms?
6. What are your methods of coping with symptoms? How do you cope with life despite your symptoms?
7. For your typical coping responses:
   a. What are the positive aspects (benefits)?
   b. What are the negative aspects (costs)?
8. What are the coping responses you want to emphasize?:
   a. In your own self-management?
   b. By utilizing significant others, family, other support systems?
   c. By activating your clinician?
9. What are the coping responses you want to replace?

Note. The work with coping responses is based on the assumption that all illness behaviors have self-perceived costs and benefits—always both. What is essential—before teaching, scolding, cajoling, motivating—is to determine this metric in the individual. What may seem ill advised, and may well be (i.e., use of substances, social isolation), has some intrinsic perceived benefit to the individual. Our task is to help the individual clarify both the benefits *and* the costs. The individual then chooses to emphasize, replace, or alter a coping response. Our professional judgment is used to guide them in this.

This Appendix represents two panels from Bauer (2003), an assessment and treatment handbook meant for generalist clinicians who deal with a variety of mental disorders. It illustrates the applicability of collaborative disease management principles, as articulated by the Life Goals Program, to the dyadic provider–patient interaction for a wide variety of disorders. Adapted from Bauer (2003). Copyright 2003 by Lippincott Williams & Wilkins. Adapted by permission.

PANEL 2: THE PROBLEM-SOLVING AGENDA AROUND LIFE DIFFICULTIES FOR SUPPORTIVE PSYCHOTHERAPY

- This function-oriented agenda focuses on social role function issues (work role, family role, social activities, health-related subjective quality of life).
- The collaborative approach to illness management is extended to life management:
  - The individual identifies functional difficulties due to illness that are of high priority to him/her.
  - Coping responses to address the difficulties are identified.
  - Costs and benefits of various strategies are made explicit.
  - The clinician serves as coach, advisor, supporter, and educator.

1. How have your symptoms prevented you from doing what you want in your life?
2. Identify a goal that is:
   a. Important, yet . . .
   b. . . . realistic (success breeds success; failure, demoralization)
3. State the goal in explicit, behavioral terms, so that both the individual, and you, know when it has been achieved, and when not.
4. Break the goal down into manageable, behaviorally identifiable steps
   a. Manageable: success breeds success
   b. Behavioral: to know when you've succeeded
5. Analyze and address "roadblocks":
   a. Strategize problem solving
   b. Consider personal costs and benefits of various options
   c. Support
   d. Destigmatize
6. Process subsequent high-priority goals iteratively
7. Recapitulate disease management skills issues (Panel 1) frequently— mastery takes time and practice, success, and failure.

INDEX